CARDIAC CELLULAR ELECTROPHYSIOLOGY

BASIC SCIENCE FOR THE CARDIOLOGIST

1. B. Swynghedauw (ed.): *Molecular Cardiology for the Cardiologist*. Second
    Edition. 1998   ISBN: 0-7923-8323-0

2. B. Levy, A. Tedgui (eds.): *Biology of the Arterial Wall*. 1999
                                                 ISBN 0-7923-8458-X

3. M.R. Sanders, J.B. Kostis (eds): *Molecular Cardiology in Clinical
    Practice*. 1999.   ISBN 0-7923-8602-7

4. B. Ostadal, F. Kolar (eds.): *Cardiac Ischemia: From Injury to Protection*. 1999
                                                 ISBN 0-7923-8642-6

5. H. Schunkert, G.A.J. Riegger (eds.): *Apoptosis in Cardiac Biology*. 1999
                                                 ISBN 0-7923-8648-5

6. A. Malliani, (ed.): *Principles of Cardiovascular Neural Regulation in Health
    and Disease*. 2000   ISBN 0-7923-7775-3

7. P. Benlian : *Genetics of Dyslipidemia*. 2001
                                                 ISBN 0-7923-7362-6

8. D. Young : *Role of Potassium in Preventive Cardiovascular Medicine*. 2001
                                                 ISBN 0-7923-7376-6
9. E. Carmeliet, J. Vereecke : *Cardiac Cellular Electrophysiology*. 2002
                                                 ISBN 0-7923-7544-0

KLUWER ACADEMIC PUBLISHERS - DORDRECHT/BOSTON/LONDON

CARDIAC CELLULAR ELECTROPHYSIOLOGY

by

Edward Carmeliet

and

Johan Vereecke

Department of Physiology
K.U.L. University Leuven
Belgium

KLUWER ACADEMIC PUBLISHERS
Boston / Dordrecht / London

Distributors for North, Central and South America:
Kluwer Academic Publishers
101 Philip Drive
Assinippi Park
Norwell, Massachusetts 02061 USA

Distributors for all other countries:
Kluwer Academic Publishers Group
Distribution Centre
Post Office Box 322
3300 AH Dordrecht, THE NETHERLANDS

Library of Congress Cataloging-in-Publication Data

The Publisher offers discounts on this book for bulk purchases. For further information, send email to [laura.walsh@wkap.com]

Dedicated to

Prof. Silvio Weidmann

and in memory of

Prof. Edouard Coraboeuf

Contents

Acknowledgements

For copyright permission to reproduce figures we should like to thank the following publishers or societies:

Acad Press: IV.13, IV.17, IV.29, IV.31, IV.32, V.24, V.28, V.29.

Am Physiol Soc: I.4, IV.5, IV.6, IV.9, IV.12, IV.20, IV.24, V.5, V.18, V.20, V.26, V.30, V.32, VII.20, VII.22.

Am Soc Clin Invest: V.33.

Am Soc Pharmacol Exp Ther: IV.14.

Brit Med J Pub Co: V.2.

Cambridge University Press, The Physiological Society: II.16, IV.1, IV.3, IV.4, IV.7, IV.9, IV.10, IV.15, IV.19, IV.23, IV.27, IV.28, IV.30, IV.38, IV.39, V.3, V.10, V.12, VIII.15.

Can Cardiovasc Soc: VII.6.

Ed. J.B. Baillière: VIII.17.

Elsevier: I.3, VII.12, VII.15, VII.17, IX.6, IX.16, IX.17.

Futura Publ Co Inc: V.7, VII.14, IX.10, IX.12.

Harwood Acad Publ: IV.17, IV.37.

Kluwer Acad Publ: V.9, V.14.

Lippincott Williams & Wilkins:

    Circ Res: II.31, III.8, IV.9, IV.11, IV.16, IV.22, IV.25, IV.33, V.15, V.16, V.21, V.25, VI.7, VII.1, VII.5, VII.8, VII.9, VII.13, VII.15, VII.16, VII.19, VIII.2, VIII.3, VIII.5, VIII.8, VIII.9, VIII 16, VIII.18, VIII.20, VIII.21, IX.2, IX.3, IX.4, IX.8, IX.11, IX.13, IX.14.

    Circulation: VI.8, VI.9, VII.7, VII.10, VIII.6, VIII.10, VIII.11, VIII.12, VIII.19, IX.1, IX.5, IX.7, IX.9, IX.18.

J Cardiovasc Pharmacol: V.27,

Nat Acad Sci USA: IV.26.

Nature Publ Group, Nature II.26: IV.1.

Nature Publ Group, British Journal of Pharmacology: V.31.

Raven Press: V.4.

Rockefeller University Press, The Journal of General Physiology: II.16, IV.4, IV.21, V.6.

Sinauer Ass: II.29, II.30.

Springer Verlag:

    Pflügers Archiv: IV.12, IV.14, IV.26, IV.38, VIII.1.

    Basic Res Cardiolol: V.5.

Preface

This book on "Cardiac Cellular Electrophysiology" appears in a series of "Basic Science for the Cardiologist". However in addition for use by clinicians needing a more thorough understanding of the electrophysiological basis of heart function, this book is also intended for a wider public, undergraduate students and medical students interested in the basis of the electrical activity of the heart, graduate students, research workers, pharmacologists, teachers in physiology, pharmacology and other biomedical sciences. Our goal in writing the book was twofold. Our first aim was to give a primer on basic electrophysiology, the cardiac action potential and the physiological basis of the electrocardiogram. For many non-electrophysiologists, original papers in cellular electrophysiology are often difficult to read. We wanted to provide the necessary background and to convince the readers that cellular electrophysiology is not so difficult to grasp after all. It was our intention to make these parts accessible to a wide audience. Our second aim, after having introduced the basic concepts, was to continue with giving an overview of the properties of the most important ionic currents in the heart, and to treat their modulation, in order to deal with the mechanisms underlying cardiac ischaemia, arrhythmias and remodeling.

A huge literature exists about cardiac electrophysiology. With the invention of the patch clamp technique by Neher and Sakmann in 1981, the field exploded, and with the more recent application of molecular biology to the study of ion channels, a large literature exists about the functioning of channels at the molecular and single channel level. However throughout the book our emphasis is on function rather than on channel biophysics, molecular biology or structure - function relations. Therefore our emphasis is much more on whole cell currents and their relation to cardiac electrical activity than on single channel studies.

Chapter I contains a brief general description of the electrical activity in the heart. It defines the different phases of the action potential and their variation in different parts of the heart.

Chapter II provides the ionic mechanisms underlying resting and action potential. After introducing some general principles of electric circuit theory and applying these principles to the movement of ions across cell membranes, in a second section it briefly describes the electrophysiological techniques used to study electrical properties at the protein, the cellular, the multicellular and the organ level, emphasising cellular electrophysiological methods. In the third section a brief overview is first given of the major types of membrane transport processes, distinguishing primary active, secondary active and passive processes, and making the distinction between channels and carriers. This is followed with the principles of description and analysis of ion channel properties, discussing ion permeation, channel gating, regulation and block, channel molecular structure and distribution.

The initiation and the propagation of the action potential is the subject of Chapter III. This chapter describes the concept and mechanisms of excitability and automaticity, and the basic mechanism underlying normal and abnormal conduction. It starts with the concept of threshold and the factors modulating excitability. Next it treats automaticity and the main determinants of 'the initiation of the heart beat'. In the last section it gives an introduction to one-dimensional cable theory and its application to propagation of the action potential. It describes the concepts of electrotonic potential, source – sink, short-circuit current and liminal length, conduction velocity and safety factor. It then deals with the complications introduced by the three-dimensional structure of the heart and provides some background information on discontinuous propagation, anisotropy, unidirectional propagation, to lay a basis for understanding reentrant arrhythmias.

Chapter IV first describes the properties of the most important ionic currents contributing to the electrical activity of the heart. The emphasis is on currents that have been identified in human cardiac cells, or that appear to be generally present in mammalian hearts. As such this chapter is somewhat encyclopaedic, and reading of the properties of some of the transport mechanisms may eventually be postponed until needed to understand some topic treated in later chapters, especially since not all transport processes have (yet) been identified in human cardiac cells. In the last section of this chapter the action potential morphology in different cardiac cells is explained in terms of the different ion transport mechanisms, as described in the previous sections.

Chapter V deals with the modulation of the electrical activity by rate, by the autonomic nervous system, by humoral, autocrine and paracrine factors and by the hormonal state. It also treats the effects of drugs, and discusses the problems related to antiarrhythmic treatment and possible future approaches.

Chapter VI handles the electrophysiological basis of the electrocardiogram and the normal electrocardiographic waves. It also briefly deals with abnormalities of ST segment, T wave and U wave. This chapter also includes the dispersion of action potential duration and its influence on the electrocardiogram.

Chapter VII successively treats acute ischaemia and reperfusion. Following a description of the biochemical alterations upon acute interruption of the coronary circulation, a detailed analysis is presented of the changes in resting and action potential, excitability and conduction, and the mechanisms involved. The second section treats the biochemical and electrophysiological changes occurring upon reperfusion, distinguishing between reversible and irreversible phases.

Chapter VIII deals with arrhythmias. In a first part an analysis is presented of the basic mechanisms, including automatism, triggered activity and reentry. Emphasis is given to recent developments, such as anisotropic reentry and spiral wave activity. In a second part we provide a description of the origin and type of arrhythmias occurring under specific conditions. We discuss arrhythmias during acute ischaemia and reperfusion, and arrhythmias at a later stage of the infarct when remodeling becomes important. We also deal with atrial fibrillation, congenital and acquired long QT syndromes, the Brugada syndrome, and arrhythmias accompanying hypertrophy and heart failure.

The final chapter in the book, Chapter IX, provides an analysis of electrical remodeling processes that develop during certain patho-physiological conditions such as hypertrophy and heart failure, atrial fibrillation, and myocardial infarction. In contrast to short-term changes described in Chapter V on Modulation, these processes include mid-term and long-term alterations of the function and structure of ionic channels, receptors and signaling pathways. Similar long-term physiological adaptations occur during preconditioning and artificial pacing. It is considered that a better knowledge of the mechanisms underlying remodeling may offer new therapeutical approaches.

We want to express our sincere and warm thanks to Mrs Lies Vereecke-Peeters, the wife of one of the authors, for her skilful work in making the numerous original figures and schemes and in adapting published figures and, in this way, fulfilling the wishes and dreams of the authors.

We want to dedicate the book to Prof. Silvio Weidmann and to the late Prof. Edouard Coraboeuf, founding fathers of cardiac cellular electro-physiology. In 1949, they were the first to register cardiac action potentials with microelectrodes during their stay in Prof. Alan Hodgkin's laboratory.

Edward Carmeliet
Johan Vereecke

Chapter I

General description of electrical activity

1.   DIFFERENT PHASES OF THE ACTION POTENTIAL

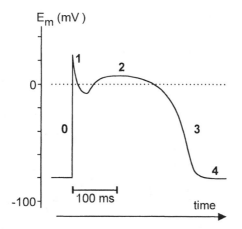

Figure I.1. The phases of the cardiac action potential.

1

The cardiac action potential can in general be subdivided into four phases, although the shapes of the action potentials show large variations between different cells, and some phases are not pronounced or may even be absent in some cell types (Fig. I.1). Phase 0 consists of the initial depolarisation phase, which brings the membrane potential quickly from a negative value during diastole to positive potentials. Following phase 0, a partial repolarisation phase (phase 1) sometimes occurs, which repolarises the membrane to potentials of about 0 mV, or even more negative values. This phase is followed by the plateau phase (phase 2). Phase 1 can eventually result in the appearance of a notch between phase 0 and phase 2. During the plateau phase the membrane potential remains for some time near 0 mV, but during this phase the membrane potential slowly becomes more negative. The plateau phase is ended by the final repolarisation (phase 3). These three phases approximately correspond to the mechanical systole. After the final repolarisation phase follows the diastole (phase 4), which can be a stable resting potential, as is e.g. the case in normal atrial or ventricular myocardium, or a slow diastolic depolarisation, eventually initiating spontaneous activity, as is the case in the sinoatrial node [for excellent books see 79,518,828,1087,1344].

2.   MORPHOLOGY OF THE ACTION POTENTIAL IN DIFFERENT PARTS OF THE HEART

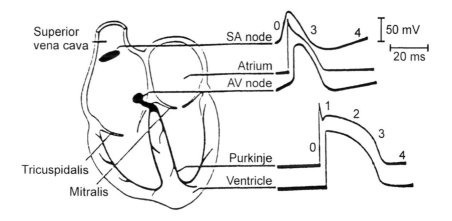

Figure 1 2. Action potential configuration in different parts of the heart.

The electrical activity in the heart is initiated by spontaneous activity in the sinoatrial node (SAN), a small mass of spindle-shaped cells near the junction of the superior vena cava and the right atrium. Since cardiac cells are electrically coupled by gap junctions, the electrical activity spreads from the SAN to the surrounding atrial tissue. Atrial cells are not electrically connected to ventricular cells, but the electrical activity from the atrial cells spreads via the atrioventricular node (AVN) to the His bundle Purkinje system and from there the excitation reaches the ventricular myocardium. These different regions of the heart show distinct electrophysiological properties (Fig. I.2). Cardiac cells can be subdivided in two groups according to the rate of depolarisation during the upstroke of the action potential. The SAN and AVN are slow response cells, while atria, His bundle, Purkinje and ventricular myocardial cells are called fast response cells. The difference is based on a difference in origin of the inward current responsible for phase 0 of the action potential. While the depolarisation of the slow response cells is caused by Ca^{2+} current, the action potential upstroke of the fast response cells is due to Na^+ current.

2.1   Sinoatrial node

Sinoatrial node cells are small with a diameter of about 5-10 μm, with distinct electrical properties. The cells are characterised by a low maximal diastolic potential from which a slow but marked diastolic depolarisation arises, resulting in spontaneous activity. The diastolic potential is in the range between −50 and −60 mV. The diastolic potential range varies with the location of the cells within the SAN. Cells located more peripherally have more negative diastolic potentials due to electrical coupling with atrial cells, which have a more negative resting potential. Phase 0 of the action potential has a low upstroke velocity of about 1 - 10 V/s, and therefore SAN cells are slow response cells, and an overshoot of about 30 mV. The action potential duration is of the order of 100 to 200 ms. Propagation velocity in the SAN is less than 0.05 m/s.

2.2   Atria

No clear boundary exists between the SAN and the atria. However atrial cells away from the boundary have a diameter of about 10-15 μm and appear somewhat larger than SAN cells. The cells are not spontaneously active and they have a more negative resting potential of about −80 mV. The upstroke velocity is 100-200 V/s and the fast depolarisation phase reaches an overshoot of about 30 mV (Fig. I.3). After the fast depolarisation phase the cells slowly return to the resting potential; a small and short plateau may be present but often there is no clear separation into a plateau and a final repolarisation phase. The duration of the action potential is about 100 to 200 ms, and shows transmural dispersion. Differences in action potential duration are also found between different parts of the atria [326,1308], and action potential duration is shorter in left atrium than in right atrium [644]. The propagation velocity in atrial tissue amounts to about 0.3 - 0.4 m/s.

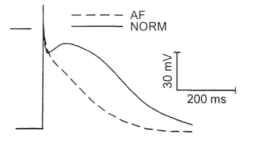

Figure I.3. Action potential in normal human atrium (full line) and from atria with atrial fibrillation (dashed line). Modified from [218].

2.3   Atrioventricular node

AVN cells have a diameter of about 5-10 μm. They have a resting potential of –60 to –70 mV. The AVN has spontaneous activity; however during the normal cardiac cycle, action potentials are triggered by electrical activity in adjacent atrial cells, before the diastolic depolarisation of the AVN reaches the threshold. The upstroke of the action potential is slow: the maximal rate of rise is about 5 – 15 V/s. Action potential is generated by Ca^{2+} current. It has an overshoot of about 20 mV and a duration around 100 – 300 ms. The action potential propagates at a speed of about 0.1 m/s.

2.4   His bundle Purkinje system

The His bundle runs from the AVN into the ventricles. It penetrates through the connective tissue separating atria and ventricles, and is normally the only electrically conducting tissue connecting atria and ventricles. In the ventricle it divides into a left and right bundle branch, and ends in a network of Purkinje fibres, which provide the electrical contact with the myocardium. The His bundle Purkinje system forms the fast conduction system of the heart, which conducts the electrical activity rapidly towards the apex of the ventricle, ensuring nearly synchronous and uniform spread of activation of the ventricles. The His bundle Purkinje systems consists of large, more or less cylindrical cells, which have a diameter of 20 - 50 μm and a length of 100 - 200 μm, which is more than three times larger than myocardial cells. The cells have a diastolic potential in the range of –80 to –90 mV, which is much more negative than the range of diastolic potentials of the SAN. The cells of the ventricular conduction system show a slow diastolic depolarisation, which may eventually lead to spontaneous activity at a low frequency, if not previously activated by electrotonic interactions from adjacent cells. In normal conditions the action potentials in the His bundle are started by electrical activity propagating from the AVN. The action potential has a fast upstroke of up to 800 V/s and shows an overshoot of about 40 mV, which is followed by a fast partial repolarisation to a plateau at potentials around 0 mV. A short notch towards a more negative potential may precede this plateau. The plateau phase evolves approximately in the potential range between 0 and –20 mV, and lasts for about 300 ms after which follows the final repolarisation phase. The duration of the action potential is very dependent on the frequency of stimulation and can vary from about 200 to about 500 ms. The cells are electrically connected by numerous end-to-end gap junctions located in the intercalated disks. The propagation velocity is very high, reaching values between 2 to 5 m/s.

2.5 Ventricle

Ventricular myocardial cells have a diameter of about 10 to 20 μm. Their resting potential is about –80 mV. The upstroke has a velocity of the order of 100 to 200 V/s and an overshoot of about 40 mV. The fast upstroke ensures a high velocity of propagation of the action potential (although it is considerably lower than in the His bundle Purkinje system), reaching values between 0.3 to 0.5 m/s. The action potential spreads through the ventricular wall from the endocardium near the apex, towards the epicardial wall at the base of the ventricle.

The upstroke is followed by a marked plateau phase. During this plateau phase the membrane potential gradually but very slowly develops in the direction of more negative potentials. The plateau phase is ended by a fast repolarisation. The duration of the action potential is very dependent on the frequency of stimulation, shortening with increase in frequency, and can vary from a few hundred ms to about half a second.

The duration of the ventricular action potential is not uniform over the whole ventricle, but depends on the location of the cells [for review see 129]. Action potential duration is shorter in cells at the apex than at the base of the ventricle [175]. Differences in action potentials configuration also exist between right and left ventricle [1222].

Studies in isolated tissues and myocytes indicated that electrical activity in transmural sections also shows marked variations in action potential duration with depth (Fig. 1.4). The duration is shortest in the subepicardial region and especially at the base of the ventricle. The subendocardial cells have longer action potentials, especially in the apical region, but the longest action potentials are found in the midmyocardial region, as was described by

Antzelevitch and collaborators [1039]. This region contains a class of cells (the so-called M cells), which have a number of characteristics in common with Purkinje cells, although they can be distinguished from Purkinje cells by their lack of diastolic depolarisation and their sensitivity to autonomic agents. M cells show a steep frequency response of the action potential duration, a spike - dome configuration and a large maximal rate of depolarisation of phase 0. They are found mostly but not exclusively in the midmyocardium of the left and right ventricle. M cells have been found in different species in including human [29,45,121,280,647,1092].

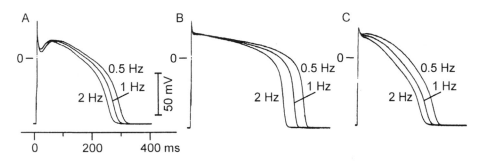

Figure I.4. Transmural dispersion of action potential duration in human ventricular myocardium at different stimulation frequencies. A: subepicardial. B: midmyocardial. C: subendocardial. Modified from [647].

Also the shape of the action potential shows marked variation (Fig. I.4). The subepicardial action potentials have a pronounced phase 1, which results in a pronounced notch, giving the action potential a spike - dome appearance The midmyocardial action potentials also have a marked phase 1 repolarisation, often resulting in a marked notch. The subendocardial cells have little phase 1 repolarisation, so that its plateau starts at more positive potentials, closer to the peak of the action potential, and is not preceded by a marked notch.

While the presence of M cells has been confirmed in humans [280,647], it is still controversial whether transmural repolarisation gradients are present in vivo and are relevant to humans. A recent study failed to find transmural repolarisation differences within the human ventricle [1121].

Chapter II

Ionic basis of resting and action potential

1.   THE CELL AS AN ELECTRIC CIRCUIT

In order to describe the electrical behaviour of a cell, electrophysiological analysis attempts to establish the electrical equivalent model of the preparation under study and to determine its parameters. This can be done by studying the response of the cell to an electrical excitation, which most often has the form of a step current, a sinusoidal current, or a voltage step.

1.1   Principles of electric circuit theory

1.1.1   Circuit elements

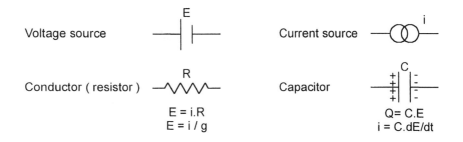

Figure II.1. Electric circuit elements.

The most important electric circuit elements for studying electrophysiology are the voltage source (E or V), the current source (i), the resistor (R) or its inverse the conductor (g) (g = 1/R) and the capacitance (C) (see Fig. II.1). Voltage and current sources are both generators of electricity. An ideal voltage source generates a potential, which is independent of the load (the rest of the circuit), whereas the current it delivers depends on the load. An ideal current source generates a current that is independent of the load, while the voltage at its output varies with the load.

Notation

In the electrophysiological literature both symbols E or V are used for potential, and their use is in general not consistent. However, while in comparison of a membrane potential with an equilibrium potential the symbol E is used (e.g. E_m-E_K) in some other equations (e.g. cable equations or some abbreviations (I-V relation, dV/dt_{max})) the symbol V is generally used as symbol for membrane potential.

Resistor.

According to Ohm's law the potential E (in Volt) across a resistor is equal to the current i (in Ampere) flowing through the resistor, times the resistance value R (in Ohm) of the resistor: E = i.R. By convention positive current flows in the direction of movement of positive charges. The conductance (g in Siemens) is a measure of the ease of flow of current and is the inverse of the resistance: $g = 1/R$. When the current is plotted as function of the potential, Ohm's law is represented by a linear current-voltage relation, with slope $di/dE = 1/R = g$ (Fig. II.2).

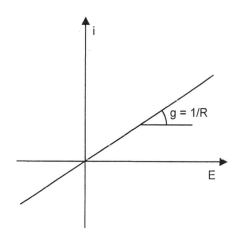

Figure II.2. Ohm's law: $E = i.R$ or $i = g.E$. Current-voltage relation.

The resistance values of conductors however are not always constant. The resistance may vary with the polarity of the current, or may depend on the size of the voltage applied to them. In this case the current-voltage relation is non-linear. Such non-linear current-voltage relations are said to show rectification.

Capacitor.

A capacitor consists of two conducting media separated by an electric insulator (Fig. II.1). The capacitance value (C) depends on the dielectric constant (ε) of the insulator, the polarisability of free space (ε_0), the thickness (d) and surface area (A) of the insulator: $C = \varepsilon\varepsilon_0 A/d$.

A capacitor permits the separation of electric charges, which provides a means of storing energy. The potential E on a capacitor is determined by the charge Q (in Coulomb) on the capacitor divided by the value C (in Farad) of the capacitor: $Q = CE$. The energy (in Joule) stored on a capacitor $U = Q^2/2C = \frac{1}{2} CE^2$. A sudden voltage step across a capacitor causes current flow, and positive charges accumulate on one side of the capacitor and negative charges accumulate on the other side. A steady–state is rapidly reached and the current drops quickly to zero. Since current is the change of charge per unit of time ($i_C = dQ/dt$), the capacitive current charging or uncharging a capacitor is proportional to the rate of voltage change: $i_C = C.dE/dt$

1.1.2   Circuit analysis

Kirchhoff's laws

Kirchhoff's laws, together with the relation between potential and current in the circuit elements (such as voltage or current sources, resistors and capacitors), determine the distribution of potentials and currents in electric circuits (Fig. II.3).

Kirchhoff's first law

At any junction the algebraic sum of the currents must be zero.

This law is simply a restatement of the conservation of charge. The number of charges coming into the junction must be exactly the same as the number of charges leaving the junction; otherwise charges (positive or negative) would be created at the junction.

Kirchhoff's second law

In any closed circuit the sum of changes in potential encountered in making a complete loop is zero.

This law is based on the conservation of energy. It is an expression of the fact that at each point only one potential can be assigned. It is the electrical equivalent of stating that any point on a mountain has a unique elevation: if one starts walking from a point and returns to the starting point via another route, the sum of the changes in elevation encountered is zero.

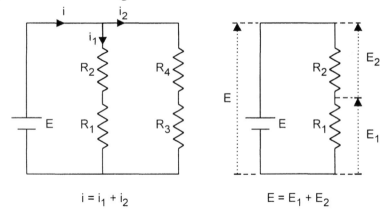

$$i = i_1 + i_2 \qquad\qquad E = E_1 + E_2$$

Figure II.3. Kirchoff's laws

Elements in series or in parallel

For resistances in series the total resistance is the sum of the resistances. Thus $R = \sum R_i$ (series resistance add up).

For resistances in parallel the total conductance is the sum of the conductances: $g = \sum g_i$ or equivalently $1/R = \sum 1/R_i$.

For capacitances in series: $1/C = \sum 1/C_i$.

For capacitances in parallel $C = \sum C_i$ (parallel capacitances add up).

1.2   The uniformly polarised cell

The lipid bilayer of the cell membrane forms a thin layer of non-conducting material separating the intracellular and extracellular solutions. The lipids of the membrane form a dielectric separating two electrically conducting media. Such an arrangement is electrically equivalent to an electrical capacitor. The specific capacity of the membranes of all cells is about 1.0 $\mu F/cm^2$; this value is determined by the dielectric constant and the thickness of the lipid bilayer. The cell membrane however does not form a perfect isolator, since it also contains proteins, some of which behave as ion permeation pathways. These pathways can be represented by an electrical conductance, or equivalently by its inverse, an electrical resistance. The membrane can thus be described as a leaky capacitor, and therefore its electrical equivalent circuit can be represented by a capacitor (with a specific capacity of 1 $\mu F/cm^2$) in parallel with a resistor (the value of which depends on the specific transport processes present in the membrane and their regulation) (Fig. II.4).

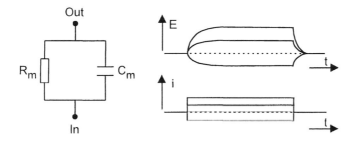

Figure II.4. Membrane electrical equivalent model and the membrane potential change during constant current pulses.

The total membrane current i_m consists of two components, the current i_c charging the capacitor (capacitative current) and the current (i_{ionic}) flowing through the resistive pathway (ionic current) (Fig. II.4 and II.5). The capacitative component will cause a change of the amount of charge separated by the membrane and hence a change in voltage, and the rate of change of the membrane potential is proportional to the size of the capacitative current. When a current i is forced through the membrane (i_m), some of the current charges the capacitor (i_c) while some of it leaks as ionic current (i_{ionic} or i_i) through the resistive pathway (Fig. II.5).

$$i_m = i_c + i_i$$
$$i_c = dQ/dt = C_m\, dE_m/dt$$
$$\text{Therefore: } i_m = C_m\, dE_m/dt + i_i$$
$$i = i_m = C_m\, dE_m/dt + i_i$$

1.2.1 The linear membrane model

The response of the cell to an application of a small amount of current i, resulting in membrane potential changes limited to a few mV from the resting potential, is called the passive response of the cell membrane. In this case the relation between potential and ionic current can be approximated by Ohm's law $i_i = E_m/R_m$ where R_m is the membrane resistance. Hence:

$i = C_m \, dE_m/dt + E/R_m$

When R_m is constant, the solution of this equation for a sudden constant current step is a simple exponential change in potential:

$E_m = i.R_m \cdot [1-\exp(-t/\tau_m)]$ in which $\tau_m = R_m \, C_m$ is called the membrane time constant; it is the time at which the membrane potential rises to $1-e^{-1}$ ($= 0.6321$ which is approximately 2/3) of its steady-state value $i.R_m$. Since R_m can be obtained by dividing the steady-state potential by the current, and τ_m can be obtained from the time course of the transient, C_m can be calculated.

The voltage and currents during a step change in i for this simple linear membrane model are graphically illustrated in Fig. II.5.

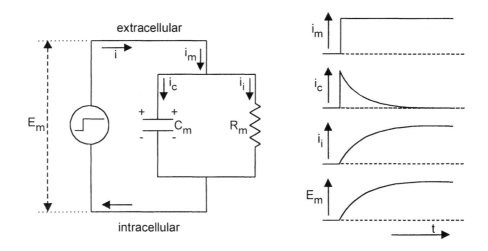

Figure II.5. Passive membrane model and the time-dependence of membrane potential change and ionic and capacitive current during a constant current pulse (i).

Following application of the current, the initial current is almost completely capacitive, charging the membrane. The capacitive current decays exponentially to zero while the potential rises. This rise in potential *causes charge to leak through the channels as ionic current. This ionic* current is proportional to the potential.

1.2.2 Non-linear membrane properties

In general the ionic current flowing through the membrane is not a linear function of potential and the linear membrane model is generally only valid for potential changes not exceeding a few mV. The net ionic current consists of several components originating from the flow of current through different types of channels, which can be regulated by different processes. Opening and closing of channels causes the ionic current to be voltage- and time-dependent. Application of a step current flowing through the membrane therefore results in a complex pattern of membrane potential changes, and the resulting changes in potential will also affect the ionic currents.

In the absence of any external current $C_m\, dE_m/dt = -i_{ionic}$ with i_{ionic} the net ionic current, which is equal to the algebraic sum of all ionic currents $i_{ionic} = \sum i_i$. The time course of the membrane potential is then fully determined by the ionic currents flowing through the membrane. The rate of change of the membrane potential is proportional to the net ionic current flowing through the membrane. The total charge transferred by the ionic current (the integral of the net current over time) determines the magnitude of the voltage change: $Q = \int i_i\, dt = \int -\sum i_i\, dt = C.E_m$.

The ionic currents are in general non-linear functions of voltage and time, and the purpose of the electrophysiological studies is to gain information about the laws governing these ionic currents.

1.3 Ion movement through membranes

The ionic composition of the cytoplasm is different from the extracellular medium. Cardiac cells, like most cells, contain high $[K]_i$ and low $[Na]_i$, while the reverse is true for the extracellular environment. The Na^+ and K^+ gradients are maintained by an active ATP-driven Na^+/K^+ pump.

The membrane contains proteins, which allow certain ions to pass passively across the membrane. These membrane proteins can have approximately the shape of a tunnel or pore through which the ions diffuse, in which case they are called channels, or they can be carriers which change their configuration subsequent to binding the ion, thereby translocating the bound ion from one side to the other side of the membrane.

1.3.1 Diffusion

1.3.1.1 Simple diffusion
Molecules in solution are constantly moving randomly due to thermal agitation. When a concentration gradient is present a net movement of molecules from the region of higher concentration to the region of lower

concentration takes place. The net transfer of molecules due to concentration gradient can be described by Fick's law of diffusion

$F = -D \, dc/dx$

where F is the flux which is the number of particles transferred per second and per unit area, D the diffusion coefficient (expressed in cm^2/s), c the concentration and x the distance, so that dc/dx represents the concentration gradient. According to the Stokes – Einstein equation the diffusion coefficient is inversely proportional to the radius of the molecule.

For diffusion of uncharged substances across a cell membrane Fick's law reduces to

$F = P \, (C_e - C_i)$

where C_e and C_i represent the extracellular and the intracellular concentrations and P the permeability of the membrane. The permeability is proportional to the diffusion coefficient of the substance in the membrane.

$P = D/d$ (with d the thickness of the membrane).

For substances which diffuse through the lipid phase of the membrane the permeability also depends on oil / water partition coefficient (β) of the substance, since this coefficient determines how easily the substance enters the membrane at the water lipid interface. Thus

$P = \beta D/d$

According to Fick's law the flux is linearly proportional to the concentration (Fig. II.6).

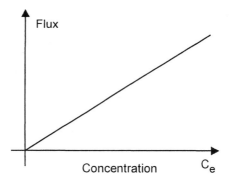

Figure II.6. Fick's law of diffusion. Concentration-dependence of transmembrane diffusion rate shows a linear relationship. In this example net transmembrane flux is shown as function of C_e with C_i assumed to be zero.

1.3.1.2   Facilitated diffusion

Large molecules (such as glucose, amino acids etc.) do not easily diffuse through the membrane. In order to transport such substances across membranes, cells make use of carriers. Carrier-mediated transport (also called facilitated diffusion) follows Michaelis-Menten kinetics. Such transport can be described by equations similar to the equations of enzyme kinetics, since it can be viewed as a catalysed reaction, where the reaction is not a change in chemical structure of the substance, but a translocation of the substance across the membrane. Carrier-mediated transport shows saturation (Fig. II.7), and competitive and non-competitive inhibition, stereo-specificity, and has a relatively slow turnover.

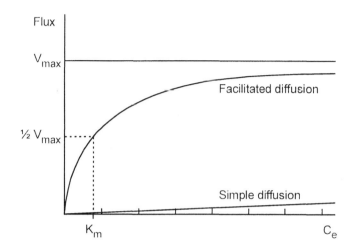

Figure II.7. Carrier-mediated transport can enhance diffusion of substances for which the membrane has a limited permeability. The concentration-dependence of transport rate shows saturation and is similar to Michaelis-Menten kinetics; it is characterised by V_{max} and half-maximum concentration K_m. The curves show net transmembrane flux as function of C_e with C_i assumed to be zero.

1.3.1.3   Electrodiffusion

For charged substances moving in a uniform electric field in the absence of a concentration gradient, the current (which is proportional to the flux) is proportional to the potential difference according to Ohm's law.

For ions moving in a concentration gradient, eventually the presence of electric field should also be taken into account. The total gradient considered is then the electrochemical gradient. The passive movement of ions in the presence of an electrochemical gradient is called electrodiffusion, which is quantitatively described by the Nernst-Planck equation [for a good overview see 449,1340]. Solving the equation for calculating the amount of current flowing through the membrane (which is a problem of kinetics) requires assumptions about the processes within the membrane. However, no such assumptions are required to calculate the potential at which the net flow (or current) of an ion will be zero, which is a purely thermodynamic property. This potential is the equilibrium potential of the ion.

1.3.2   Equilibrium potential and the Nernst equation

Consider two compartments, which in analogy to a cell we will call the i (intracellular) and e (extracellular) compartment, separated by a membrane selectively permeable for ion X (such as K^+) that is present at a higher concentration in one compartment (e.g. in the cell). Due to the concentration gradient for K^+, some positively charged K^+ ions will leak out of the cell. This outward movement of positive charges will leave the cell interior negatively charged, counteracting further outward movement of K^+ ions. As more and more K^+ ions are leaving the cell, the potential difference across the membrane rises, opposing further K^+ efflux. When the electrical potential gradient, created by K^+ ions leaving the cell, becomes exactly equal to the opposite K^+ concentration gradient, net K^+ flux becomes zero, and the system is in equilibrium (Fig. II.8). The potential at which equilibrium occurs is the "Equilibrium potential".

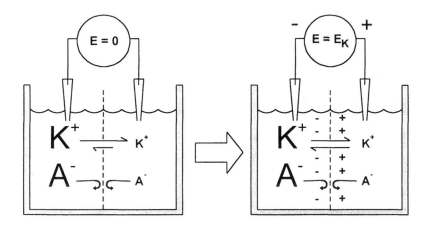

Figure II.8. Diffusion of ions and equilibrium potential. A concentration gradient of an ion across a selectively permeable membrane leads to a net ion flux, which will cause a potential difference across the membrane. Net ion movement will stop when the transmembrane potential reaches a value equal to the equilibrium potential (given by the Nernst equation).

The equilibrium potential for an ion X (E_X), can be obtained by equating the Gibbs free energy contained in the concentration gradient ($RT \ln [X]_e /[X]_i$) and the free energy in a potential gradient (zFE), and is given by the Nernst equation:

$$E_X = \frac{RT}{zF} \ln \frac{[X]_e}{[X]_i}$$

At 37 °C (310 °K) the Nernst equation can be written as:

$$E_X = 61 \log \frac{[X]_e}{[X]_i} \text{ mV}$$

T = absolute temperature in degree Kelvin

R = universal gas constant, = 8.31 Joule/°K-mol

z = charge number of ion (+1 for monovalent cations)

F = Faraday const.: charge per mol monovalent ion: 96.480 Coulomb/mol

RT/F = 27 mV at 37 °C

ln = natural logarithm (base e = 2.718) and log = base 10 logarithm

$[X]_e$ and $[X]_i$ extracellular and intracellular concentrations of ion X^+.

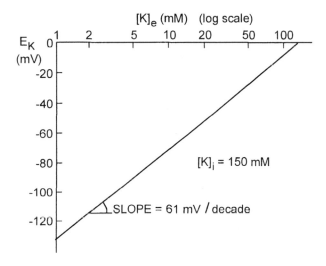

Figure II.9. Nernst equation. Equilibrium potential as function of concentration (here shown for K^+). When the concentration is plotted on a logarithmic scale a linear relation is obtained with a slope of 61/z mV per 10-fold change in concentration (at 37 °C).

The equilibrium potential of an ion is the potential at which thermodynamic equilibrium will occur (which can be obtained by solving the Nernst-Planck equation for zero net flux [see 449]). At the equilibrium potential no <u>net</u> movement of this ion will occur, independent of the membrane permeability. However equilibrium does not mean that transmembrane movement of this ion is absent, but only that the rate of movement (flux) from inside to outside (unidirectional efflux) will be exactly equal to the unidirectional influx. Both unidirectional fluxes can eventually be measured using radioactive tracers.

A cardiac cell at rest contains approximately 140 mM K^+, and 4 mM K^+ is present in the extracellular medium. With these concentrations the equilibrium potential for K^+ ions equals $E_K = -94$ mV (by convention membrane potentials are given as potential of the cytoplasm (intracellular potential E_i) with respect to the extracellular medium (E_e); thus $E_m = E_i - E_e$; negative membrane potentials therefore mean that the potential of the cytoplasm is more negative than the extracellular space). For a cardiac cell selectively permeable for K^+, a potential difference of -94 mV would exist across the cell membrane. The equilibrium potential can also be calculated for other ions (Table II.1), and is dependent on the intra- and extracellular concentration of the ion according to the Nernst equation e.g. E_{Na} is approximately $+60$ mV, since an approximately tenfold lower concentration of Na^+ is present in the cell than in the extracellular solution.

Table II.1. Typical concentrations and equilibrium potentials in mammalian cardiac cells. Actual concentrations vary between cell types and species. The cytoplasmic concentration for Ca^{2+} refers to free calcium ion concentration. The total intracellular Ca^{2+} concentration is much higher due to Ca^{2+} binding and sequestration in intracellular stores, and is of the order of several mM.

	Plasma	Cytoplasm	E_{ion}
Ion	mM	mM	mV
Na^+	145	10	+67
K^+	4	150	-94
Ca^{2+}	1.8	10^{-4}	+130
Mg^{2+}	1.5	0.8	+8
Cl^-	120	20	-47

It is important to realize that the number of ions that have to cross the membrane to cause physiological membrane potential changes of the order of 100 mV is very small, and that the resulting small concentration changes are most often negligible (except for transmembrane Ca^{2+} movements).

From the relation $Q_m = C_m E_m$ it can be calculated that in a cell with a diameter of about 20 μm, a 100 mV potential difference is obtained by a transmembrane movement of monovalent ions of about 10^{-17} mole, which would result in a concentration change of the order of only a few μM. For Na^+ and K^+ ions (which are present in the cell at concentrations of the order of 10 respectively 100 mM) this would have negligible effects on the concentrations (on the long term eventual concentration changes are compensated by active transport processes). However for Ca^{2+} ions, which are present at submicromolar concentrations in the cytoplasm, the cytoplasmic concentration changes produced by Ca^{2+} ions flowing through the membrane can be very important. This enables the cell to use Ca^{2+} for cellular signalling.

Changing the extracellular ion concentration and measuring the change in membrane potential is the best method to investigate whether a membrane or ion channel is selectively permeable for one type of ion. If this is the case the Nernst equation predicts that the membrane potential must be a linear function of the concentration with a slope of 61/z mV per unit increase in the logarithm of the concentration. E.g. for a membrane selectively permeable for K^+ ions, changing $[K]_e$ will give a linear relation between E_K and log $[K]_e$ with a slope of 61 mV per 10 fold change in $[K]_e$. For a membrane selectively permeable for some ion, the equation can also be used to determine the intracellular concentration of this ion: the extracellular concentration of the ion at which the membrane potential becomes zero is equal to the value of the intracellular concentration of the ion.

1.3.3   Stationary membrane potential and the Goldman equation

Cardiac cell membranes at rest are highly permeable to K^+ ions, which together with the large K^+ concentration gradient across the membrane is responsible for the generation of an electrical gradient across the membrane, which is close to the K^+ equilibrium potential. The cells show a small but finite permeability for other ions, e.g. Na^+. Therefore, due to the important Na^+ concentration gradient and electrical gradient across the membrane, Na^+ ions will tend to enter the cell passively, thereby depolarising the cell. This depolarisation will bring K^+ ions out of equilibrium, resulting in passive outward movement of K^+, counteracting the electrical effect of Na^+ entry. When the K^+ efflux equals the Na^+ influx, a steady-state occurs since the net charge transfer across the membrane is zero. The potential at which steady-state occurs is given by the **Goldman-Hodgkin-Katz potential equation** (often simply called the Goldman equation or GHK equation) which is shown here for a membrane permeable to K^+ and Na^+ ions only, with P_K and P_{Na} the K^+ and Na^+ permeability:

$$E_m = \frac{RT}{F} \ln \frac{P_K [K]_e + P_{Na} [Na]_e}{P_K [K]_i + P_{Na} [Na]_i} = 61 \log \frac{[K]_e + \alpha [Na]_e}{[K]_i + \alpha [Na]_i} mV$$

The stationary membrane potential thus depends on the extracellular and intracellular Na^+ and K^+ concentrations and on the ratio $\alpha = P_{Na}/P_K$. Since the membrane at rest is mainly permeable for K^+, but has also some permeability for Na^+, the resting potential of the membrane (E_r) is therefore dependent on ratio of P_{Na}/P_K at rest. In case the membrane is selectively permeable for one ion (P_K or P_{Na} being equal to zero) the Goldman equals reduces to the Nernst equation giving the equilibrium potential for that ion.

The Goldman equation can be used to relate the resting membrane potential to the existing concentration gradients and permeabilities. It is also very useful to determine the selectivity of membranes or channels. Changing the concentration of a monovalent ion will only result in a 61 mV change in potential if the membrane is selectively permeable for the ion (Fig. II.9 and II.10). If the membrane is permeable to more than one type of ion, a change in concentration of an ion will not result in a linear relation. However from the shape of the relation of the membrane potential as function of the concentration one can calculate the permeability, without requiring knowledge of the intracellular concentration (providing the change in extracellular concentration did not affect the intracellular concentrations).

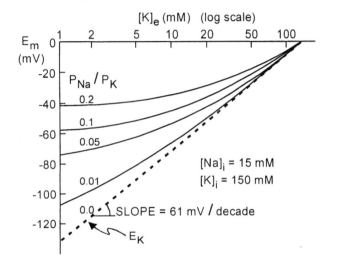

Figure II.10. Goldman potential. When the membrane is permeable for more than one ion, a stationary state will be established at the potential where the sum of the currents carried by all ions is zero. The Goldman potential is shown as function of $[K]_e$ for different values of P_{Na}/P_K for a cell at 37 C, with $[Na]_e = 150$ mM, $[Na]_i = 15$ mM and $[K]_i = 150$ mM. $[K]_e$ is plotted on logarithmic scale.

If also Cl⁻ is included the Goldman equation becomes:
$$E_m = \frac{RT}{F} \ln \frac{P_K [K]_e + P_{Na} [Na]_e + P_{Cl} [Cl]_i}{P_K [K]_i + P_{Na} [Na]_i + P_{Cl} [Cl]_e}$$
It is important to realise that the potential calculated by the Goldman equation only predicts the potential at which no net movement of electric charge will occur, and is not a thermodynamic equilibrium potential but depends on kinetics of passive transport processes:
− At the Goldman potential the different ions are not in equilibrium across the membrane. Therefore net transmembrane fluxes of the ions will occur.
− In the long run the net movement of ions occurring at the Goldman potential will cause concentration changes in the cytoplasm, which would cause the Goldman potential to

change if not active transport processes such as the Na^+/K^+ pump would keep the cytoplasmic concentrations of these ions at a constant level.
– The stationary potential calculated by the equation depends on the transport kinetics: the equation contains the permeabilities, which characterise the rate of ion transport.
– The potential calculated by the equation will only be a stationary potential if the permeabilities as well as the concentrations do not change with time.
– The Goldman equation does not include the contribution of electrogenic active transport.

1.3.4 Contribution of electrogenic pump current to the membrane potential

Since net passive movements of K^+ and Na^+ occur, the Na^+/K^+ pump has to transport Na^+ and K^+ to compensate for these net passive fluxes in order to keep the intracellular concentrations constant. Since the pump transports 3 Na^+ out of the cell for 2 K^+ ions entering the cell, for each cycle of the pump a net positive charge is transported from inside to outside, which tends to hyperpolarise the cell. The hyperpolarisation (ΔE_m) due to such an electrogenic pump is equal to the product of the pump current (i_p) and membrane resistance $\Delta E_m = i_p.R_m$. Also other passive electrogenic transporters, such as the Na^+/Ca^{2+} exchanger will contribute a current, eventually resulting in some effect on the membrane potential.

1.4 Electrically equivalent circuit of the cell

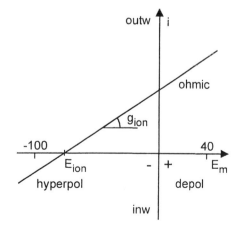

Figure II.11. Ionic current as function of potential in the presence of a concentration gradient. $i_{ion} = g_{ion} (E_m - E_{ion})$. The current is zero at the equilibrium potential of the ion.

   Different ion channels with different properties are present in the membrane. For an accurate electrically equivalent description of the ionic current pathway, the conductive pathway must be split into several components in parallel, each representing the contribution to the ionic current of one type of channel. Each ion channel contributing to the net current is then represented by a resistance (or its inverse conductance $g = 1/R$), which may not be constant, and therefore is represented by a variable resistor.

   The existence of concentration gradients of different ions across the membrane causes the current flowing through a channel not being zero at zero membrane potential, but at the equilibrium potential of the ion (Fig. II.11). In order to describe ionic currents flowing through the membrane in the presence of an ion concentration gradient, Ohm's law must be adapted to take into account the flow of ions driven by the concentration gradient, which results in a shift of the current-voltage relation. The ionic current can then be described by $i_{ion} = g_{ion} \cdot (E_m - E_{ion})$.

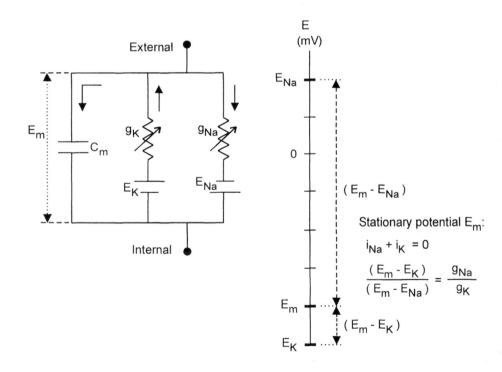

Figure II.12. Electrical equivalent circuit for a membrane permeable to Na^+ and K^+ (left) and interpretation of the stationary potential as weighed average of equilibrium potentials (right). Larger values of g_{Na}/g_K result in E_m to deviate more from E_K and to become closer to E_{Na}.

   The ion concentration gradient has an effect equivalent to a battery (electromotive force). The electrical equivalent representation of each of the ion permeation pathways across the membrane therefore consists of a battery in series with a resistance (or equivalently a conductance). The battery representing the electrical equivalent effect of the ion concentration gradient generates a potential equal to the equilibrium potential of the ion across the membrane. The resistance represents the permeability of the membrane for the ion. The simple electrical equivalent circuit shown in Fig. II.4 must therefore be replaced by a circuit like the one illustrated in Fig. II.12.

Conventions:

According to the normal convention for describing electric currents, direction of electric current flow refers to the direction of movement of positive charges. Outward current flowing through the membrane therefore is defined as positive charges leaving the cell. Therefore current due to K^+ ions leaving the cell is referred to as outward current while Na^+ entering a cell produces inward current. Influx of Cl^- into the cell causes negative charges entering the cell, which is electrically equivalent as positive charges leaving the cell, and therefore is represented as outward current. By convention in the nowadays electrophysiology literature (unlike in the early literature) outward currents are considered positive and shown as upward deflections, while inward currents are negative and shown as downward deflections.

Membrane potentials are given as potential of the cytoplasm (E_i) with respect to the extracellular medium (E_e); thus $E_m = E_i - E_e$. At the normal resting potential the cell is thus negatively polarised. Making the potential more negative is called hyperpolarisation, while changing the potential in the opposite direction (to less negative or positive values) is called a depolarisation. The return of the membrane potential in the direction of its normal resting potential after a depolarisation is called repolarisation.

2. ELECTROPHYSIOLOGICAL METHODS

A large variety of electrophysiological techniques are available to measure potentials or ionic currents flowing through a whole cell membrane or through single channels. For a good overview see [794,818].

2.1 Potential measurements

2.1.1 Intracellular potential measurements

The membrane potential of cardiac cells can be measured by inserting a glass microelectrode into the cell. A microelectrode consists of a very fine pipette-shaped glass capillary filled with a conducting electrolyte solution (often a 3 M KCl solution). Such an electrode has an open tip with a diameter of the order of 1 μm and has a resistance typically of the order of 10 MΩ. The microelectrode tip is inserted through the membrane into the cell, and the potential at the tip is measured with respect to an extracellular reference electrode. Membrane potentials are expressed as the potential inside the cell minus extracellular potential: $E_m = E_i - E_e$.

Cardiac cells at rest or during diastolic depolarisation have membrane potentials of the order of −50 to −90 mV, depending on cell type. Measuring the resting potential at different ion concentrations provides information about the permeability of the cell for different ions. Since in the absence of external current flow, the rate of change of the potential (dE_m/dt, mostly named dV/dt) is directly proportional to the net ionic current, the net ionic current flowing during the action potential can be derived from the shape of the action potential.

2.1.2 Extracellular potential measurements

Differences in membrane potential between different parts of the tissue cause redistribution of electric charges resulting in current flowing in the intracellular as well as in the extracellular medium (local circuit currents). These currents give rise to potential differences in the extracellular space surrounding the tissue.

2.1.2.1 Extracellular field potentials

Extracellular field potentials show a marked resemblance with the first time derivative ($\partial V/\partial t$) of the action potentials, although it is important to note that the situation in a complex non-uniform structure like the heart can markedly deviate from this relation (see e.g. Chapter VI).

The extracellular current flow between two parts of a tissue at different potential is proportional to the potential difference between these two sites. If an action potential is conducted as a wave at constant speed, the distance travelled in a given time is dependent on the conduction velocity (θ) so that the shape of the curve relating the potential V to t at constant x, and that of V to x at constant t, is identical:

$$\partial V/\partial x = (1/\theta) \, \partial V/\partial t$$

Since the extracellular potential difference is proportional to the current and the current is proportional to the spatial gradient of the membrane potential, and the spatial membrane potential gradient is proportional to the time derivative of the potential, a marked resemblance between extracellular potential registrations and rate of change of membrane potential under the recording electrode can be expected, although detailed analysis shows that the relation is more complex [1074].

2.1.2.2 Monophasic action potentials

Measurements of extracellular potentials in appropriate conditions can approximately reproduce the resting and action potential. Such extracellular recordings of action potentials, called monophasic action potentials or MAPs, have been obtained for more than a century, either by applying a laesion or injury, by suction electrode, or by pressing an electrode against the myocardium. A contact electrode technique that enables stable MAP recordings, lasting several hours, from human endocardium or epicardium was developed by Franz (Fig. II.13) [for review see 345].

MAP registrations are usually made in a so-called close bipolar MAP electrode arrangement. This is obtained by pressing non-polarisable contact electrode, electrically isolated except at its tip, against the heart. The potential difference between this MAP electrode (E1) and an indifferent electrode (E2), a few mm proximal to the depolarising tip electrode, is measured using a direct current (DC)-coupled amplifier. Pressing an electrode against the tissue causes local depolarisation (to a level estimated at −30 to −20 mV in clinical MAP recordings), but does not cause 'injury' as was the case with the older techniques. A potential gradient between depolarised cells and the adjacent normal cells is thus created. The depolarisation inactivates Na^+ and Ca^{2+} channels, making the cells under the MAP electrode unexcitable, so that excitation of the normal tissue causes reversal of the spatial electric gradient. The spatial gradients during rest and activity are at the basis of the MAPs, which reflect the potential of the cells in the immediate vicinity of the cells under the contact electrode.

According to the Schütz hypothesis, developed to explain the MAPs recorded with suction electrodes, the MAP is the voltage drop between the different electrode in contact with the 'injured' myocardium and the indifferent electrode (at the uninjured myocardium). Franz however explains the origin of the MAP potentials based on the 'volume conductor hypothesis' [345]. However the approach by Schütz (when correctly applied to the contact electrode technique) yields a simple and very good quantitative description of close bipolar MAPs, as explained below.

When the MAP electrode is brought in close contact with the tissue and pressure is applied, a 'seal' is obtained: the close contact between the electric isolation surrounding the electrode and the membrane surface provides a high extracellular seal resistance (R_s) between the part of the membrane under the contact electrode and the extracellular space. The existing spatial difference between the membrane potential of the cells under the electrode and the potential of the adjacent cells causes a short-circuit current (i), which causes voltage drops across R_i and R_s (respectively equal to $i.R_i$ and $i.R_s$) (Fig. II.13). When the seal resistance (R_s) between the measuring electrode (1) and the reference electrode (2) is large compared to the intracellular resistance (R_i) between the two electrodes, the potential difference (E1 – E2) between the recording electrode and the reference electrode approaches the true difference in membrane potential between the recording site ($E_m(1)$) and the adjacent site ($E_m(2)$). Since the depolarised cells are unexcitable, the close bipolar MAPS reflect the shape of action potentials of the cells adjacent to the electrode, although the MAP amplitude is smaller by a factor $R_s/(R_s+R_i)$, and the baseline is somewhat shifted (see equations in Fig. II.13).

While MAP recordings underestimate the amplitude of the potentials and the rate of rise of the action potential, the technique is very useful to study timing relations such as activation time and action potential duration and its dispersion.

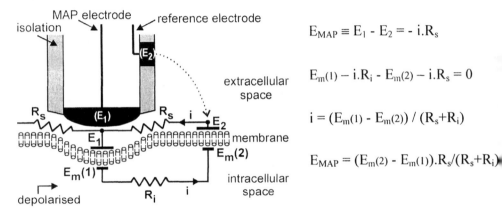

$$E_{MAP} \equiv E_1 - E_2 = - i.R_s$$

$$E_m(1) – i.R_i - E_m(2) – i.R_s = 0$$

$$i = (E_m(1) - E_m(2)) / (R_s+R_i)$$

$$E_{MAP} = (E_m(2) - E_m(1)).R_s/(R_s+R_i)$$

Figure II.13. MAP registration. Simplified equivalent circuit.

2.1.3 Potential measurement using fluorescent dyes

Voltage-sensitive fluorescent dyes have become powerful tools for optical registration of resting membrane potentials and action potentials. They enable measurements of potentials in subcellular organelles and in cells that are too small to allow the use of microelectrodes, and, in conjunction with imaging techniques, can be used to map spatial distribution of membrane potentials. Two classes of voltage-sensitive fluorescent dyes can be distinguished [1,1055].

– Fast-response dyes (usually styrylpyridinium dyes such as di-4-ANEPPS) change their electron shell structure, and consequently their fluorescence properties, in response to a change in the surrounding electric field. These dyes have been extensively used to study electrical activity in cardiac muscle and cell cultures, and to visualise excitation waves inside cardiac tissues, in whole heart and in vivo heart [for references see 64].

– Slow-response probes, which include cationic lipophilic compounds, exhibit potential-dependent changes in transmembrane distribution according to the Nernst equation, accompanied by a fluorescence change. Slow-response probes, such as carbocyanines (such as JC-1), rhodamines and rosamines, can be used to detect changes in average membrane potentials of nonexcitable cells and mitochondria. While several of these compounds have been used to study the membrane potential of cardiac mitochondria [249,391,750] [see 392], it was concluded from studies comparing a number of slow potentiometric dyes that only JC-1 stained cardiac mitochondria in a potential-dependent way [714].

2.2   Constant current

In addition to an intracellular potential measuring electrode, a second intracellular microelectrode can be inserted into the cell, and this electrode can be used to inject a constant current. Small positive currents applied through this electrode inject positive charges into the cell and thereby charge the membrane capacitance and depolarise the cell. The time course of the ionic current follows an exponential with a time constant that is equal to the product of the membrane capacitance times the membrane resistance. In steady-state, the amount of depolarisation is proportional to size of the current pulse and the membrane resistance (see Fig. II.5).

2.3   Voltage clamp

2.3.1   Principle

Current injection can be used to study membrane electrical properties. However the investigated properties may be affected by the change in membrane potential resulting from the injected current. The basic problem in studying the properties of ionic currents is that the ionic current is dependent on membrane potential, and that the ionic current itself also changes the membrane potential. The problem could be avoided if the membrane potential somehow could be kept constant despite the flow of ionic current through the membrane. This can be achieved by the voltage clamp technique.

The technique was invented by Marmont and Cole and extensively applied by Hodgkin and Huxley [460,461] to voltage clamp the squid axon. The purpose of this technique is to hold the potential difference across the membrane at a known and controlled value during the time and over the areas in which the membrane current is measured. In the classical voltage clamp technique two electrodes are inserted in the cytoplasm (in their experiments Hodgkin and Huxley used two long thin wires inserted along the axoplasm of a squid axon), while the extracellular medium is kept at zero potential by a ground electrode (Fig. II.14).

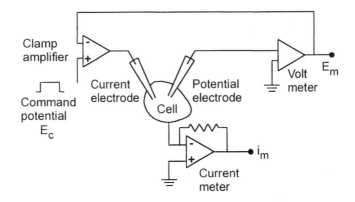

Figure II.14. Voltage clamp technique. Principle: deviations between membrane potential and command potential, caused by ions flowing through the membrane, are measured and are automatically compensated by injecting current. The amount of current that needs to be injected to keep the potential constant equals the ionic current flowing through the membrane.

One of these intracellular electrodes is used to inject current while the other electrode measures the intracellular potential. The two electrodes are connected by a negative feedback circuit: the difference between the membrane potential (E_m) and the desired value (Command potential E_c) is amplified by means of a feedback amplifier, and the output of the amplifier is connected to the current electrode. Any difference between E_m and E_c gives rise to a non-zero output potential of the amplifier, and therefore causes current flow through the membrane which changes the membrane potential, reducing this difference between E_m and E_c. The current injected can be measured and is equal to the sum of the current charging the membrane capacitance plus the net ionic current, as mentioned before. During a fast voltage step a rapid surge of current that decays very rapidly is initially seen. This current represents the capacitative current charging the membrane, and this component is over as soon as the membrane potential has reached a constant value: when the membrane potential is constant, $dE_m/dt = 0$ and therefore no capacitative current flow is present. The measured current is then equal to the net ionic current i_i flowing through the membrane (Fig. II.14).

2.3.2   Measurements

Under voltage clamp conditions, a number of different types of measurements can be done.

2.3.2.1   Membrane current measurement

In the standard voltage clamp experiments, the total membrane current flowing through the whole membrane of the cell or multicellular preparation is measured. This current is composed of a capacitative current and the net ionic current. The capacitative current during a clamp step is present only during the brief time interval during which the membrane potential is suddenly changed to another level. By using fast changes of membrane potential, the resulting capacitative current is made as short as possible, in order to avoid that it interferes with the time course of the ionic current. The ionic current is the sum of the currents flowing through all ion channels and electrogenic transporters (carriers). In order to separate the net ionic current in its components, and thereby to gain information on the current flowing through one type of channels, different experimental procedures are used:
- Procedures can be used to make the contribution of other currents negligible
- Ion substitution.
   Ions flowing through other channels are substituted by non-permeant ions; eventually chelators are used in addition (e.g. a Ca^{2+} chelator such as EGTA can be added to buffer Ca^{2+}).
- Pharmacological separation.
   Specific channel blockers or activators can be added to the solution (e.g. tetrodotoxin (TTX) can be used to specifically block voltage-dependent Na^+ channels).
- Voltage protocols.
   Known properties of channels can be used to make the contribution of a channel to the measured net current negligible by applying specific voltage protocols. Voltage protocols can be used to inactivate a current (e.g. the potential steps can be started from a holding potential at –60 mV, which is known to inactivate voltage-dependent Na^+ channels), or measurements can be done at the equilibrium potential of a current.
- The previously mentioned procedures can be also used to make the contribution of current under study negligible. Subtracting the currents measured under this condition from the currents in control solution yields a so-called "difference current" which is equal to the contribution of the current under study to the net ionic current, if the interventions change the amplitude but not the kinetics of the currents.

In addition to the isolation of an individual ionic current component from the total membrane current, these procedures (especially the use of specific voltage protocols) can also be used to study specific parameters of an ionic current.

2.3.2.2   Gating current

Voltage-gating of channels requires a voltage sensor in the channel. Such a voltage sensor must be a charged particle or a dipole in the channel protein that is displaced when an electric field is applied to the membrane, and thereby generates a small electric current. In order to measure this current, all ionic currents are blocked so that only the capacitative current is left. The capacitative current during a voltage step in the range of activation is then compared with voltage steps in a potential range where the process under study has no voltage-dependence. The difference between the capacitive currents in both conditions reflects the gating current. This gating current directly measures the movement of voltage-dependent gating particles in the channel protein, and yields information of the transition of the channel between different states. It can give information about the processes governing the voltage-dependent steps involved in the channel kinetics, eventually also giving information about state transitions between closed states which cannot be measured with most other techniques [for review see 87].

2.3.2.3   Noise

The currents recorded under voltage clamp conditions contain noise that is partially due to opening and closing of channels in the membrane.

Measurement under *stationary* conditions of the noise power variance or the frequency spectrum of the noise together with the mean current can yield important information about the underlying electrophysiological processes, such as channel density, open state probability and kinetics [201,795]. Power spectral density of the noise can be obtained by Fourier analysis of the current fluctuations. The frequency at which the power is reduced to half-maximum yields information about the channel kinetics.

Even in *non-stationary* conditions information on single channel current and density can be obtained by measuring average current and variance of the current from a large ensemble of responses to an identical stimulus [1042].

Fluctuation analysis has in most cases been replaced by single channel analysis, but the technique is useful for studying channels or carriers with single channel current too low or channel density too high for single channel events to be resolved.

2.3.2.4 Single channel current

Single channel current measurements are a specific type of voltage clamp experiments, where, by using the patch clamp technique (see section 2.3.3.2), the current flowing though a small membrane area (the patch) of the order of a few μm^2 is measured while the membrane potential is controlled by the clamp amplifier [794]. Since such a small area of membrane typically contains only a limited number of channels, this technique often allows to resolve single channel events (depending on the channel density). The composition of the pipette solution and/or bathing solution is chosen to optimise the chance of recording only the type of channel under investigation.

2.3.3 Clamp techniques

In most preparations inserting a large wire electrode, as has been done in squid axons, is not feasible. Other methods must be used to inject current and to ensure uniformity of membrane potential over the preparation. Spatial uniformity of the potential can be reached using sufficiently small multi-cellular preparations, or using single cells isolated by enzymatic dissociation.

According to the method used for current injection and voltage measurement several types of voltage clamp are possible.

2.3.3.1 Microelectrode techniques
2.3.3.1.1 Two microelectrode techniques

The two microelectrode technique uses one intracellular microelectrode to measure the membrane potential and one electrode to inject current. The current electrode is connected to the output of a feedback amplifier that compares the membrane potential with the command potential (Fig. II.14). Any difference between the two potentials causes an output voltage, which results in current flowing into the cell, which keeps the membrane potential at the level of the command potential.

2.3.3.1.2 Single microelectrode techniques

The single microelectrode technique uses one normal intracellular microelectrode for both current injection and voltage measurement. Current injection however causes a voltage drop across the microelectrode, which according to Ohm's law, is the product of the injected current times the electrode resistance. Therefore the measured potential is not equal to the membrane potential, unless this voltage drop is somehow compensated. Two general methods, the Wheatstone bridge method and the switched clamp, can be used to avoid the problem.

- In the bridge method, the voltage drop across the electrode is compensated by adding a voltage equal to the membrane current times the electrode resistance to the command signal.

For correct measurement of the membrane potential this extra potential is subtracted from the measured potential using a circuit equivalent to a Wheatstone bridge.

- In the switched clamp method, a sample-and-hold technique is used, whereby the current is interrupted at a high frequency. During these short periods of no current flow the voltage is measured. This potential is then used to determine the amount of current injection during the next short period of current injection. Typically the frequency of alteration between voltage measurement and current injection is of the order of several kHz.

2.3.3.2   Patch electrode techniques

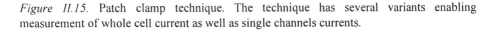

Figure II.15. Patch clamp technique. The technique has several variants enabling measurement of whole cell current as well as single channels currents.

In the patch clamp technique, invented by Neher and Sakmann [414], a special type of electrode with a large mouth (diameter of a few micrometers) and a short shank is used. Such a patch-electrode has a relatively low resistance. The electrode tip is fire polished to make a smooth tip and the electrode is filled with a solution with an ionic composition on the basis of the composition of either cytoplasmic or extracellular solutions. The tip is slightly pressed on the membrane surface. Small suction pulses are applied to the electrode, (hence the name suction pipette) which then seals to the membrane, providing a good electrical isolation between the inside of the electrode and the outside medium. The resistance of the seal is typically of the order of 10 GigaOhm (thus the name gigaseal), ensuring that current leaking between the electrode and the extracellular medium is negligible.

The patch clamp technique can be used in different configurations that basically fit in two categories. In whole cell methods the patch clamp technique is used to measure the total current flowing through the whole membrane of the cell. In single channel techniques only the current flowing through the small patch of membrane located at the tip of the electrode (size a few μm^2) is measured, enabling the measurement of current through single channels (Fig. II.15).

2.3.3.2.1 Whole cell techniques

The *whole cell clamp* is a single electrode method based on the patch clamp technique to measure the total current flowing through the membrane of a cell. After making a gigaseal further suction is used to destroy the membrane patch underneath the electrode tip, so that the pipette interior and the cell interior are in direct contact. This way the electrode can be used in a way similar to an intracellular microelectrode. The patch pipette is electrically connected to the patch clamp amplifier, which senses the potential of the cell and maintains the potential at the desired value, set by the command pulse, by injecting current using a feedback mechanism. Since the potential is measured by the same electrode that passes the current, the voltage-drop across the electrode resistance needs to be compensated by series resistance compensation.

Since after rupturing the patch of membrane under the electrode, the patch pipette is in direct contact with the cytoplasm, the cytoplasmic solution will be exchanged with the pipette solution. The whole cell clamp technique offers the advantage of controlling to a large extent the intracellular medium. However important substances normally present in the cytoplasm may have been diluted by perfusing the cell.

The *permeabilised patch* (also called perforated patch) is a variant of the classical whole cell clamp technique, the only difference being that the patch of membrane under the pipette is not destroyed by suction, but made leaky by using channel-forming substances (such as nystatin or amphotericin B) added to the pipette solution. The incorporation of the pore-forming substances enables passage of monovalent inorganic ions through the patch membrane. The pores thereby ensure a low resistance electrical pathway to the interior of the cell, but dilution of large organic ions and molecules from the cell is avoided and $[Ca^{2+}]_i$ is not affected, so that the cell remains in a more normal physiological condition.

2.3.3.2.2 Single channel techniques

In contrast to the whole cell techniques, which measure the total membrane current of the whole cell, the single channel techniques measure only the current flowing through the small patch of membrane under the tip of the pipette. The technique is very sensitive and allows recording of currents with amplitudes less than 1 pA, depending on the thermal noise of the patch - seal combination. Single channel currents can be recorded using different patch clamp configurations.

2.3.3.2.2.1 Cell-attached patch

The patch clamp configuration obtained immediately after a giga seal is established is called the *cell-attached patch* configuration. If voltage clamp is done in this configuration, all current flowing through the pipette passes through the small patch of membrane under the pipette into (or depending on the polarity of the current out of) the cell, and leaves (or enters) the cell through the rest of the membrane.

Since the membrane area under the patch is extremely small in comparison with the whole cell area, the resistance of the whole cell membrane is negligible compared to that of the patch. Therefore any potential change applied to the pipette drops almost completely across the membrane patch. Clamping in this configuration thus gives the relation between current and potential of a small patch of membrane that is still attached to the rest of the membrane. The outer side of the patch membrane sees the solution in the pipette, while the inner side of the membrane faces the normal cytoplasmic environment. In this configuration: $E_m = -E_{pipette} + E_{cell}$ (where E_m is the membrane potential of the patch, $E_{pipette}$ is the potential applied to the pipette and E_{cell} the potential of the cell).

The *macro patch* is a form of cell-attached patch whereby the diameter of the pipette is much larger than in normal cell-attached patches. By measuring the current flowing through a number of channels under a relatively small area of membrane, this technique is sometimes used for studying channels with very small conductance, or for carriers, which have single channel currents that are too small to resolve.

2.3.3.2.2.2 Cell-free patch

After gigaseal formation the contact between the cell and the pipette is mechanically very stable, and the pipette can be withdrawn from the cell surface, ripping off a patch of membrane from the rest of the cell membrane, thus establishing an "excised patch" also called a cell-free patch. Depending on the procedure, two excised patch configurations are possible whereby either the cytoplasmic face or the external face of the patch membrane faces the bathing solution.

2.3.3.2.2.2.1 Inside-out patch

In inside–out patch techniques a procedure for ripping off the patch is used that results in an excised patch whereby the cytoplasmic side of the patch membrane faces the bathing solution. This configuration makes it easy to expose the cytoplasmic side of the membrane to different solutions. Eventually pipette perfusion techniques can be used to change the solution facing the extracellular side of the membrane.

Pulling the pipette away from the cell after giga seal formation (eventually in Ca^{2+}-free solution or after air exposure to avoid vesicle formation) a patch of membrane remains at the tip of the electrode. The cytoplasmic side of the patch membrane faces the external medium while the external side of the membrane is exposed to the pipette solution. Since the inner side of the membrane now faces the bath (outside) solution, this configuration is called an inside-out patch. This configuration makes it easy to expose the cytoplasmic side of the membrane to different solutions. Eventually pipette perfusion techniques can be used to change the solution facing the extracellular side of the membrane. In this configuration: $E_m = -E_{pipette}$

2.3.3.2.2.2.2 Outside-out patch

In outside-out patch configuration, a patch isolation procedure is used that results in a patch whereby the outer side of the patch membrane faces the bathing (outside). Outside-out patches enable easy change of the solution at the extracellular side of the membrane.

If the membrane under the pipette is ruptured before slowly withdrawing the pipette from the cell, a neck-like structure forms, which becomes narrower and eventually breaks of from the rest of the cell but reseals forming a patch of membrane under the pipette. In this configuration: $E_m = E_{pipette}$

3. ANALYSIS AND PROPERTIES OF ION TRANSPORT MECHANISMS

3.1 Types of transport processes

The cytoplasmic concentrations of many molecules and ions are different from the concentrations in the extracellular medium, and the plasma membrane acts a barrier separating the intracellular medium from the extracellular compartment. However the membrane also serves as a pathway for exchange of material and information between the cell and its environment. Therefore the plasma membrane contains a number of mechanisms for transporting ions and molecules. Some of these processes (active transport processes) are needed to build and maintain the transmembrane gradients and require energy, while other processes (passive transport) do not require energy consumption, since the movement occurs in the direction of the existing transmembrane gradient.

3.1.1   Active transport

Passive diffusion tends to destroy any gradient. In order to maintain the cell out of equilibrium with its environment several substances need to be transported across the cell membrane in a direction opposite to the existing gradient. Such transport occurs though carrier proteins and requires energy. It is called active transport. Energy for such a transport against the gradient can be obtained from metabolic processes, by directly coupling the transport process to ATP hydrolysis. This type of active transport is called primary active transport (e.g. Na^+/K^+ ATPase). However energy can also be obtained by coupling the reaction to a passive transport process, whereby the energy released by the passive transport, which would normally be wasted as heat, is now used to do work to drive the carrier. The potential energy of an existing gradient of one substance is therefore used to drive a process of transporting another substance against its gradient. This type of transport is called secondary active transport. Although it does not directly use metabolic energy, it receives its energy from an existing gradient, which must be built up and maintained by processes consuming metabolic energy. When the direction in which the two transported substances move is the same the carrier is called a cotransporter or symport (e.g. Na^+-HCO_3^-), otherwise it is called an exchanger or antiport (e.g. Na^+/Ca^{2+} exchanger).

Passive as well as active transport can be electroneutral or electrogenic. Transport is electrogenic whenever the transport results in net translocation of electric charges across the membrane. If this is the case the transport results in net transmembrane current, and thereby influences the membrane potential, while it also is influenced itself by changes in membrane potential. Electrogenic processes, whether active or passive, are therefore not only influenced by concentration gradients but are determined by the so-called electrochemical gradient. The electrochemical gradient is the difference between the membrane potential and the reversal potential. The reversal potential is the potential at which the free energy of the chemical gradient and the potential gradient are exactly equal but opposite, so that at this potential no net transport takes place.

3.1.2   Passive transport

Some substances are transported through the membrane in a purely passive way. This type of transport occurs in the presence of transmembrane gradients and is driven by diffusion. This transport does not require energy, and net movement is in the direction as to decrease the existing gradient. According to Fick's law the rate of transport of uncharged molecules is proportional to the existing chemical gradient and the diffusion coefficient, which is inversely related to the molecular radius. Some substances will diffuse through the membrane lipid. These substances include uncharged non-polar substances, or small uncharged polar molecules, such as O_2, CO_2, NO, H_2O, urea. In order to permeate through the membrane, they must first enter the lipid phase of the membrane Therefore their permeation also depends on lipophilicity, as expressed in the oil/water partition coefficient.

Several substances which are too large, or charged (ions) or strongly polar are unable to permeate through the membrane lipids but can permeate via integral membrane proteins. Passive transport via proteins can occur via diffusion through channels or pores that form a permeation pathway through the membrane. This is the case for inorganic ions such as Na^+, K^+, Ca^{2+} and Cl^-. Channels and pores however are limited in size; the presence of very large channels in the membrane would enable many different types of molecules to pass, which would eventually lead to the disappearance of the transmembrane gradients necessary for cellular function. For permeation of large molecules, cells make use of 'facilitated diffusion'. In this type of transport, the diffusion is facilitated by carrier proteins, which bind the molecule to be transported. The binding is followed by a conformation change of the carrier, which causes translocation of the bound molecule from one side to the other side of the membrane. Facilitated diffusion is characterised by substrate specificity and a low turnover rate as compared to permeation via channels, Michaelis-Menten kinetics and competitive and non-competitive inhibition. The transport is passive, driven by the existing gradient, but is facilitated: the rate of diffusion (which would be very low in the absence of a carrier) is largely enhanced by the presence of the carrier.

3.2 Channels

As in most other cells electrophysiological effects in cardiac cells are mainly due to ions moving through channels. Channels are pore-like structures formed by proteins embedded in the lipid bilayer membrane. The channel proteins are not static structures, but can dynamically alter their configuration depending on factors in their environment. The pores can be in the open or closed state, and in the open state they allow specific types of ions to translocate between the extracellular and intracellular medium.

For understanding the contribution of different channels to the electrophysiological properties of cells, it is imperative to understand the fundamental properties of channels. Four basic properties that characterise channels are important for their function in the membrane:

1. Channel distribution in the membrane.
– Where are the channels located?
– What is their density?
2. Channel permeability.
– Which ions can permeate through the channels, in other words what is the channel selectivity?
– What is the rate of permeation for permeating ions?
3. Channel kinetics.
– What regulates or modulates opening of the channel?
– What is the kinetics of this regulatory process?
– Which substances inhibit current flow through the channel?
4. Molecular structure.
– What is the primary, secondary, tertiary and quaternary structure?
– How does structure correlate with function?
– What is the effect of structural defects?

A major breakthrough in understanding ionic currents came in 1952 from Hodgkin and Huxley [461]. These authors investigated the mechanism of the generation of the action potential by voltage clamp experiments on squid axons and provided a full analysis of voltage-dependent sodium and potassium currents. The model they introduced was able to predict the shape of the action potential and had important mechanistic implications for channel functioning. However, while it now is clear that the Hodgkin – Huxley model does not fully describe channel functioning at the molecular level, most of its fundamental properties and many of its functional implications are still valid, and the model is still a very good approximation for understanding the role of channels in physiological and pathological conditions. Therefore the Hodgkin – Huxley model and its variants are still widely used as the simplest models that can describe many ion channels in cardiac (and other) membranes. A thorough understanding of the Hodgkin – Huxley model is therefore required for the interpretation of many electrophysiological data. For this reason, we will first summarise the Hodgkin – Huxley model and describe the kinetic processes of Na^+ current and delayed K^+ current in terms of this model.

As more and more detailed data became available on ionic currents in many cell types, a large number of variants, extensions and refinements of the Hodgkin – Huxley model were introduced. Finally the invention of the patch clamp and single channel analysis, and the application of molecular biology, required description of channels on a deeper level. Therefore, following the description of the Hodgkin – Huxley model we will describe the general properties of ion channels, first on the whole cell and then at the single channel level.

3.2.1 Hodgkin – Huxley model

Hodgkin and Huxley in collaboration with Katz first described the time course of the ionic current during different voltage steps (Fig. II.16 upper left panel) and determined the relation between membrane current and potential (Fig. II.16 lower left panel). Hodgkin and Huxley then demonstrated that they could separate the net ionic current into a Na^+ and a K^+ component (by lowering Na^+ concentration) (Fig. II.16 upper right panel). They showed that an inward Na^+ current first increases with time during a depolarising voltage step, and after reaching a peak it decays to zero. The outward K^+ current on the other hand shows a slower rise towards a maximum value at the end of the clamp step, without showing a decay. This outward current only decreases after clamping back the membrane to the original potential.

Clamping back the membrane to the resting potential after a depolarising step results in a sudden change of the ionic current, which is followed by a gradual decay. By comparing the amplitude of the current during depolarising and repolarising steps Hodgkin and Huxley concluded that each component of ionic current could be described as the product of two factors: one factor is an instantaneous function of potential and represents the driving force, while the other factor is a continuous function of voltage and time due to a gradual permeability change.

To investigate the first factor they studied the relation between membrane potential and ionic current in situations where the permeability does not change (doing a clamp step to open channels and then suddenly changing the potential and measuring the instantaneous current). They found that the relation between potential and current in this condition ("instantaneous current-voltage relation") is linear and could thus be approximated by Ohm's law, the current passing through zero at the equilibrium potential of the ion. The first factor is therefore the driving force, which is equal to $(E_m - E_i)$, the difference between the membrane potential and the equilibrium potential of the ion.

Applying Ohm's law by dividing the currents by the driving force gives the second factor: a conductance g_i defined as $g_i = i_i / (E_m - E_i)$. This conductance describes the membrane permeability and is a continuous function of voltage and time, as is shown for g_{Na} and g_K in the lower right panel of Fig. II.16.

Based on their extensive analysis of the conductance changes, Hodgkin and Huxley found that the decrease in g_K during a repolarising step could be described by a first order kinetic process, while its rise during a depolarising step needs a fourth order equation. They concluded that a useful simplification could be achieved by assuming that g_K is proportional to the

fourth power of a variable obeying first order kinetics and which they called
the activation. To describe the onset and decay of g_{Na} they introduced two
different variables (activation and inactivation). Based on these assumptions
they proposed a mathematical model to describe the kinetics of Na^+ and K^+
currents in terms of a number of voltage-dependent gates controlling the
channels [for an overview see 449].

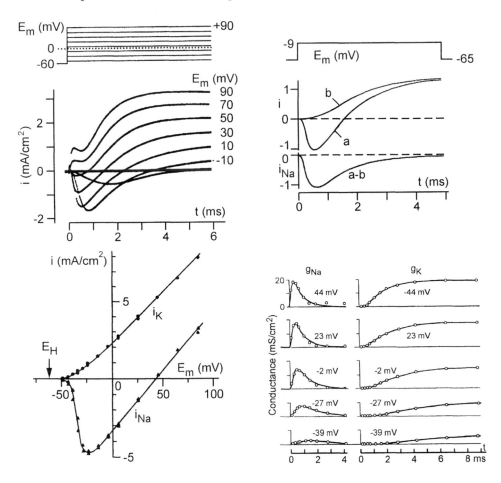

Figure II.16. Analysis of ionic currents. Upper left: net ionic current in the squid giant axon as
a function of time during different voltage steps. Modified from [33]. Upper right: separation
of Na^+ and K^+ current; current in control (a) and in conditions that remove the Na^+ current
such as TTX or Na^+-free solution (b); i_{Na} = difference current (a) - (b). Lower left: peak Na^+
current and steady-state K^+ current as a function of membrane potential. Modified from [197].
Lower right: time course of Na^+ and K^+ conductance at different membrane potentials.
Modified from [461].

This mathematical model introduced by Hodgkin and Huxley to describe the membrane conductance for Na^+ and K^+ can be visualised by assuming that one or more mutually independent gates control the channels in the membrane. These gates thus modulate the flow of ions through the membrane channel. Such a gate can be in one of two positions, either open (O) or closed (C), and the transitions between open and closed states are governed by voltage-dependent rate constants α and β.

$$C \underset{\beta(E)}{\overset{\alpha(E)}{\rightleftharpoons}} O$$

From this simple model, which describes the transitions between open and closed position of the gates, we can calculate the equilibrium of the gating reaction, as would be done in conventional chemical calculations by calculating the equilibrium constant. However since the rate constants depend on the potential, the equilibrium cannot be represented by a single equilibrium constant, but is a function of membrane potential. Therefore the equilibrium of the reaction is represented by an equation or a curve showing the voltage-dependence of the equilibrium. The description of the equilibrium of the reaction determining the state of the gate by electrophysiologists also uses a different convention than is usual in classical chemistry. Instead of representing the equilibrium of the reaction by an equilibrium constant K which is equal to the ratio n_O/n_C (the number of gates in open and closed position) in steady-state, electrophysiologists describe the fraction (n) of gates in the open state and its steady-state value (n_α), where $n = n_O/(n_C+n_O)$ with n_O and n_C the number of gates in open and closed position.

The net rate of change in fraction of open gates (dn/dt) can be calculated as the difference of the rate of opening (which equals the product of the fraction of channels in the closed state times the rate constant of opening) minus the rate of closing (fraction of channels in open state times rate of closing):

dn/dt = $\alpha.(1 - n) - \beta.n$

At steady-state dn/dt = 0 and thus

$n_\alpha = \alpha/(\alpha + \beta)$

Since the rate constants are voltage-dependent, a change in membrane potential will affect the fraction of gates in the open state. For the simple two state models the fraction of gates in the open state is a sigmoid function of the membrane potential.

$n_\alpha = 1 / (1+ \exp[-zF(E-E_{1/2})/RT])$

where $E_{1/2}$ is the potential at which half of the gates are in open position.

The sigmoid voltage-dependence of the steady-state distribution (steady-state activation or inactivation) originates from the famous Boltzmann distribution: given a particle, which exists in an environment with a given certain thermal energy, and which can be present in a number of states which differ in energy level, the Boltzmann equation describes the probability of finding the particle in each of the different energy states.

In a system of a population of independent identical particles (such as gating particles) which can be in two different states (positions), the distribution of the particles over the two states depends on the energy difference ($U_2 - U_1$) between the two states and the thermal energy according to the Boltzmann distribution ($n_2/n_1 = \exp-[(U_2-U_1)/kT]$, where $U_2-U_1 = w$ (with w the work that must be done to move the particle from state 1 to state 2). For electrically charged particles moving in an electric field, w includes a component of electric energy, which depends on the charge of the particle (ze_0, with e_0 the elementary electric charge and z the number of elementary charges of the particle) and on the potential difference between the two positions ($w = w_0 + ze_0E$).

Also the time course of the net change in fraction of open gates (dn/dt) can be calculated by solving the equation $dn/dt = \alpha.(1 - n) - \beta.n$

In response to a step voltage, n changes to a new steady-state value:

$n(t) = n_\infty + (n_0 - n_\infty).\exp(-t/\tau)$

where n_0 is the initial value of n at the time of the voltage change, n_∞ is the steady-state value, t is the time after the voltage change, and τ is the time constant.

The time course of n, after a step voltage, is thus a simple exponential with time constant $\tau = 1/(\alpha + \beta)$

and steady-state $n_\infty = \alpha/(\alpha + \beta)$

The parameters α and β can thus be directly obtained from the steady-state value of n and the time constant: $\alpha = n_\infty/\tau$ and $\beta = (1 - n_\infty)/\tau$.

Experimentally it is generally found that the rate constants α and β are monotonic functions of membrane potential, one having a positive and the other a negative slope. If α increases (and β thus decreases) upon depolarisation, then depolarisation causes opening of the gates. Gates that open upon depolarisation are called activation gates. Gates that close upon depolarisation are called inactivation gates (or gates activating upon hyperpolarisation).

Hodgkin and Huxley found that they could describe the properties of the currents by assuming that one or more gates, acting independently of each other, control each channel and that a first order voltage-dependent process governs each gate. They described the kinetic factor governing the Na^+ channel as m^3h indicating the presence of three independent and identical activation gates (m being the proportion of open activation gates) and one independent inactivation gate (h the proportion of open inactivation gates). The K^+ channel kinetics could be described by assuming 4 independent activation gates, which they called n and thereby the kinetics of the K^+ channel was described as n^4 (Fig. II.17).

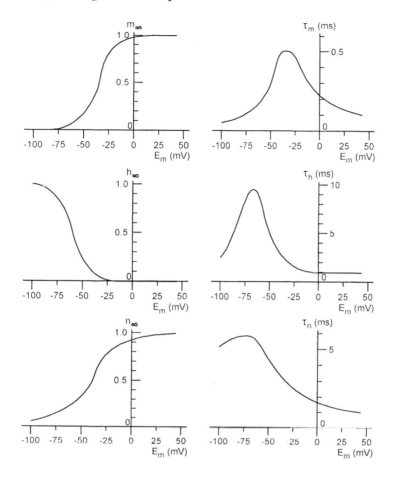

Figure II.17. Hodgkin – Huxley model of the kinetics of voltage-dependent Na^+ and K^+ channels. Upper and middle rows: steady-state activation (m_∞) and inactivation (h_∞), and time constants of activation (τ_m) and inactivation (τ_h) of i_{Na}. Lower row: steady-state activation (n_∞) and time constants (τ_n) of activation of i_K

A cartoon illustrating the Hodgkin – Huxley model is shown in Fig. II.18. The figure shows the state of the activation and inactivation gates for a cell at rest, during the peak inward Na^+ current and in steady-state during a depolarising step to a potential large enough to activate Na^+ channels.

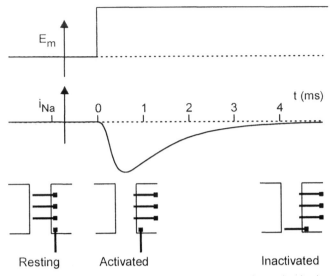

Figure II.18. Hodgkin – Huxley model of independent first order activation and inactivation of i_{Na}: correlation of time course of i_{Na} with the state of the activation gates and inactivation gate. The model assumes the presence of three identical fast activation gates opening upon depolarisation, and one slower inactivation gate closing upon depolarisation.

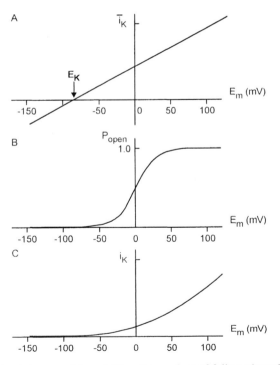

Figure II.19. Steady-state current (panel C) as the product of fully activated current (panel A) and steady-state activation (panel B) for a channel without inactivation gate.

From the fully activated current and the activation (and eventually inactivation) kinetics, the ionic current during a voltage step can be predicted as is shown in Fig. II.19 for the steady-state current through a hypothetical K^+ channel without inactivation gate.

For channels with activation as well as inactivation gating, steady-state current is in general absent over most of the potential range. However when steady-state activation and inactivation have an overlapping potential range, at these potentials a small current will be present in steady-state: this is the so-called window current (Fig. II.20).

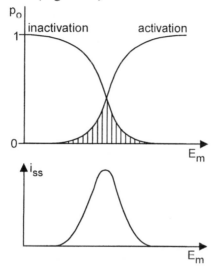

Figure II.20. Window current. When the potential range of steady-state activation and inactivation overlaps, a steady-state current exists in a limited potential region. This window current is proportional to the product of steady-state activation and inactivation.

3.2.2   Properties of Channels

After having introduced the principles of the analysis by Hodgkin and Huxley of the voltage-dependent currents in squid giant axons, the next sections describe the general properties of ionic currents in terms of ion permeation, kinetics and regulation.

3.2.2.1   Description of whole cell currents

For thermodynamic reasons the net current carried by each ion species must change sign at the equilibrium potential (E_i) of that ion. The ionic current through the membrane is therefore a function of the driving force, which is the difference between the membrane potential and the equilibrium potential of the ion: $i_i = f(E_m - E_i)$. The exact shape of this function and the magnitude of the current are determined by the kinetics of the ion translocation process. They depend on permeability characteristics of the membrane, which are determined by the nature of the ion permeation process. The permeability characteristics of the membrane can be described in analogy with Ohm's law by dividing the current by the driving force. The conductance (g) thus defined as the ratio of the current and the driving force $g_i = i_i / (E_m - E_i)$ is a measure of the membrane permeability. When measurements are made so rapidly that the channels have no time to change their state, the relation between current and voltage is often linear, yielding a constant conductance. However no fundamental law of nature dictates that this function must be linear. But even when the ionic currents are non-linear functions of the membrane potential this approach is useful, but in that case the conductance itself is potential-dependent.

In cases where the relation between ionic current and membrane potential is non-linear two kinds of conductance are generally defined. Chord conductance (g_m), is the ratio of the ionic current to the difference of the potential and the reversal potential ($g_m = i_i/(E_m - E_{rev})$. The reversal potential is the potential at which the current reverses direction. In case of a perfectly selective channel or membrane, the reversal potential corresponds to the equilibrium potential of the ion and is given by the Nernst equation. In case of incomplete selectivity, the reversal potential is given by the Goldman equation. The derivative (di_i/dE_m) is called the slope conductance ($G_m = di_i/dE_m$). The slope conductance may be positive or negative. The chord conductance of an individual ionic current, however, must always be positive, because the direction of the individual currents is only dependent on the sign of the driving force.

The ion transport processes in the membrane may be modulated, and thereby change as function of time. Opening of ion channels (gating) can be governed by changes of potential across the membrane, but also by the presence of agonists in the extracellular environment, by mechanical forces, by phosphorylation of the channel or by binding of intracellular or membrane-bound ligands. Since conformation of the channels cannot change instantaneously but requires some time, this regulation introduces time-dependence of the currents. Therefore an additional kinetic factor $k_i(E_m, \text{ligand}, ..., t)$, often called the gating factor, describing the modulating effect of the membrane potential, ligand concentration, or other regulatory factors on the flow of ions must be included. The kinetic factor can be expressed as a dimensionless quantity varying between 0 and 1. This quantity represents the fraction of channels in the open state. Therefore the ionic current can be expressed as: $i_i = k_i(E_m, \text{ligand}, ..., t).f(E_m - E_i)$, or as $i_i = \bar{g}_i.k_i(E_m, \text{ligand}, ..., t).(E_m - E_i)$, where $\bar{g}_i$ represents the fully activated channel conductance, which is the conductance when all channels are in the open state.

To describe voltage- and time-dependent ionic currents, the current is often plotted as a function of potential. Several kinds of current-voltage relationships are defined: the steady-state current-voltage, $i_\infty = f(E, \infty)$, the current-voltage relation measured at a particular moment, e.g. the peak inward current-voltage relation or the instantaneous current-voltage relationship at time t^*, $i_{inst} = f(E,t^*)$, which is obtained by measuring the current in response to a voltage step before the kinetic processes have time to proceed.

3.2.2.1.1   Ion permeation

If the kinetic factor for ionic currents equals 1 (all channels are open), then $i_i = f(E_m - E_i)$; the current carried by ion i, in this case therefore equals the value of the ion transfer function; thus the ion transfer function is often called the fully activated current-voltage relation and denoted by $\bar{i}_i$.

For the squid axon in normal seawater Hodgkin and Huxley found that the ion transfer processes are linear functions of the driving force, with the ionic channels behaving like simple ohmic conductors. The ion transfer process could therefore be described as $\bar{i}_i = \bar{g}_i \cdot (E_m - E_i)$, where $\bar{i}_i$ is the fully activated current and $\bar{g}_i$ is the fully activated conductance for ion species i that is independent of membrane potential. In general, however, the relationship between the fully activated current and the membrane potential may be non-linear, and the conductance calculated in this way is potential-dependent. When the fully activated current-voltage relation is non-linear (the conductance is not a constant but is a function of membrane potential), the current is said to show rectification (Fig. II.21).

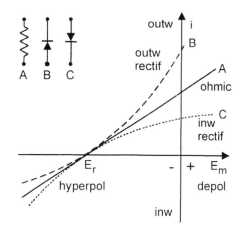

Figure II.21. Current–voltage relation. Linear I-V relation (Ohm's law) and non-linear I-V relations (rectification). The inset shows symbols for ohmic resistors and for rectifiers.

Non-linearity is characterised according to the direction in which the channel most easily passes current. A channel passing outward current more easily than inward current is called an outward rectifier: the slope of the current-voltage relation increases with depolarisation (conductance for outward current is larger than the conductance for inward current). Inward rectification is the opposite phenomenon, whereby the slope of the instantaneous current-voltage relation decreases with depolarisation.

3.2.2.1.2   Kinetics and regulation

3.2.2.1.2.1 Voltage-dependent channels

Generalising we can describe Hodgkin Huxley kinetics $k_i(E_m,t) = x^p.y^q$, where x denotes an activation and y an inactivation variable, and p and q are the number of activation and inactivation gates that act independently in series to control the channel. If inactivation is not present, then $q = 0$.

From the description of the ion transfer process $\bar{i}_i$ and gating processes, the net current carried by one ion species may be described, according to the Hodgkin – Huxley model, by the equations

$i_i(E_m,t) = x^p(E_m,t).y^q(E_m,t).\bar{i}_i(E_m - E_i)$

$dx/dt = \alpha_x(E_m).(1 - x) - \beta_x(E_m).x$

$dy/dt = \alpha_y(E_m).(1 - y) - \beta_y(E_m).y$

The first equation describes the amplitude of the current as the product of kinetics (activation and inactivation gating) times the current which would flow if all channels were in the open state. The second equation describes the kinetics for the activation gating. It states that the net rate of opening of gates is the difference between the rate of opening of closed gates and the rate of closing of open gates. The rate of closing equals the fraction of open channels (x) times the rate constant of closing, while the rate of opening equals the fraction of closed channels (1 - x) times the rate constant of opening. The third equation describes the kinetics of the inactivation process.

A full description of a time-dependent ionic current in terms of Hodgkin-Huxley requires knowledge of $\bar{i}_i(E_m - E_i)$, p and q, $\alpha_x(E_m)$, $\beta_x(E_m)$ and if inactivation is present $\alpha_y(E_m)$ and $\beta_y(E_m)$. Instead of α and β, the time constant and steady-state value of the gating variable are often given as a function of potential.

While the Hodgkin – Huxley model is very useful in describing voltage-dependent channels, it is clearly only an approximation of the kinetics of voltage-dependent channels.

– Channel activation and inactivation may not be independent. In contrast to the original formulation of Hodgkin and Huxley, activation and inactivation are now known to be linked. While channels can inactivate from a closed state, the inactivation may be facilitated by previous opening of the channel.

– Channel opening may be governed by a more complex reaction scheme eventually consisting of several closed and open states. Channel kinetics is described by Markow processes. Fig. II.22 shows a few examples of possible simple kinetic schemes for a channel showing activation and inactivation.

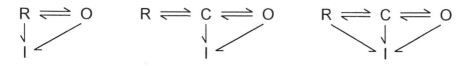

Figure II.22. Examples of possible state diagrams for a channel showing activation and inactivation. R resting state; O: open state; I: absorbing inactivated state; C pre-open closed state. Left: inactivation can proceed from resting and open state. Middle: Inactivation can proceed from C or O. Right: inactivation can proceed from R, C and O.

– Channels may also be regulated by several different factors in addition to potential.
– Voltage- and time-dependence is not always due to conformational changes of the channel but may be caused by block of the channel by charged particles, such as Mg^{2+}.
– Block of channels may be state-dependent, resulting in use-dependence, frequency-dependence and voltage-dependence.
– Ions passing through a channel may not move independently of each other, but could eventually move in single file.

3.2.2.1.2.2 Other channels

While the ionic current flowing through all channels is voltage-dependent because of the electrochemical gradient driving the transmembrane ion movement, not all channel have voltage-dependent kinetics. Channel opening can be controlled by binding of extracellular, intracellular or membrane-bound ligands, or by covalent modification such as phosphorylation, or by mechanical forces, which e.g. can be produced by stretch or cell swelling. These factors change the fraction of open channels by affecting the rate constant of opening or of closing of the close – open state reaction. Many channels are governed by more than one factor such as ligand binding and membrane potential. Conversely most factors affect more than one channel. Therefore extensive interaction of different pathways causes important convergence of several stimuli influencing the same effectors, as well as divergence, so that one stimulus modulates many effectors. The multiple interactions also result in the presence of feedback pathways.

3.2.2.1.2.3 Regulation of channels

3.2.2.1.2.3.1 Regulation by direct binding of ligand

Some channels can be directly activated by binding of an extracellular agonist to the channel molecule. Ligand-gated channels form an important class of channels, occurring in different tissues. Standard examples of this category are the nicotine acetylcholine-receptor in the neuromuscular junction of skeletal muscle and the AMPA and NMDA glutamate-receptors and the GABA$_A$-receptors in neuronal cells. Also cardiac cells contain ligand-gate channels, such as the P2X ATP-receptor. These receptors form non-selective cation (NSC) channels that are activated by binding of ATP to the channel molecule.

3.2.2.1.2.3.2 Regulation via G proteins

G proteins are membrane bound proteins that are activated when ligands bind to receptors belonging to category of G protein-coupled receptors (also called 7 transmembrane segment (7TM) receptors). G proteins are hetero-trimeric proteins consisting of α, β and γ subunits. At least twenty α, five β and six γ subunits have been described, giving rise to a large number of different combinations.

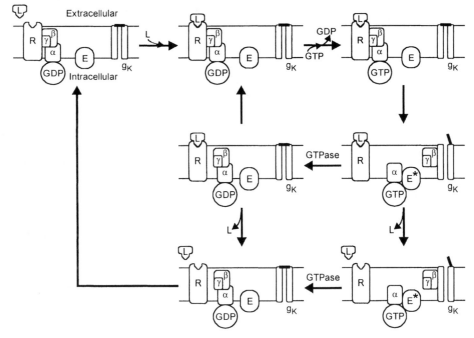

Figure II.23. G protein cycle. Example showing activation of an enzyme by the α subunit and of a K$^+$ channel by the $\beta\gamma$ complex.

The α subunit contains a guanine nucleotide binding site and has intrinsic GTPase activity. In the inactive state the G protein forms a trimer with GDP bound to the α subunit. Binding of a ligand (L) to the 7TM-receptor (R) results in exchange of GDP with GTP, which is followed by dissociation of the trimer in αGTP and a βγ complex. αGTP as well as the βγ complex can interact with effectors (E), causing activation or inhibition of the effector (E*). The effector can be an enzyme (e.g. adenylate cyclase) or a channel (e.g. a K^+ channel). The dissociation of βγ from the α subunit enables the GTPase activity of the α subunit, resulting in dissociation of the α subunit from the effector and reassociation with the βγ complex (Fig. II.23).

A typical example of a channel regulated via G protein interaction is the ACh-sensitive K^+ current $i_{K.ACh}$ in the sinoatrial node. This channel is activated when acetylcholine binds to the M2 (muscarinic type 2) receptor resulting in dissociation of a G_i protein into α_i and βγ. Binding of the βγ complex to this K^+ channel causes opening of the channel [see 762].

3.2.2.1.2.3.3 Regulation via intracellular messengers

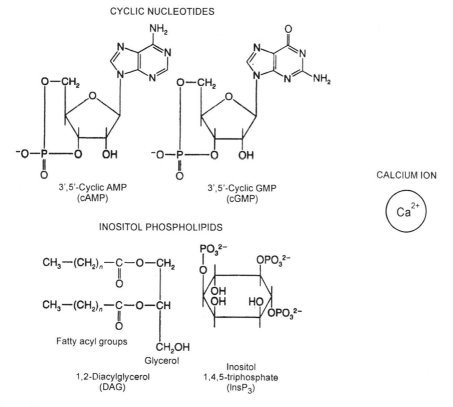

Figure II.24. Intracellular messengers.

The activity of many channels is regulated via intracellular messengers (second messengers), which either directly bind to the channels or affect channel phosphorylation via effects on protein kinases or protein phosphatases. Important intracellular messengers are the cyclic nucleotides cAMP and cGMP, lipid-derived second messengers such as diacylglycerol (DAG) and arachidonic acid (AA) and its metabolites, and intracellular Ca^{2+} (Fig. II.24).

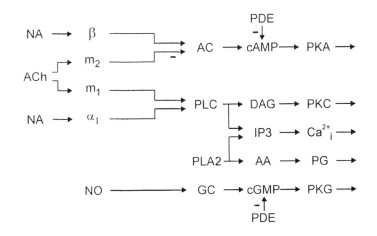

Figure II.25. Most important transduction cascades activating intracellular messengers that affect activity of ion channels.

cAMP

Adenylate cyclase (which can be activated via a G_s protein by binding of (nor)adrenaline to a β1-receptor, and inhibited via a G_i protein by binding of ACh to an M2-receptor) catalyses cAMP formation. Degradation of cAMP is catalysed by phosphodiesterases. cAMP can directly bind and activate some channels belonging to the category of cyclic nucleotide gated (CNG) channels like the i_f channel in sinoatrial node and Purkinje fibres. cAMP also activates cAMP-dependent protein kinase (PKA), which causes phosphorylation of a number of proteins including channels such as the L-type Ca^{2+} channel (Fig. II.25).

cGMP

cMGP is formed from GTP in a reaction catalysed by guanylate cyclases. Membrane-bound guanylate cyclases are activated by natriuretic peptides, such as the atrial natriuretic peptide (ANP), while cytosolic guanylate cyclases can be activated by nitric oxide and related vasodilators. cGMP can directly activate CNG channels, cGMP-dependent protein kinase (PKG) and cyclic nucleotide phosphodiesterases, which convert cAMP or cGMP to 5'-nucleoside phosphates (Fig. II.25).

Lipid-derived second messengers

Phospholipases, such as PLC, PLD, PLA_2, generate a wide variety of second messengers by breaking down membrane phospholipids.

Membrane-bound phospholipase C (PLC) is activated by binding of ligand to a receptor such as the α1-adrenergic receptor or the M1 muscarinic receptor. PLC hydrolyses phosphatidylinositol bisphosphate (PtdIP2) into inositol trisphosphate (IP3) and diacylglycerol (DAG). DAG can activate protein kinase C (PKC) while IP3 can cause Ca^{2+} release from IP3-sensitive intracellular stores, thereby increasing free cytoplasmic concentration of Ca^{2+}, which controls or modulates many processes, including the activity of a number of ion channels (Fig. II.25).

Phospholipase D produces phosphatidic acid by releasing the polar head group of the phospholipid. Phosphatidic acid can be further metabolised to DAG.

The result of PLA2 activation is the production of arachidonic acid (AA) and lysophospholipids, which can act as important elements in signal transduction, but also as precursors of other mediators such as prostaglandins (PG) and leukotrienes, which can activate channels or activate PKC.

Ca^{2+}_i

Intracellular Ca^{2+} is a key player in activation of most cell types. It is involved in many important cellular processes such as contraction, secretion, metabolism, cell proliferation and remodeling. The free cytoplasmic Ca^{2+} concentration is therefore tightly regulated. It can be enhanced by Ca^{2+} influx through the plasma membrane or via release from intracellular stores. Ca^{2+} influx can occur via voltage-gated, ligand-gated, stretch-activated channels or store-operated channels. Two families of intracellular channels can cause Ca^{2+} release from intracellular stores: ryanodine receptors (RyR) or IP3-receptors (IP3R). $[Ca^{2+}]_i$ can be decreased by Ca^{2+} ATPases in the plasma membrane or endoplasmic reticulum, or by a plasmalemmal Na^+/Ca^{2+} exchanger (Fig 24).

Many enzymes, channels and Ca^{2+} binding proteins are targets for intracellular Ca^{2+}. An important class of Ca^{2+} binding proteins are the so-called EF-hand proteins such as calmodulin. As these proteins bind Ca^{2+}, they change their conformation, which enables them to activate a large variety of downstream targets, such as some protein kinases or phosphatases, phosphodiesterases, NO synthase etc., thereby influencing several transduction cascades.

3.2.2.1.3 Channel block

Binding of a drug to a channel can influence either the channel kinetics or the permeation of ions.

3.2.2.1.3.1 Open channel block

A number of substances cause inhibition of channels by occluding the pore, resulting in a reduction of the current due to a decrease of the fully-activated current. If the decrease of the conductance is the same at all membrane potentials, the block is said to be voltage-independent.

Channel block can also be voltage-dependent. Charged substances may be able to bind to the channel molecule within the electrical field of the membrane (this can e.g. be the case when a pore contains a binding site which can be occupied by an ion or charged drug that is able to enter the pore but is too large to cross the selectivity filter). This way movement of the blocking substance from either extracellular medium or cytoplasm to its binding site in the pore is influenced by the transmembrane potential. Membrane potential changes will therefore affect the occupancy of the site. A hyperpolarisation will e.g. enhance the probability that a positively charged ion or drug present in the extracellular medium will bind to the binding site in the channel. The rate constant will depend on the fraction of the electrical field (the so-called electric distance) that is sensed by the blocker. The K_d of a charged drug thus depends on the membrane potential [1295]. Voltage-dependent block can also occur by intracellular ions, such as is the case for Mg^{2+}, which blocks outward current through the inward-rectifying K^+ channel, thereby producing inward rectification (Fig. II.26). This type of voltage-dependent block is called true voltage-dependent block, since voltage-dependence of block can be due to mechanisms different from open channel block (e.g. state-dependent block, see section 3.2.2.1.3.2).

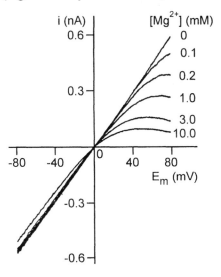

Figure II.26. Voltage-dependent block of a weak inward-rectifying K^+ channel by intracellular Mg^{2+}. In the absence of Mg^{2+} the I-V relation is linear. Intracellular Mg^{2+} blocks outward current; block is more pronounced at more positive potentials. Modified from [680].

3.2.2.1.3.2 State-dependent block

Channels can occur in different conformations (classically the resting, activated and inactivated state are considered) and the conformation of the channel may affect the interaction of inhibitors with the channel, causing the affinity of the channel to depend on the state, as proposed in the "modulated receptor hypothesis" of Hondeghem and Katzung [468] and Hille [448] (Fig. II.27). This phenomenon has been demonstrated for the interaction of local anaesthetics with Na^+, for Ca^{2+} channel blockers with the L-type Ca^{2+} channel, as well as for class III antiarrhythmic drugs with K^+ channels. The state-dependence of the affinity may be a real change of affinity of the interaction site, or alternatively it may be an apparent change in affinity due to a change in the accessibility of the binding site for the drug, as was proposed in the "guarded receptor hypothesis" by Starmer et al. [1093].

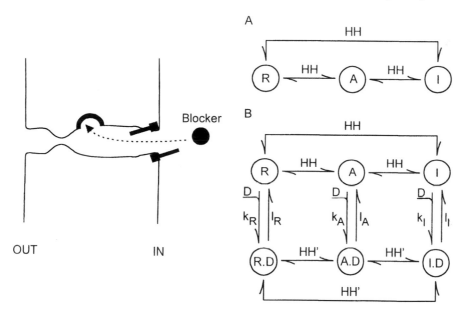

Figure II.27. State-dependent block. Left panel: Simplified model of a Na^+ channel with the drug binding site for class I antiarrhythmic agents (local anaesthetics). Upper right panel: Hodgkin – Huxley state diagram of the Na^+ channel. Lower right panel: Drug (D) interaction with the channel according to the modulated receptor hypothesis: reaction rate constants (k and l) are different for the resting (R), activated (A) and inactivated (I) state of the channel. HH refers to changes of the state of the channel according to the Hodgkin – Huxley model.

In the Hodgkin – Huxley state diagram the affinity of the channel for a drug can be largest in the activated open state (such a drug is called an activated state blocker), or for the inactivated state (inactivated state blockers. When the drug that has previously entered the channel cannot escape when the channel is in the resting state, trapping is said to occur

(Fig. II.28). Since the Hodgkin – Huxley model is only one of several possible state diagrams, the modulated receptor hypothesis can also be applied to other state diagram models of channels, as is illustrated in Fig. II.28, where a pre-open activated state is included.

Since for voltage-dependent channels the time the channel spends in each state depends on the membrane potential, state-dependent block can make the effect of a blocker voltage-dependent. Since during electrical activity the fraction of time a channel spends in the resting, activated (and eventually inactivated) state, the amount of block can eventually vary with action potential frequency, resulting in so-called frequency–dependence. When the amount of block changes with time when the stimulation frequency is suddenly changed to a new value, the block is said to be use-dependent. Fig. II.29 shows the development of the effect of the local anaesthetic lidocaine on a nerve fibre during trains of depolarisations at different frequencies after a period at rest. Higher frequencies causes a more pronounced block.

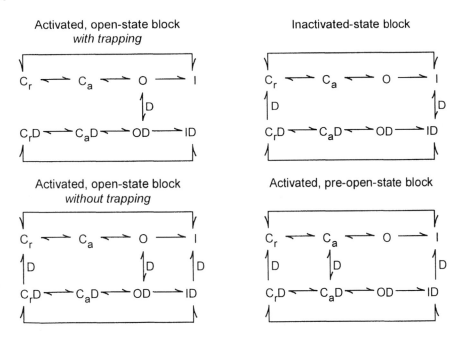

Figure II.28. Different kinds of state-dependent block. In this figure a pre-open activated state (C_a) of the channel is included in the Hodgkin – Huxley diagram in addition to the closed resting state (C_r), the open state (O) and the inactivated state (I).

While state-dependent block results in voltage-dependence of the block, state-dependent blockers can eventually also cause true voltage-dependent block. This is the case when the binding site of a charged state-dependent blocker is within the electric field of the membrane. The voltage-dependence resulting from state-dependence and that from true-voltage dependent block can even be opposite, as is the case for bradycardic agents (see Chapter IV section 1.1.5.3).

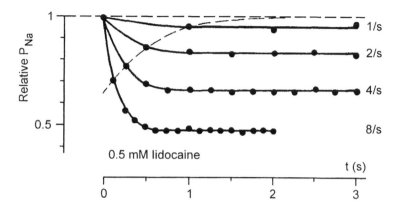

Figure II.29. State-dependent block. The effect of lidocaine on a nerve fibre is shown during repetitive depolarising pulses after a period of rest. The experiment is repeated at four different frequencies from 1 to 8 pulses per second. The stimulation causes a gradual decrease of the Na^+ current (use-dependent block). In steady-state the block is more pronounced at higher frequencies (frequency-dependence). Modified from [449].

3.2.2.2   Description of single channel properties

With the advent of the patch clamp technique, it became possible to study the electric current flowing through individual ion channels. While in whole cell clamp experiments the time-dependence of the kinetic processes results in currents gradually changing with time, the current through a single channel does not gradually change as a function of time, but is characterised by sudden jumps, which represent the opening and closing of the channel. The gradual change of the amplitude of the whole cell current is due to a change in the number of open channels. The total current flowing through all channels of one specific type (e.g. through all voltage-dependent Na^+ channels in the membrane) can be expressed in terms of single channels properties. This total current (i_{tot}) is the product of the number of channels (N) times the open channel current (i) times the open state probability of the channel (p_o), which depends on the kinetics and regulation of the channel.

$$i_{tot} = N.i.p_o$$

A full description of channels therefore requires a description of channel density (or number of channels), of open channel current and of the kinetics of the processes governing the open probability. The time course of the whole cell current can be obtained by averaging the currents obtained from repeated measurements on a single channel (ensemble average), since it can be demonstrated that the average of a population of one type of channels has the same time course as the ensemble average (Fig. II.30).

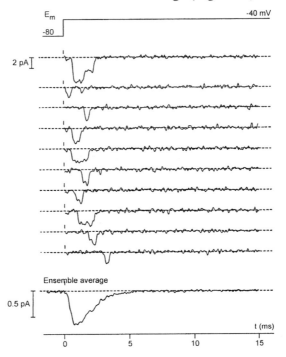

Figure II.30. Relation between whole cell current and single channel current, as shown for the Na^+ current. While single channel current shows sudden jumps between open and closed state, the ensemble average current of repeated single channel measurements changes gradually in time. The time course of the ensemble average is the same as the time course of the whole cell i_{Na} current. Modified from [449].

3.2.2.2.1   Distribution

Channels can be distributed uniformly across the whole area of the membrane or they can be clustered in specific areas of the membrane. The distribution of channels can e.g. be different in surface membrane or T-tubules. In case of uniform distribution the number of channels is generally expressed per unit membrane area (most often per μm^2) as channel density.

Channel density can vary from less than 1 μm^{-2} to more than 10000 μm^{-2}, depending on channel and cell type. Even densely spaced channels leave ample room for many other membrane proteins and lipids in the membrane. The type of channels expressed in cardiac cell membranes and the channel density varies with cell type, and must therefore obviously be tightly regulated. Expression of channel density as well as type of channels is known to vary with the stage of development and can also change in pathological conditions (remodeling). Thus far only limited information is available on the cellular processes governing channel expression.

3.2.2.2.2 Ion permeation

Channels are a very efficient means for translocating electric charges across the membrane, thereby changing the membrane potential. Single channel conductances vary largely from femtoSiemens (10^{-15} S = 1 fS) to about 300 picoSiemens (10^{-12} S = 1pS). For a 100 mV driving force, a single channel with a conductance of 20 pS will pass 2 pA of current through the membrane, which corresponds to about 10^7 ions/s. Such a current flowing through a single channel would change the membrane potential of a cell with a diameter of 20 µm at a rate of about 150 mV/s.

Most channels are also highly selective, allowing only certain types of ions to pass. Combining a high rate of permeation with a high selectivity puts strict requirements on the structure of the pore, and channel regulation is generally governed by different processes than the processes regulating permeation and selectivity, although the distinction between permeation and gating is not always clear cut (e.g. voltage-dependent block).

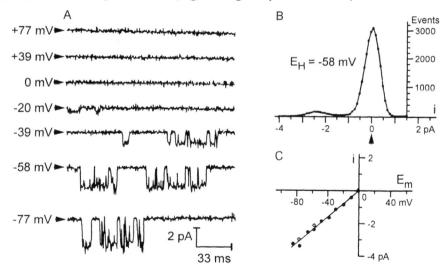

Figure II.31. Single channel currents, amplitude histogram and current–voltage relation. Results showing the currents through single acetylcholine-sensitive K^+ channels in human atria. Modified from [438].

Single channel amplitudes are small, of the order of pico ampere (pA) (Fig. II.31A), and are often not much larger than the baseline noise levels, which are mainly due to thermal noise in the seal resistance. Accurate measuring of the amplitude of the current flowing through open channels therefore requires averaging. Therefore single channel amplitudes are most often obtained by constructing amplitude histograms, whereby the number of data points for each current level is plotted as a function of the current level (Fig. II.31B) (often the ordinate is normalised to express the probability density). In case only a single channel (which does not have substates) is present in the patch, the distribution will be a sum of two Gaussian peaks.

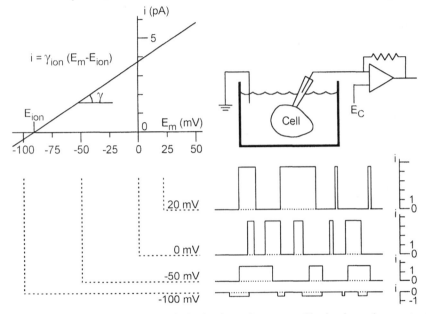

Figure II.32. Potential-dependence of single channel currents. Single channel current often shows a linear current-voltage relation, and is characterised by the single channel γ_{ion} conductance and the reversal potential (E_{ion}), which depends on the selectivity of the channel and the concentrations of the permeating ions.

The distance (difference in current) between the two peaks gives the single channel current, while the width of the peaks corresponds to the noise. The area of the peak of the open state relative to the total area under both peaks represents the open state probability of the channel. In case more than one channel is present in the patch several equidistant peaks at distances that are integral multiples of the single channel current can be present. Instead of all or nothing opening of channels, a number of channels are known to have substates. Substates are states of the channel with smaller conductance levels than the fully open state. Also the presence of substates results in additional peaks in the amplitude histogram, which often appear as small peaks in between the open and closed state peaks.

Measuring the single channel current at different membrane potentials and plotting this current as a function of membrane potential yields the single channel current-voltage relation (Fig. II.32). The slope of this relation (di/dE) gives the single channel conductance (γ). The potential at which the single channel current is zero is called the reversal potential. For an ideal perfectly selective channel the reversal potential corresponds to the equilibrium potential of the permeating ion according to the Nernst equation. For a channel that passes several types of ions the reversal potential follows the Goldman equation. By varying ion concentrations and using the Goldman equation the investigator can determine the selectivity ratios for different ions.

3.2.2.2.3 Channel kinetics

From the amplitude histogram the open state probability of the channel can be determined. In case a single channel is present in the patch the area of the peak of the open state relative to the total area under both peaks represents the open state probability of the channel. When multiple independent channels are present in the patch the areas under the different peaks should follow a binomial distribution, from which the open state probability and the number of channel can be estimated [202,203].

When voltage clamping a single channel molecule in steady-state conditions the channel is seen to alternate between the closed state and an open state, which is characterised by current flowing through the channel. Opening and closing are random events. The durations of all these individual open and closed states can be measured and summarised in distributions (or more strictly speaking in probability density functions), nl. the open time distribution and the closed time distribution (Fig. II.33). The distribution of the open and closed time duration can be interpreted when the channel is assumed to be governed by a Markow process that can be described as a model in which channels are viewed to switch between n different states with rate constants describing the probabilities per unit time of transitions between pairs of those states. The distribution of open and closed time follows a sum of exponentials, the time constants of which are related to the transition probabilities per unit time.

In the case of a channel with one open and one closed state,

$$C \underset{\beta}{\overset{\alpha}{\rightleftharpoons}} O$$

the time constant of the open times is equal to the average open time of the channel, and this value is equal to the inverse of the rate constant of the open to close transition $\tau_o = 1/\beta$ of the channel, while the average close time equals the inverse of the rate constant of close to open transition $\tau_c = 1/\alpha$.

Most channels have more complex kinetics. The channel can have a number of different closed or open states. The presence of several closed states is often reflected in channel openings being grouped in bursts. The number of exponentials in the open and closed time distribution is equal to the number of distinguishable open (respectively closed) states [202].

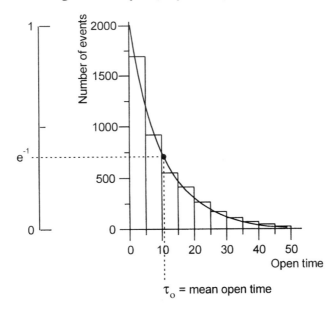

Figure II.33. Single channel current kinetics. Open and close time histograms consist of a sum of exponentials. In this example an open time histogram is shown consisting of a single exponential. The time constant of the exponential is equal to the channel mean open time.

Often several closed states are present covering a wide range of close time intervals. In this case it is more convenient to use "log binning" as was suggested by McManus et al. [729] and Sigworth and Sine [1043]. The histograms presented this way use a logarithmic time axis and have constant bin width on the log scale. The log-binned histograms are sums of skewed bell shaped curves. The number of peaks corresponds to the number of exponentials, and the peaks occur at time equal to the time constants of the exponentials.

While different open states can have the same conductance, many channels are known to have substates. Substates are open states of the channel with smaller conductance levels than the fully open state. In addition to transitions between the closed and the fully open state, the channel can make transitions between the fully open state or closed state and a substate or transitions between different substates. Like the probability of opening or closing transitions the transition to and from substates may be voltage-dependent or dependent on the presence of agonists or antagonists.

Often two or more channels are present in the patch. The presence of a second channel can eventually be seen as a transition from a single open state to a higher current level at twice the single channel current. Multiple channels can show up by currents at levels that are multiples of the single channel current. The transitions are nearly always to consecutive levels, since the probability of two channels opening at exactly the same time is very small. It should be noted that the presence of more than one channel does not always show by the presence of double current levels. If the open probability of the channel is low, the closed periods will be much longer than the open periods. In this case the probability that the second channel will open at a time when the first channel is open, is very low, and double openings may not occur for long periods of time.

3.2.2.2.4 Molecular structure

Substantial progress has been made in understanding channel functioning at the molecular level by combining electrophysiological techniques with molecular biological methods, but treatment of the molecular biology, structure and biophysical properties of ion channels is beyond the scope of this book [for an excellent overview of properties and molecular biology of ion channels in disease see 36]. Complete amino-acid sequences have been obtained for many types of channels. From these studies important homologies have been shown to exist. These homologies enable to classify channel proteins into a number of families and super families, such as voltage-gated channels, the ligand-gated channels, the cyclic nucleotide gated channels, the connexon family etc.. Ligand-gated channels are formed as heteropentamers of different subunits. Connexon channels in gap junctions consist of two hemi-connexons (one in each membrane of the cells that make contact), each consisting of 6 connexins (Fig. II.34).

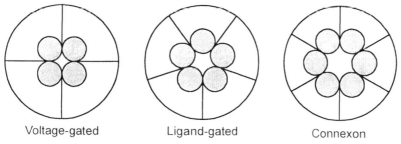

Voltage-gated   Ligand-gated   Connexon

Figure II.34. Voltage-gated, ligand-gated channels and connexons. Voltage-gated channels are tetrameric structures, ligand-gated channels are formed from 5 subunits while connexons forming gap junctions are juxtapositions of two hemi-channels each composed of six subunits.

The voltage-gated channel superfamily contains the Na^+ and Ca^{2+} channels and a large variety of K^+ channels. In addition to the pore-forming unit many channels contain one or more additional subunits. Na^+ and Ca^{2+} channels contain four internal domains (repeats) each consisting of six transmembrane segments. Using site-directed mutagenesis the structure of the channel has been correlated with function. It was demonstrated that the activation of the voltage-gated channels is governed by the fourth transmembrane segment (S4) of these channels. The loop (H5 or P loop) between S5 and S6 of each domain lines part of the ion permeation pathway (pore) of the channel (Fig. II.35 upper panel). Originally it was thought that the four subunits surround a central pore; however recent evidence indicates that the voltage-sensitive sodium channel is a bell-shaped molecule with several cavities [976] [for a cartoon of the 3 D structure see 154].

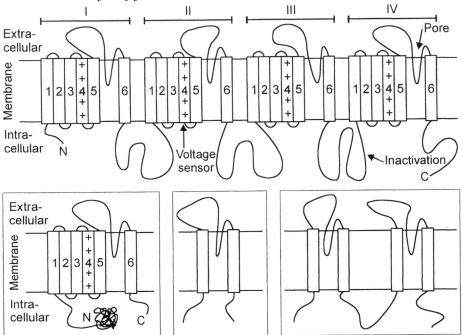

Figure II.35. Structure of Na^+, Ca^{2+} and K^+ channels. Upper row: Voltage-gated Na^+ and Ca^{2+} channels consist of four homologous domains each with six transmembrane segments. Lower left panel: Voltage-gated K^+ channels are formed as tetramers of proteins containing a single domain with 6 transmembrane segments, which is homologous to the domains of the Na^+ and Ca^{2+} channels. Lower middle panel: Inward-rectifying K^+ channel proteins consist only of two transmembrane domains separating the pore domain. Lower right panel: Two pore type K^+ channel subunits consist of four transmembrane domains and two pore domains.

A number of different K^+ channel families exist, which can be subdivided in four classes, three of which are present in mammals [see 1058].

The voltage-gated K^+ channels [see 796] are made up of pore-forming subunits that may be associated with an accessory subunit that regulates channel activity. A large variety of pore-forming subunits exist. Each of these pore-forming subunits has a size of about a quarter of the size of the Na^+ channel, and is very homologous to one internal repeat of the Na^+ and Ca^{2+} channels. The channel itself is made up of four subunits, and can be a homo- or a hetero-tetramer, which contributes to the huge variety of K^+ channels. Like in the Na^+ an Ca^{2+} channels, the outer part of the pore is formed by a P loop between S5 and S6, and the voltage-dependent activation is also mediated by the S4 segment. Voltage-dependent K^+ channels display two main modes of inactivation. A fast inactivation is governed by the amino terminus of the channel and is therefore called N-type inactivation. This type of inactivation is due to the distal part of the N terminus acting as a ball that can occlude the pore. The ball is tethered to the channel by the proximal region of the N terminus, which acts as a chain. N-type inactivation is therefore also called ball-and-chain type inactivation. Another type of inactivation is often slower and is called C-type inactivation; it involves a conformational change near the outer mouth of the pore [580,669].

Inward-rectifier K^+ channels are also tetramers, but each of the four peptides consists of only two transmembrane segments separated by a P loop.

A third category of K^+ channels are the two-pore domain K^+ channels with four transmembrane domains (2P/4TM), such as TASK-1, which are thought to be dimers [for review see 95,380,845] (Fig. II.35 lower panels).

3.2.3   Channel nomenclature and classification

A large variety of ion channels exist. They may be identified by their permeation and selectivity properties, by mode of activation and kinetics, or by selective block by drugs, toxins or ions. Channels can be classified according to different criteria and the nomenclature in the literature is far from uniform, while in some cases the name does not even reflect a property.

Channels can be classified according to their
− Distribution
  human, cardiac, …
− Ion permeation properties
− Selectivity:
  Na^+, K^+, Ca^{2+}, Cl^-, cation-selective, anion-selective, non-selective
− Rectifying properties:
  inward-rectifying, outward-rectifying
− Single channel conductance:
  50 pS, large conductance, maxi
− Kinetics and gating
− Regulation of the gating:
    - Voltage-gated,
      Voltage-activated channels show activation and eventually
      inactivation upon depolarisation. i_{Na}, i_{Ca}
    - Ligand-activated
      Channels can be activated by extracellular or intracellular agonists.

Extracellular agonists can activate ligand-activated channels by binding of ligands to receptors. These receptors, can form part of the channel molecule, or can be separate proteins which can activate the channel indirectly via a G protein, or via an intracellular messenger which can either bind to the channel (and thus act as an intracellular ligand) or cause a change in channel phosphorylation state.

Ligand-gated channels are identified according to the physiological ligand or a selective agonist:

ACh-activated, Ca^{2+}-activated, ATP-inhibited, IP3R, RyR

  - Other mechanisms of activation

    stretch-activated, volume-regulated, store-operated

— Time-course of the current:

delayed, transient, instantaneous

— Others

funny current (i_f), L-type Ca channel

— Structure, family, gene and encoded protein [for nomenclature see 163,309,378]

K_v, Kir, CLC, CFTR, HCN,

SCNA, KCNQ, KCNJ2

Table II.2. Most important human cardiac ion channel pore-forming subunits and exchangers and genes encoding them.

Current	Protein	Gene
i_{Na}	$Na_v1.5$	*SCN5A*
i_{CaL}	$Ca_v1.2$ ($\alpha1C$)	*CACNA1C*
i_{CaT}	$Ca_v3.2$ ($\alpha1H$)	*CACNA1H*
i_f	HCN2 / HCN4	*HCN2 /HCN4*
i_{to}	$K_v4.3$	*KCND3*
i_{Ks}	K_vLQT1	*KCNQ1*
i_{Kr}	HERG	*KCNH2*
i_{Kur}	$K_v1.5$	*KCNA5*
$i_{K.Ach}$	Kir3.1 / Kir3.4	*KCNJ3 / KCNJ5*
$i_{K.ATP}$	Kir6.2	*KCNJ11*
i_{K1}	Kir2.1	*KCNJ2*
$i_{Cl.PKA}$	CFTR	*CFTR*
i_{Clvol}	ClC-3 ?	*CLN3 ?*
$i_{Cl.ir}$	ClC-2 ?	*CLN2 ?*
Na^+/K^+ ATPase	NaKa1	*ATP1A1*
Na^+/Ca^{2+} exchanger	NCX1	*NCX1*

Often the channel protein is identified in the literature by different names. However as more and more structural data become available, channels are classified into families, and the naming becomes more standard. Table II.2 shows the most important human cardiac ionic currents, the corresponding channel pore-forming subunits and the genes encoding them.

Chapter III

Excitability, pacemaking and conduction

1.   INTRODUCTION

The initial event starting the normal heartbeat is the spontaneous activity in the SA node. Most cardiac cells do not possess normal automaticity, but must be excited by electric current flow. In order to generate an action potential, the cells must be depolarised to a critical potential (the threshold potential E_t or V_t): sufficient channels carrying inward current (Na^+ or Ca^{2+} current) must be opened to overcome the outward current. If this is the case, the cells generate a net inward current, which will cause further depolarisation and thereby start a regenerative action potential. Excitability of the cell depends on the balance of ionic currents flowing in the potential region between resting and threshold potential. Excitability is therefore influenced by many different factors affecting individual ionic currents.

Cardiac cells are electrically coupled by gap junctions, which provide a low resistance pathway for current flowing from cell to cell, providing a mechanism for exciting the adjacent cells. Electrical activity starting by spontaneous activity in the SA node can thereby spread to the rest of the heart. Electrical activity in one cell causes electrotonic currents (also called short-circuit or local currents), carried by ions flowing to electrically coupled adjacent cells. The short-circuit current causes depolarisation of the neighbouring cells, which eventually can be sufficient to electrically excite them, causing conduction of the action potential through the whole heart. The propagation of the electrical activity depends on the current-generating capacity of the cells that provide the short-circuit current, on the excitability of the neighbouring cells and on the coupling resistance between the cells [for reviews see 34,515,518].

2.   THRESHOLD AND EXCITABILITY

2.1   Threshold potential

In order to generate an action potential the membrane of the cell must be depolarised to a critical potential (the threshold potential E_t). Depolarisation will result in opening of Na^+ channels (for slow response cells (SAN and AVN) the mechanism is similar, except that the inward current is carried by Ca^{2+}). The inward current flowing through these channels tends to further depolarise the cell, opening more Na^+ channels and thereby causing more inward current. This results in a positive feedback mechanism, which produces a regenerative action potential, depolarising the cell towards the Na^+ equilibrium potential. However the depolarisation also causes an increase of outward current flowing through K^+ channels. Therefore at small depolarisations that only activate a small number of Na$^+$ channels, the limited increase in Na$^+$ current is too small to overcome the repolarising effect of the K$^+$ current. In order to generate a regenerative action potential, enough Na$^+$ channels must be opened so that the Na$^+$ current dominates, resulting in a net inward movement of positive charges. While at small depolarisations the outward K$^+$ current is larger than the inward Na$^+$ current, and hence the net current is outward, at depolarisations above threshold the Na$^+$ current is larger than the outward current, and the net current is inward, causing further depolarisation. The threshold potential is the potential at which the net current changes direction from outward to inward with increasing depolarisation. In a current-voltage relation it is a point of zero net current in a negative slope region of the current-voltage relation, and corresponds to an unstable equilibrium point. At the threshold no net current flows, and therefore there will be no change in potential. However any small disturbance will result in flow of current in such a direction, that it will cause the potential to deviate even further from the threshold value (Fig. III.1).

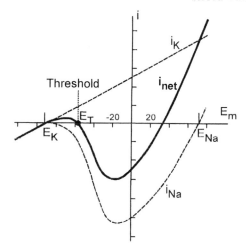

Figure III.1. The threshold potential is the potential at which the polarity of the net ionic current (in this example shown as the sum of i_K and i_{Na}) during a depolarising step changes from outward to inward.

Since the threshold is not a property of a particular channel (voltage-dependence of channels follow a smooth curve), but is due to a balance of the currents flowing through different channels, the threshold potential can be changed by changes in properties of outward (in cardiac cells mainly i_{K1}, see Chapter IV) as well as inward current, and is dependent on conductance, kinetics, channel density, ion concentration etc. Since many channels are voltage-dependent, the threshold potential also depends on the resting potential. Therefore many factors such as hormones, neurotransmitters, drugs, ion concentrations etc. can influence the threshold potential.

2.2   Threshold current

In order to be able to excite a cell, electrical stimulation must cause a depolarisation large enough to overcome the threshold. The depolarisation required equals the difference between the actual membrane potential and the threshold potential (E_m-E_t). For evoking an action potential by constant current stimulation a minimum amount of current (the threshold current) is needed to reach the threshold potential.

The amplitude of the current required to stimulate the cell depends on the duration of the current pulse: for longer duration pulses less current is needed. The intensity – duration curve relates the minimum current intensity for reaching the threshold, to the duration of the constant current pulse. For homogeneously polarised fibres, the curve has approximately an exponential shape, while a minimum intensity is needed even at very long durations. The curve can be approximately described by two parameters. The minimum intensity required for pulses of long duration is called rheobase (R). The minimal duration of a pulse with current amplitude twice the rheobase intensity is called the chronaxy (C) (Fig. III.2). The value of the rheobase in homogeneously polarised cells is equal to the current amplitude times membrane resistance ($R = i.r_m$), while the chronaxy is related to the time constant of the membrane ($C = \tau_m . \ln 2 = r_m.c_m . \ln 2$).

This type of intensity – duration curve can be expected if one assumes that the membrane behaves as a resistance and capacitance in parallel, and that its potential must be brought to a fixed threshold. For short pulses, approximately a constant amount of charge is needed to charge the membrane capacitance to the threshold potential. Since for constant current pulses the charge (Q) provided by the current is equal to the product of current intensity (I) times duration (D) of the current pulse, the intensity required is inversely proportional to the duration of the pulse ($I = Q/D$). For long pulses a minimum amount of current is required to compensate for current loss through the resistor. Intensity – duration curves for long cable-like structures, such a Purkinje fibres, have been derived by Fozzard *[342]*.

Since the intensity of the current is dependent on the difference between resting membrane potential and threshold potential, the excitability is affected by factors influencing the resting membrane potential or the threshold potential. Also any changes in resting membrane resistance or properties of ionic currents flowing in the potential range between E_m and E_t will affect excitability [see e.g. 480].

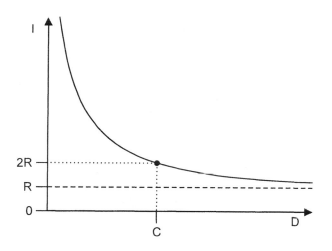

Figure III.2. Intensity-duration curve. Stimulus intensity (I) required to reach threshold is plotted as function of the duration (D) of the stimulus. The minimal intensity required even at very long duration is called Rheobase (R). The minimal stimulus duration for reaching the threshold when I is twice the Rheobase intensity is called Chronaxy (C).

2.3 Factors affecting excitability

Since excitability is determined by the balance of ionic currents, it can acutely be affected by a large variety of factors, such as ion concentrations, hormones and neurotransmitters, amphiphiles and fatty acids, free radicals and stretch and volume changes. It is therefore not surprising that cardiac excitability is affected in a large number of physiological, pharmacological or acute pathological circumstances such as ischaemia, while it can also be affected by altered expression of ion channels as can occur during disease-induced remodeling [for reviews see 145,148,790,869,1150].

2.3.1 Ions

2.3.1.1 Potassium

Altering the extracellular K^+ concentration changes the K^+ equilibrium potential according to the Nernst equation. Since cardiac cells at rest have a high permeability for K^+ due to the presence of the inwardly rectifying K^+ channel (see Chapter IV), the resting potential of cardiac cells (with the exception of the sinoatrial node) approaches E_K. Therefore increasing the external K^+ concentration causes depolarisation, while decreasing K^+ has the opposite effect. The depolarisation caused by important increases in $[K^+]_e$ will partially inactivate Na^+ channels and thereby decrease excitability in the myocardium. However a small increase of external K^+ concentration has only a limited effect on Na^+ channel availability, but moves the membrane potential closer to the threshold potential, so that excitability may be increased. This effect causes "supernormal conduction". However increasing $[K^+]_e$ also results in an increased conductance of i_{K1}: the resulting increased outward current partially counteracts the effect of the decreased E_m - E_t.

Loss of intracellular K^+, as can occur e.g. in ischaemia, will decrease the K^+ gradient across the membrane and depolarise the cell, causing effects which are qualitatively similar to the effects of increasing $[K^+]_e$ resulting in cell depolarisation.

2.3.1.2   Calcium

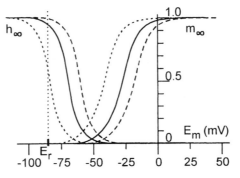

Figure III.3. Increasing the extracellular Ca^{2+} concentration (dashes) results in a shift of the steady-state activation and inactivation curve of the Na^+ current in depolarising direction, causing a decrease in excitability, because of the shift of the activation curve to more positive potentials. A small decrease of $[Ca^{2+}]_e$ has the reverse effect (dotted lines), causing hyper excitability. A large decrease of $[Ca^{2+}]_e$ causes decreased excitability, because the effect of the shift of the inactivation curve dominates.

Changes in $[Ca^{2+}]_e$ do not have a major influence on the resting potential, but have important effects on the kinetics of the Na^+ channels, by shifting the potential-dependence of the steady-state activation and inactivation curves, by shielding negative surface charges on the membrane [344]. Increasing $[Ca^{2+}]_e$ results in a shift of both curves in the depolarising direction. In this situation the shift of the activation curve dominates the effect. The shift of steady-state activation causes a depolarising shift of the threshold potential of the Na^+ channels, resulting in decreased excitability (the effect of the shift in the inactivation curve in the depolarising direction is negligible since the fraction of channels in the inactivating state in both cases is near 100 %) (Fig. III.3).

A decrease of external Ca^{2+} results in a shift of the two curves in the hyperpolarising direction. Upon a limited decrease of $[Ca^{2+}]_e$ the effect of the activation curve dominates, causing a more negative threshold potential, and resulting in hyperexcitability. A large decrease of $[Ca^{2+}]_e$ on the other hand causes a decreased excitability, since the shift of the inactivation curve in the hyperpolarising direction causes partial inactivation of Na^+ channels at the resting potential E_r. Since this causes a decrease of the availability of the Na^+ channels, the threshold potential is shifted towards more positive values, making it more difficult to activate the myocardial cells.

2.3.1.3   pH

Extracellular acidosis inhibits Na^+ channels, and shifts the potential-dependence of the kinetics to more positive values [1347]. Both effects reduce the excitability of the fast response cells. Intracellular acidosis causes a decrease of the open probability of Na^+ channels; it also inhibits the inward-rectifying K^+ current, which results in a fall in the resting potential, causing a reduction of the availability of Na^+ channels. Therefore also intracellular acidification reduces excitability of myocardial cells and cells in the ventricular conduction system.

2.3.2   Hormones and transmitters

Excitability depends on several ionic currents and can therefore be influenced by changes in different ionic currents. Since many ionic currents are modulated by transmitters and humoral factors, most of these substances have an effect on excitability (see Chapter V). The most important chemical agents affecting excitability are agents secreted by the autonomic system.

β-adrenergic stimulation enhances the L-type Ca current by stimulating adenylate cyclase, which results in PKA-mediated phosphorylation of the channel. Adrenaline thereby increases the excitability of the sinoatrial node (SAN) and the atrioventricular node (AVN). This results in enhanced spontaneous activity of the SAN (positive chronotropic effect), and in an increase in conduction velocity of the AVN (positive dromotropic effect).

ACh and adenosine bind to M2 muscarinic, respectively A1 purinergic receptors, in the SAN and AVN and in atrial cells. These receptors are coupled by inhibitory G proteins to adenylate cyclase, and their activation thereby counteracts the effects of β-adrenergic stimulation. ACh and adenosine also activate $i_{K.ACh}$ channels in SA and AV node and in atrial cells, and thereby hyperpolarise the membrane. The effects on Ca^{2+} and K^+ currents causes a decrease of the excitability of supraventricular cells, which mainly results is a slowing of the rate of spontaneous activity in the SA node and of conduction in the AV node.

2.3.3   Drugs

Local anaesthetics (class I antiarrhythmics) block Na^+ channels and thereby reduce excitability of myocardial cells and cells in the His Purkinje system. Ca^{2+} channel blockers reduce the excitability of slow response cells such as the AVN (see Chapters IV and V). Block of the channels by these agents is state-dependent, and therefore the effect of the drugs on excitability depends on membrane potential and frequency.

2.3.4   Refractoriness

During the plateau and a large part of the repolarisation of the myocardial action potential the Na^+ channels are in the inactivated state and the cells are non-excitable. The period of non-excitability is called the absolute refractory period. The final repolarisation of the cell causes the Na^+ channels to recover from inactivation (de-inactivation or repriming). The time interval during which channels slowly recover from inactivation is called the relative refractory period. The relative refractory period corresponds to the late phase of final repolarisation and part of diastole. During this interval excitability is reduced, since the availability of Na^+ channels during the refractory period is less than in steady-state, which causes the threshold potential to be shifted to less negative potentials. The effective refractory period is the time interval during which stimulation fails to induce propagation of regenerative action potentials, but only results in decremental conduction, producing a wave of potential changes with amplitude gradually decreasing with distance.

3.   PACEMAKING

An action potential can be initiated in a cell by an electrical stimulus from an external source, or via conduction from adjacent cells that are electrically coupled via gap junctions. However some cells do not need an external source of current to initiate an action potential, but are spontaneously active. Several types of cardiac cells possess pacemaker activity (see Chapters I and IV). While the SAN acts as the primary pacemaker, the AVN, the His bundle Purkinje system also have spontaneous activity, although at a slower rate. These cells are subsidiary pacemakers, and provide a safety mechanism in case of failure of the primary pacemaker, respectively of AVN conduction. Ventricular or atrial myocardial cells can also be spontaneously active in pathological circumstances (see Chapters VII, VIII, IX).

Pacemaker activity is a form of an oscillatory process (the attractor in a phase plane is not a stable point, but a "limit circle"). In order for the membrane potential to have a stable value (E^*), the rate of potential change must be zero ($dE^*/dt = 0$) at that potential. Since the rate of change of the membrane potential is directly proportional to the net ionic current ($c_m.dE^*/dt = i_{net}(E^*)$), a stable membrane potential requires the net ionic current to be zero, and to remain zero ($i_{net}(E^*) = 0$ and $di_{net}(E^*)/dt = 0$). Even though at some moment during the action potential cycle the net ionic current may be zero, the conductance of some time-dependent ion channels may not have reached a stationary value at the potential and time at which the net current is zero (this happens e.g. at the peak of the action potential or at maximum diastolic potential). Therefore the conductance is still changing at that moment, resulting in a change of the net current with time, so that the potential where the net current is zero is not stable.

From the previous argument it is clear that the essential feature required for cellular pacemaker activity is that the rate of change of the net ionic current during the cardiac cycle is out of phase with the amplitude of the current. Delays introduced by the time-and voltage-dependent kinetics of ion channels provide the basis for the mechanism underlying spontaneous activity. At the maximum diastolic potential (E_d), the net ionic current is zero ($i_{net}(E_d) = 0$). At that moment however ion conductances are still changing, and net ionic current, which is outward during the repolarisation, changes with time from outward to inward. This can be due to a time-dependent increase of conductance of channels carrying inward current (such as i_f, which is activating due to the repolarisation) or a time-dependent decrease of conductance for outward current (such as i_K) which is deactivating due to the repolarisation. The inward current causes the cell to gradually depolarise, and eventually the threshold for an action potential can be reached, starting the cycle all over again.

4.   CONDUCTION

An action potential initiated at one site in a cardiac cell propagates throughout the cell. Since cardiac cells are electrically coupled through gap junctions, the action potential also spreads to the adjacent cells, causing an electrical wave of action potentials throughout the whole heart. The basis of the action potential propagation is the passive charge redistribution (electrotonic potential), which depends on the cable properties of the cardiac tissue. When the electrotonic potential at a more distant site reaches the threshold potential, an action potential is initiated, causing propagation.

4.1   Mechanism

4.1.1   Cable properties

The spread of the electric signal in a cell or multicellular preparations resembles the spread in an electric cable or transmission line. The so-called cable equation, originally derived by Lord Kelvin, is the equation that describes the passive properties of non-uniformly polarised cells [462]. Application of the cable equations to cellular structures, in particular cardiac tissue, is a simplification of the real situation, since in its standard form the cable equation treats the cell as an ideal infinitely long linear one-dimensional cable. However, it is a very useful model: it provides the framework for understanding electrical propagation; it very well describes the propagation in long cylindrical structures, such a nerve axons; it is applicable to multicellular systems which are organised in bundles and in which the cells are electrically coupled by gap junctions, such as Purkinje cells; it can be extended to three-dimensional systems such as the myocardial wall; it can also be applied to non-linear systems and time-dependent systems (although in general no analytic solutions of the equations exist in this case, a number of approximations have been described [see 34,339,507,515,518]).

4.1.1.1   The one-dimensional cable
4.1.1.1.1   The cable equation

The cell (or a bundle of electrically coupled cells) can be represented as a cylinder of electrically conducting cytoplasm separated from the conducting external medium by the membrane, which behaves as an imperfect insulator. Viewed this way the cell is like an undersea cable: a conducting wire surrounded by an insulator from the conducting seawater.

The cell can be subdivided in small sections (which in the limit are made infinitely small). Each section represents a small membrane patch (represented as membrane capacitance (c_m) in parallel with membrane resistance (r_m)) separating the extra and intracellular medium. Consecutive patches of membrane are electrically connected via a small amount of resistance (r_a), which represents the resistance of the cytoplasm (and in electrically coupled multicellular preparations also the gap junctional resistance). The equivalent electrical circuit (Fig. III.4) provides the basis for the understanding of the cable equation .

Current injected at one point in the cable will cause local accumulation of electric charge and a change of the membrane potential at the point of injection. The excess charge will spread out along the cable, causing current flow in the longitudinal (axial) direction (x) (see Appendix). This current will produce changes in potential across the intracellular resistance of the cytoplasm of the cell. However some of the charge will leak out of the cell through conductive pathways in the cell membrane. The leaking out of current through the membrane will cause a gradual decrease of the axial current flow, resulting in a gradual decline of the potential with distance along the cable (for a brief overview of the equations and their derivation see Appendix).

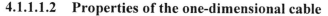

Figure III.4. The cell as a passive linear cable.

4.1.1.1.2 Properties of the one-dimensional cable

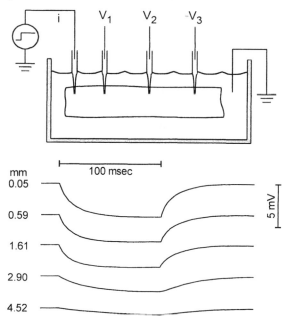

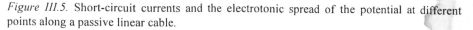
Figure III.5. Short-circuit currents and the electrotonic spread of the potential at different points along a passive linear cable.

The exact mathematical form of the solutions of the cable equations is rather complex. From the solution of the one-dimensional linear cable equation a number of important conclusions can be made. A constant current step produces gradual changes of potential at the point of injection as well as at other points along the cable. The change in potential is smaller and slower for more distant points (Fig. III.5) [1264].

4.1.1.1.2.1 Steady-state properties

In steady-state the potential in an infinite cable decays exponentially as a function of distance (Fig. III.6):

$V(t=\infty) = R_{in}.I_o.\exp(-x/\lambda)$

with input resistance $R_{in} = \sqrt{r_m r_a}/2$ and length constant $\lambda = \sqrt{r_m/r_a}$,

where r_m is the membrane resistance per unit length in Ohm cm,

and r_a intracellular resistance per unit length in Ohm cm^{-1}.

The input resistance is the total resistance faced by the current; it is the ratio of the steady-state potential change at the site of current injection to applied current amplitude.

The length constant λ can be interpreted as the distance at which the potential in steady-state will drop to $1/e$ (which is about 0.37) times the potential at the point current injection ($V_{x=\lambda} = V_{x=0} . e^{-1}$).

The resistances and capacitance per unit length of fibre (r_m and r_a and c_m) depend on the cell diameter according to

$r_m = R_m/2\pi a$

$r_a = R_a/\pi a^2$

$c_m = C_m.2\pi a$

with R_m (Ohm cm^2) the membrane resistance per square cm membrane area, R_a (Ohm cm) the resistivity of the cytoplasm, C_m (F/cm^2) the membrane capacitance of one cm^2 membrane, and a the cell radius.

Therefore also the length constant increases with cell diameter:

$\lambda = \sqrt{aR_m/2R_a}$

In cardiac cells the length constant is of the order of 0.5 to 2 mm, depending on the cell type. Since these values are much longer than the length of a single cardiac cell, these data provided the first evidence for electric communication between cardiac cells [1264]. Additional evidence was obtained by the demonstration that radioactive K^+ loaded into cells spread intracellularly over many cells.

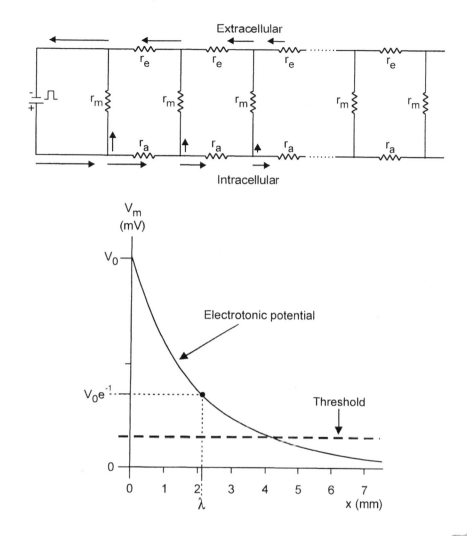

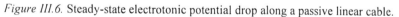

Figure III.6. Steady-state electrotonic potential drop along a passive linear cable.

4.1.1.1.2.2 Transient properties

The cell membrane does not behave like a pure resistor. Its capacitance introduces time-dependence in the response to injection of current. The generated electrotonic potentials therefore are not instantaneous, but take some time to develop (Fig. III.5). The transient response is not an exponential process but a so-called error function [see 507]. The potential rises relatively fast at the point of current injection, but more slowly at more distant sites.

4.1.1.2   The three-dimensional cable

While the one-dimensional cable theory is very useful for understanding the principles governing the spread of electric charge in cells and the conduction of the action potential, for most cells, including cardiac tissues, it can only be a first approximation. The treatment of multi-dimensional conduction presents a much more complicated mathematical problem; e.g. the electrotonic potential around a point source in two or three dimensions decays much faster as a function of distance than in a one-dimensional cable [see 507].

4.1.2   Propagation of the action potential

One of the most important properties of the cell is the non-linearity of the electrical phenomena, without which no action potentials could be generated. By generating electrotonic potentials, the cable properties of cells provide the mechanism for all-or none propagation of the action potentials to distant sites. This propagation of the action potential is due to a combination of the passive spread of electric charges along the cable, and the existence of a threshold phenomenon.

4.1.2.1   Source, sink and propagation of the action potential

An action potential initiated at a site not only causes depolarisation of that site, but also creates an electrical gradient between the cells and its neighbours, and thereby provides a source of current spreading to the adjacent tissue. The current flowing into the neighbouring cells provides the electric charges that cause depolarisation of these cells by charging their membrane capacitance. The adjacent cells therefore act as a current sink: the depolarisation in these downstream cells causes outward current flowing through their membranes, and also short-circuit current depolarising cells located further downstream (see Fig. III.7 upper panel). The neighbouring cells therefore draw current from the source and have a loading effect on the source, drawing charges away from the membrane capacity at the site of the source. The current by the source therefore acts as excitatory current for the sink, while the sink counteracts the depolarisation of the source.

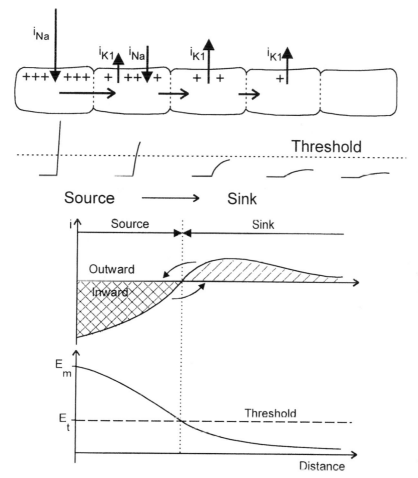

Figure III.7. Source, sink and liminal length. Upper panel: Relation between ionic currents, short-circuit currents and membrane potential changes in source and sink. Lower panel: Conduction requires that a minimum length of fibre (the liminal length) is depolarised so that the total number of positive charges (cross-hatched area) entering cell in the source region (where potential during depolarisation phase is above threshold), exceeds the total number of positive charges (hatched area) leaving the cell in the sink (non-excited region).

Wherever at a distant site the electrotonic potential caused by the passive redistribution of charges exceeds the threshold potential, the inward Na^+ current becomes larger than the outward current. Therefore net inward current will flow, which will further depolarise the cell, initiating a regenerative action potential at this site. This action potential will also cause charge redistribution causing initiation of action potentials at more distant sites. When the electrical properties of the tissue are uniform along the cable, an all-or-none action potential will propagate along the cable at constant velocity (see Appendix).

4.1.2.2   Liminal length

The outward current flowing through the membrane of the sink draws current away from the membrane capacitor at the site of the source, and thereby opposes the depolarisation of the source during the action potential. In the same way as drawing a large current from a battery can result in an important voltage drop of the battery, the generation of a full scale action potential could be prevented when the load provided by the sink is large compared to the current-generating capacity of the current source. In order to describe the interaction between source and sink in a one-dimensional cable, Rushton [951] introduced the idea that it is necessary to excite a minimum length of fibre in order to initiate a propagated action potential. He therefore provided the concept of liminal length, which is defined as the length of fibre that needs to be raised above threshold so that the depolarising influence of the inward currents generated in that length of fibre exceeds the repolarising influence of the rest of the fibre. Whether an action potential will be propagated depends on whether the total net inward current provided by the source (integrated over the whole membrane area of tissue generating net inward current) will be larger than the total net outward current generated by the rest of the tissue (the sink) (Fig. III.7).

4.1.2.3   Safety factor

The reliability of the propagation of the action potential depends on the ratio of the net inward current generated by the source to the current required to excite the sink. If the current delivered by the source is too small, all-or-none propagation of the action potential may fail: the sink may not reach threshold, or decremental conduction may occur, producing a wave of potential changes with amplitude gradually decreasing with distance. The reliability of action potential propagation can be described by the "safety factor for conduction (SF)" defined by Rushton [951] and others [507,1011,1246]. This safety factor is the ratio of the amount of charge generated by cell excitation to the minimal amount of charge required to cause the excitation. A SF >1 indicates that more charge was produced during cellular excitation than charge required to cause excitation [1011].

In the fast response cells of the heart in normal condition, the safety factor for conduction is relatively large, due to the large density of Na^+ channels. It was estimated to be about 1.5 (see Fig 8). The safety factor is much smaller in the AVN where the inward current during the Ca^{2+} action potential is more than an order of magnitude smaller than in the fast response cells. This explains the vulnerability of the heart to AVN conduction block.

4.1.2.4   Factors determining conduction velocity

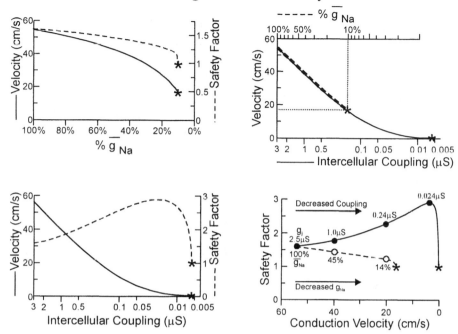

Figure III.8. Simulation of the effect of decreasing Na⁺ conductance (upper left panel) and intercellular coupling conductance (lower left panel) on conduction velocity and conduction safety factor in ventricular myocardium. The * mark the occurrence of conduction block. Comparison of the effect of a reduction in intercellular coupling and Na⁺ conductance on the conduction velocity (upper right panel) (note the logarithmic scale of the abscissa). Correlation between safety factor and conduction velocity for a change in Na⁺ conductance or a decrease intercellular coupling conductance (lower right panel). Modified from [1011].

Conduction velocity depends on the properties of the ionic currents and on the passive electrical properties of the cells. Since it is determined by the complex non-linear time-dependent properties of the ionic currents, no simple equation relates the conduction velocity to cell properties, although several authors provided approximations [see 339,481,507].

In general, factors determining conduction velocity can be viewed as belonging to three groups: source factors, sink factors and coupling resistance between source and sink.

– The source for electrical propagation in cardiac tissue is the action potential itself. The net inward current provides the charges for depolarising the membrane and provoking an action potential at the site of initiation. This causes an excess of positive charges in the cell, which generates the action potential and provides a spatio-temporal potential gradient; the spatial redistribution of charges provides the short-circuit current for propagation. Therefore the amplitude of the action potential and the total net inward current are important factors for action potential propagation. The total net inward current is a function of ionic gradients and channel characteristics. It also depends on the area of membrane that is simultaneously active, and therefore depends on geometrical factors of the cells and tissue.

– The source must excite the sink. The short-circuit current generated by the source must therefore bring the membrane potential at a site in the sink from its diastolic value (E_m) to the threshold (E_t). It therefore must charge the membrane capacitance of the sink, by providing the current to impose a potential change (E_t - E_m), and it must also overcome the net outward current flowing during this depolarisation. In addition to the difference between threshold and diastolic potential, the membrane capacitance and resistance of the sink and the properties of the ionic currents in the potential region between E_t and E_m determine the excitability of the sink. The current distribution in the sink of course also depends on the size and geometry of the cells and tissue in the sink.

– Current provided by the source must reach the sink. The pathway between source and sink includes intracellular resistance provided by the cytoplasm, and in multicellular tissue also the intercellular resistance provided by the gap junctions. Extracellular resistance plays a role, but can often be neglected. The coupling resistance is mainly determined by the resistance of the gap junctions. Therefore, the number and distribution of gap junctions is an important factor for conduction of the action potential. Also the conductance of the gap junction proteins (connexons) is important, because it can be changed in pathological conditions such as ischaemia, since gap junctional conductance is modulated by factors such as pH, and [Ca^{2+}].

Since depolarising currents, excitability of the cell, the spatial pattern and degree of gap junctional coupling, and geometrical factors all have an effect on conduction velocity, conduction can be compromised by a reduction in any of these factors. Which of these factors is most important is still controversial (and is an ill-defined question), since it depends on the conditions and on the parameters measured. From simulations [1009] as well as from experiments [931], it is clear however that cellular uncoupling and decrease in excitability can have different effects on conduction velocity and on the safety factor of conduction.

4.1.2.4.1   Importance of membrane conductances

The local action potential is the source of the electrotonic potential. Net current during the action potential is proportional to dV/dt, and this net current provides the charges for the local circuit current. In fast response cells the maximum net inward current is dominated by the Na^+ current, which is much larger than the outward currents.

Simulations of ventricular conduction demonstrate that reducing the maximum Na conductance causes a reduction of dV/dt_{max} and maximum i_{Na} during the action potential, as well as a decrease of conduction velocity and safety factor. Reduction of g_{Na} could reduce conduction velocity only to about one third of control (about 10 cm/s) before conduction failure [1011,1246]. These authors concluded that reduced excitability (e.g. during acute ischaemia) cannot support very slow conduction (even if transition to i_{CaL} supported inward current occurs), but is mostly associated with conduction failure.

Reducing g_{Na} not only decreases the current-generating capacity of the source, but also reduces the excitability of the sink. Reducing the excitability of the sink will also result in a decrease of conduction velocity and safety factor. However the processes determining the excitability of the sink are not identical to the processes providing the charges for the local circuit currents which cause the electrotonic potentials. To reach the threshold in the sink the short-circuit current provided by the source must load the capacitance of the sink and overcome the net outward current flowing in the potential region between resting and threshold potential. Excitability of the sink is therefore not only dependent on the inward current, but it also strongly depends on the outward currents (especially i_{K1}). Factors affecting outward currents have therefore a more pronounced effect on the excitability of the sink than on the maximum inward current provided by the source. Therefore in addition to the amplitude of inward currents, many factors affect the excitability of the sink by affecting ionic current (see Chapters IV and V) and have an influence on conduction. E.g. small increases in $[K^+]_e$ may result in supernormal conduction in fast response cells, because the depolarisation of the membrane brings the potential of the sink closer to the threshold. More pronounced hyperkalaemia on the other hand will decrease excitability and conduction velocity by shifting the threshold potential to less negative values (due to inactivation of the i_{Na}, and increase of the conductance of i_{K1}).

4.1.2.4.2 Importance of coupling resistance

Comparison of measured intracellular longitudinal resistance (r_a) in cardiac tissue, with predictions on the basis of cytoplasmic resistivity provides strong evidence that the most important element within the longitudinal resistive pathway is located in the junctional membrane, nl. in the gap junctions, which electrically couple adjacent cardiac cells. Many factors influence gap junctional coupling (see Chapter IV), and effects of gap junctional coupling on conduction can be important in pathological conditions [for reviews see 145,856,1090]. Cardiac myocytes may uncouple rapidly and completely in acute ischaemia, isolating viable cells from damaged cells. Coupling may also be altered by stretch, heart failure and remodeling [292,533,687,759,790,955,958,1245,1355]. Changes in number of gap junctions or reduction of expression of connexins such as Cx43, and also changes in distribution and lateralisation of the gap junctions have been found in virtually all cardiac diseases predisposing to arrhythmias [see 533].

Effect on conduction velocity

Experiments as well as simulations demonstrated that conduction velocity is reduced by a decrease in gap junctional conductance. However relatively large changes in gap junctional conductance are required to markedly affect conduction velocity (Fig. III.8 lower left panel: note the logarithmic scale of the abscissa). Simulations showed that a reduction by as much as 40% in total gap junctional content (as observed in diseased human hearts [856,858]) may have only moderate effects on conduction velocity [533,1009,1082]. Studies on heterozygous $Cx43^{+/-}$, or double heterozygous $Cx43^{+/-}/Cx40^{+/-}$ knockout mice revealed no significant changes in conduction velocity, or activation of the ventricular myocardium [578,760] [see 673]. Differences in cell size may be more important than gap junction distribution [1082].

Effect on safety factor and dV/dt$_{max}$

Very large reduction of intercellular coupling results in a decrease in safety factor for conduction. However simulations show that a decrease of coupling conductance over a wide range of values can cause an increase of the safety factor, and that a decrease of intercellular coupling can decrease conduction velocity to extremely low values (< 1 cm/s) before conduction fails (Fig. III.8 lower left panel), making microreentry possible. The L-type Ca^{2+} current played a major role in sustaining this very slow conduction upon decreased cellular coupling [1011]. The simulations further demonstrated that with reduced gap junction coupling conduction failure occurs at much lower conduction velocities than with reduced Na^+ conductance (Fig. III.8 upper right panel) [945,949]. These findings can be explained by the effect of coupling on the load presented by the sink on the source: when coupling is reduced less current is shunted to downstream cells, effectively increasing inward current available for local depolarization [1011], thus facilitating excitation. Experiments confirmed the increase of safety factor with partial uncoupling:

– Experiments Kléber's group demonstrated that a decrease of the gap junctional coupling can slow conduction velocity substantially more than reducing excitability before block occurs, thus indicating that the safety factor for conduction block is larger than the one for reduction of i_{Na} [931].

- In discontinuous cardiac tissue showing unidirectional block, uniform partial cellular uncoupling could restore bi-directional conduction. This was due to a larger effect of uncoupling on the load than on the source [930].
- In adult ventricular myocytes dV/dt_{max} of action potentials propagating in transverse direction is larger than for propagation in the longitudinal direction [1082]. No such difference was found in neonatal preparations [320,1082]. Model studies indicated that this phenomenon was correlated with the distribution of the gap junctions, which in the adult, in contrast to neonates, are restricted to the intercalated disk at the end of the cells, causing a smaller load in lateral than in longitudinal direction [1082].
- While computer simulations have also shown that a progressive decrease of conduction velocity during uncoupling is accompanied by a transient increase in dV/dt_{max} due to the cellular architecture of cardiac tissue [517,948,1011], these findings could not be experimentally confirmed [320,517,930], expect by one group [198].

The safety factor decreases sharply for propagation into regions of increased electrical load (expansion of tissue, increased gap junctional coupling, reduced excitability, hyperkalaemia). Reduced coupling enhances the safety factor, and thereby can compensate for effect of tissue expansion. Although it can also augment the safety factor that is reduced by depressed membranes, the effect is too small to overcome conduction failure at high levels of membrane depression [1246].

4.2 Properties of propagation in cardiac tissue

The structure of the cardiac tissues introduces several deviations from one-dimensional continuous cable theory: cardiac cells are not continuous, and they form a complex three-dimensional structure.

4.2.1 Propagation is discontinuous

While the action potential in cardiac cells appears to travel in a continuous way at constant speed, the propagation in cardiac tissue is discontinuous, and resistive discontinuities have an important influence on cardiac conduction.

While the His bundle and Purkinje system can be approximated as a one-dimensional cable, it cannot be considered uniform. It is a highly branched structure, which gives rise to macroscopic discontinuities in the electrical properties at the branching points. Also at the junction between Purkinje fibres and myocardium a sudden change in geometry takes place from a bundle to a three-dimensional structure.

The propagation in the myocardial wall is also discontinuous, and discontinuity can change with age and during disease and remodeling [250,515,584,948,1070,1073,1077-1079,1081,1085]. This discontinuous character is due to the multicellular nature of cardiac tissue:

– The gap junctions form a site with higher resistance than the cytoplasm, resulting in microscopic discontinuity of r_a. While the effect of the multicellular nature of cardiac tissue resulting in gap junctional discontinuity does not appear to disturb the continuous propagation of the action potential in otherwise uniform bundles, it can be a source of macroscopic discontinuities, which can give rise to non-uniform propagation of the action potential.

– Macroscopic discontinuities can be due to structural properties of the heart, such as non-uniform three-dimensional distribution of gap junctions, differences in cell geometry and cell types, or geometrical arrangement of the cells, such as branching of cell bundles, anatomical obstacles, such as capillaries, connective tissue, or large intercellular clefts.

– Macroscopic discontinuities may also originate from functional properties of cardiac cells. Discontinuities may be due to the active properties of the cells. Zones of impaired excitability may be encountered due to incomplete recovery of Na^+ channels or to pathological state of the tissue. They may also be due to altered passive properties, such as reduced intercellular communication, which may be present in pathological states affecting gap junctional conductance.

Discontinuities appear to affect action potential shape and conduction velocity, and can result in decremental conduction or propagation failure [198,536,948,1070,1073,1076,1081,1084,1085], but the exact effects remain controversial [938].

4.2.2 Propagation is three-dimensional

While the His Purkinje network of the heart can be rather well described as a branching one-dimensional cable, the myocardium is complex three-dimensional structure, and the one-dimensional cable theory, although a very valuable tool for understanding propagation of the action potential, can only be a first approximation. The myocardium itself must be considered a three-dimensional mass of tissue. The main effect of this organisation is that the electrotonic decay and the spread of current in more than one dimension will depend on many factors: it will be different depending on whether the excitation wave behaves more or less as a plane wave or shows a pronounced curvature in two or three dimensions. The geometry of the wave will depend on the three-dimensional electrical properties of the tissue, but also on the source of excitation. A ventricular extrasystole originating within the myocardium will provide a point source of excitation, resulting in wave fronts that are very different from normal activation, which depends on the exact locations of the Purkinje - muscle junctions.

a) Propagation is anisotropic

Besides the fact that the myocardium forms a three-dimensional structure, its passive electric properties are different in the transverse versus the longitudinal direction of the cells: the myocardial wall is anisotropic. The anisotropy is due to the rod-like shape of adult cardiac myocytes, and depends on the number, properties and distribution of the gap junctions, which in adult ventricular myocytes are mainly located at the intercalated disk at the ends of the myocytes. The lateral spread of excitation mainly occurs via intercalated disks of laterally overlapping cells [531,1061,1079]. Since in the transverse direction the number of barriers (intercalated disks) encountered for the same distance is larger than in longitudinal direction, the transverse resistance is larger than the longitudinal resistance, resulting in non-uniform spread of the electrotonic potential [190,973]. The conduction is faster in longitudinal than in transverse direction (anisotropic propagation) so that excitation spreads in an ellipse-like pattern [53,1070,1083]. Not only is conduction velocity anisotropic, but propagation may be more likely to fail in one direction than in the other. However whether propagation will fail in longitudinal or transverse direction varies depending on the conditions [see 515].

b) Anisotropy is not uniform over the myocardium

The three-dimensional structure of the ventricular myocardium presents even more complications. The orientation of the cells varies with position along the myocardial wall as well as in transmural sections [1108]. Frazier et al. [348] demonstrated that epicardial propagation was different in the presence or absence of deeper layers of myocardium. The elliptic epicardial activation fronts were asymmetric, and the orientation of the axes of the elliptic activation fronts were different in planes parallel to the epicardium taken at different depths (distance from the epicardial surface). The main reason for this difference is that the axes of the myocardial fibres rotate transmurally as much as 120 degrees [482,1108].

− Electrical properties and conduction may not be uniform. Transverse non-uniform propagation is a feature of normal myocardium, which is related to the sparsity and irregularity of the gap junctions providing connections to lateral cells. Non-uniformity of conduction can be enhanced in pathological conditions when longitudinal pathways are damaged.

− Transmural changes in intercellular resistivity in the transverse direction have been described, especially between the midmyocardial region and the ventricular epicardium, but also between endocardium and midmyocardium [1314].

– The excitation pattern depends on macroscopic discontinuities, such as blood vessels, connective tissue separating muscle bundles, and eventually scar tissue. Branching micro-architectures might contribute to slow conduction in tissue with discontinuous geometry, such as infarct scars and the AV node [605].

4.2.3   Propagation can be unidirectional

Unlike chemical intercellular transmission, electrical coupling by gap junctions is bi-directional, and propagation of the cardiac action potential can therefore proceed in either direction. While refractoriness ensures that in normal heart propagation of the action potential proceeds in one direction, pathological conditions can eventually cause the conduction to fail in one direction, while it can still proceed in the opposite direction, thereby providing a substrate for unidirectional conduction and for reentry-based arrhythmias (see Chapter VIII) [231-233]. Different ways of generation of unidirectional block have been discussed in the literature:

a) Source – sink impedance mismatch

Geometrical factors can produce an impedance mismatch between source and sink, e.g. when the size of the current sink is larger than the size of the source. Such impedance mismatch can result from geometrical factors, and can occur at branching points (such as the origin of the pectinate muscle from the larger crista terminalis), or at junctional sites (such as the interface between Purkinje fibres and ventricular myocardium). Impedance mismatch can cause a slowing of conduction and can eventually result in unidirectional block of action potential propagation (Fig. III.9).

More recently it was realised that also curvature of the wave front is an source of impedance mismatch and can be an important factor contributing to unidirectional propagation of the action potential. With a convexly curved wave front the area of the wave front becomes progressively larger. Propagation of a convexly curved wave front is therefore hampered by the larger area that needs to be excited for propagation to continue. Conduction failure can result at wave fronts with very small radius of curvature.

The curvature of the wave front depends on many factors. It is initially large when the myocardium is stimulated by a point source of current or during an extrasystole. Non-excitable regions or regions of decreased excitability can alter the shape of the wave front. When a wave front e.g. meets a line of block for action potential propagation (which can be due to an anatomical, pathological or functional (e.g. refractoriness) obstacle) the wave curls around the end of the line of block so that its curvature increases. For wave fronts with positive curvature there is a value of curvature at which propagation is impaired; this value depends on the excitability of the medium [513-516,518].

Particular perturbations of the excitation wave, such as zone of block, or of reduced excitability or coupling, may result in phenomena of self-organisation, in which the wave becomes a spiral wave or vortex. E.g. when the activation wave encounters a zone of block, the wave front can separate in two parts that circumnavigate the obstacle. Behind the obstacle the wave fronts can eventually fuse again. However at low levels of excitability the waves may curl into a pair of counterrotating spiral waves. Spiral waves form an important mechanism of reentry based arrhythmias (see Chapter VIII) [see 514,518,791].

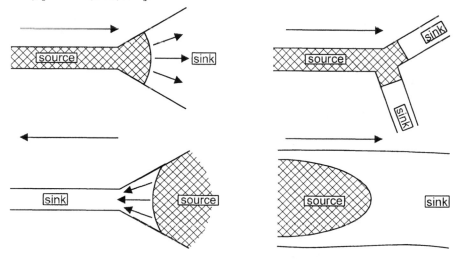

Figure III.9. Possible sources of impedance mismatch in the heart

b) Vulnerable Window

Each action potential is followed by a critical time- (and voltage-) window, during which an extra stimulus can induce unidirectional conduction. Stimulation during this vulnerable period results in block of conduction in the anterograde direction, because the cells are still refractory, whereas recovery of the Na^+ conductance has proceeded far enough to allow conduction in the retrograde direction [1009].

c) Dispersion in the action potential duration

Dispersion in action potential duration increases the likelihood to generate a temporary region of functional block due to tissue refractoriness which can cause unidirectional conduction. Spatial dispersion of action potential duration and refractoriness is normally present in the transmural direction [27,279], but also exists between apex, septum and free wall, between right and left ventricle [381,1222] and between apex and base [175].

APPENDIX: THE CABLE QUATION

The one-dimensional cable equation.

The cell (or a bundle of electrically coupled cells) can be represented as a cylinder of cytoplasm separated from the external medium by the membrane. Cytoplasm and extracellular solution are conducting media, while the membrane behaves as an imperfect insulator. Viewed this way the cell is like an undersea cable: a conducting wire surrounded by an insulator from the conducting seawater. The cell can be subdivided in small sections (which in the limit are made infinitely small). Each section represents a small membrane patch (represented as membrane capacitance in parallel with membrane resistance) separating the extra and intracellular medium. Consecutive patches of membrane are electrically connected via a small amount of resistance (the resistance of the cytoplasm and for electrically coupled multicellular preparations also the resistance of the gap junctions). The analogue equivalent circuit provides the basis for the understanding of the cable equation (Fig. III.10).

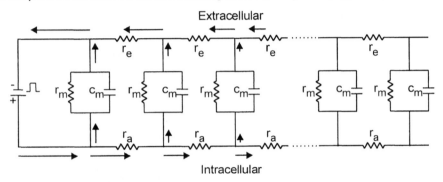

Figure III.10. The electrical equivalent circuit of a cell during current injection.

Current flow (i_a in μA) in longitudinal (axial) direction (x) will produce a voltage drop across the intracellular (and eventually intercellular) longitudinal resistance:

$$\partial V/\partial x = -r_a \cdot i_a \ (r_a \text{ intracellular resistance per unit length in Ohm cm}^{-1})$$

Since the volume of outside solution is relatively large, the extracellular resistance (r_e) is normally small. We can therefore neglect the voltage drop in the extracellular space, which is normally much smaller than the intracellular potential gradient, and the intracellular potential can be considered to represent the membrane potential. Radial voltage drops in the cytoplasm will be neglected as well as voltage drops in the extracellular medium, since both are small compared to the potential differences in the longitudinal direction of the cable which exist in the intracellular medium.

Current leaving the cell through the membrane will decrease the current in longitudinal direction:

$$\partial i_a/\partial x = -i_m \ (i_m \text{ membrane current per unit length in } \mu A \text{ cm}^{-1})$$

Combining both equations:

$$\partial^2 V/\partial x^2 = -r_a \cdot \partial i_a/\partial x = r_a i_m$$

The membrane current is the sum of ionic current (i_i) plus capacitative current (i_C) charging the membrane capacity:

$$i_m = i_C + i_i$$

The potential (V in volt) across a capacitor with capacitance C (in Farad) is proportional to the charge (Q in Coulomb) on the capacitor (Q = C.V). Since the rate of change of the capacitative charge is equal to the capacitative current ($i_C = dQ/dt$), the rate of change of the membrane potential will be proportional to the capacitative current charging the membrane capacity:

$i_C = c_m \, \partial V/\partial t$ (c_m capacitance per unith length μF cm^{-1})

Therefore the total membrane current equals:

$i_m = c_m \, \partial V/\partial t + i_i$

After combining equations we obtain the cable equation:

$$(1/r_a). \, \partial^2 V/\partial x^2 = c_m. \, \partial V/\partial t + i_i$$

where the net ionic current i_i may be a function of V and t

In the **linear cable model** the ionic current is approximated as a linear function of membrane potential according to Ohm's law:

$i_i = V/r_m$ (with r_m the membrane resistance per unit length in Ohm cm)

The cable equation in the linear approximation can then be written as:

$(1/r_a). \, \partial^2 V/\partial x^2 = c_m. \, \partial V/\partial t + V/r_m$

If we define $\lambda = \sqrt{r_m/r_a}$ (in cm) and $\tau_m = r_m c_m$ (in s) the cable equation becomes:

$$\lambda^2. \, \partial^2 V/\partial x^2 = \tau_m. \, \partial V/\partial t + V$$

In these equations τ_m is the membrane time constant of the membrane, and λ is the length constant of the cell.

Solution of the equations for a one-dimensional infinite linear cable for a current step is a rather complex. From the solution of the cable equation a number of important conclusions can be made.

In **steady-state** the potential in an infinite cable decays exponentially as a function of distance

$$V(t=\infty) = R_{in}.I_o.\exp(-x/\lambda)$$

with I_o the magnitude of the current step applied at $x = 0$
with input resistance $R_{in} = \sqrt{r_m r_a}/2$ and length constant $\lambda = \sqrt{r_m/r_a}$
where r_m is the membrane resistance per unit length in Ohm cm,
and r_a intracellular resistance per unit length in Ohm cm^{-1}.

The input resistance is the total resistance faced by the current; it is the ratio of the steady-state potential change at the site of current injection to applied current amplitude.

The length constant λ can be interpreted as the distance at which the potential in steady-state will be dropped to $1/e$ times the potential at the point current injection ($V_{x=\lambda} = V_{x=o} . e^{-1}$).

Propagation of the action potential

For an action potential conducting with constant velocity (θ) across a uniform cable the shape of the the the curves relating V to t, at constant x, and V to x, at constant t, are identical, from which follows:

$\partial^2 V/\partial x^2 = (1/\theta^2) \, \partial^2 V/\partial t^2$

In this case the cable equation for a conducted action potential becomes [462,507]:

$(1/(r_a \, \theta^2)). \, \partial^2 V/\partial t^2 = c_m. \, \partial V/\partial t + i_i(V,t)$

Mathematics tells us that $\partial^2 V/\partial t^2$ is zero when $\partial V/\partial t$ reaches its maximum value. Therefore during the propagated action potential (like in an action potential in homogeneously polarised tissue) $\partial V/\partial t_{max}$ is proportional to the maximum net inward current flowing during the action potential. $\partial V/\partial t_{max}$ or "V dot max" as it is generally called is often used as a indirect measure of the maximum inward current flowing during the upstroke of the action potential. Conduction velocity θ depends on the exact voltage- and time-dependent properties of the net ionic current.

Chapter IV

Ionic currents and action potentials in cardiac cells

1.   IONIC CURRENTS IN CARDIAC PLASMA MEMBRANES

Many different types of channels have been found in cardiac tissue [see 145,754,1087,1340,1356], and a huge literature exists on cardiac ion channels since cardiac electrophysiology started around 1949, when Coraboeuf and Weidmann registered the first cardiac action potentials with an intracellular electrode [209]. However, for obvious reasons most of the investigations have not been performed on human hearts, but on hearts from different types of animals. Data from human cardiac cells or from channels cloned from human hearts have only recently become more abundant. From the electrophysiological studies it is clear that large interspecies variability exists and that caution must be exerted when extrapolating data obtained in animals to the human heart. In this chapter we provide a general, though far from exhausting overview of the properties of ion channels that have been found in mammalian hearts. Our aim is to give a general overview of cardiac ion channels in order to provide insight in the mechanisms governing electrical activity, and to discuss how ion channels determine electrical and mechanical activity of the heart. Our emphasis is on channels that have been described in human hearts or are found to be present in most mammalian species investigated, and which appear to have an important role in physiological and pathological conditions. The channels which are most important for normal electrical activity in the heart are the voltage-dependent Na^+ channel, the L- and T-type Ca^{2+} channels, the inward-rectifying K^+ channel, the delayed rectifying K^+ channels, the transient outward current, the i_f pacemaker current and the acetylcholine-sensitive K^+ current. Modulation and pharmacological properties of channels [for review see 148] and also changes in disease [145] and remodeling [790,1116] are only briefly mentioned in this chapter, since they are treated more extensively in later chapters.

The reader may want to skip parts of the data presented in this chapter, and return to the description whenever needed for better understanding of later chapters, which often refer to properties described in this chapter.

1.1   Ion channels in the plasma membrane of cardiac cells

1.1.1 Na^+ channels

The most important Na^+ channel in cardiac tissue is undoubtedly the tetrodotoxin-sensitive voltage-dependent Na^+ channel responsible for the upstroke of the action potential in atrial and ventricular myocardium and in the ventricular conduction system [for review see 47,152,340,704,821,925]. More recently a sustained inward current carried by Na^+ has been found to be present in spontaneously active SAN cells, and this current could play a role in pacemaking. Cardiac cells also contain a small component of an ill-defined Na^+ background current.

1.1.1.1   Fast voltage-dependent Na^+ channel
1.1.1.1.1   Distribution

A voltage-operated Na^+ channel that shows activation and inactivation, and can be specifically blocked by tetrodotoxin (TTX) is responsible for the upstroke and the conduction of the action potential in many excitable cells. It provides the inward current underlying the upstroke (phase 0) of the action potential in atria, ventricles and His bundle Purkinje system. The density of the channel is highest in Purkinje cells. Although the channel is present at low density in the sinoatrial node (SAN) and atrioventricular node (AVN) cells, it does not play a role in these cells in physiological conditions, since it is inactivated by the low diastolic potential. However in neonatal (but not in adult) SAN pacemaker cells a TTX-sensitive Na^+ current can contribute to the total inward current [56].

1.1.1.1.2   Kinetics.

When a cardiac cell is depolarised an inward current is generated which rises rapidly [195,607,747] and decreases afterwards on a slower time course (Fig. IV.1 upper panel). The time to peak shortens with depolarisation [694].

The peak inward current flowing through Na^+ channels is not a monotonic function of membrane potential. Depolarisations to values between −60 and −10 mV cause an inward current that increases with depolarisation, due to the voltage-dependence of activation. With depolarisation to potentials positive to −10 mV the amplitude of the current decreases due to the reduction in driving force. The current reverses at about +50 mV (Fig. IV.1 lower left). The amplitude of the Na^+ current also depends on the holding potential previous to the clamp step, the current becoming smaller for less negative holding potentials, due to inactivation.

The time course and the voltage-dependence of the current can be explained in terms of voltage-dependent activation and inactivation. Steady-state activation and inactivation can be described by a Boltzmann distribution, with slopes around 6 mV. Activation starts at about −60 mV. Midpoints voltages in multicellular preparations are typically about -30 mV for the activation and -75 mV for the inactivation process (Fig. IV.1 lower right).

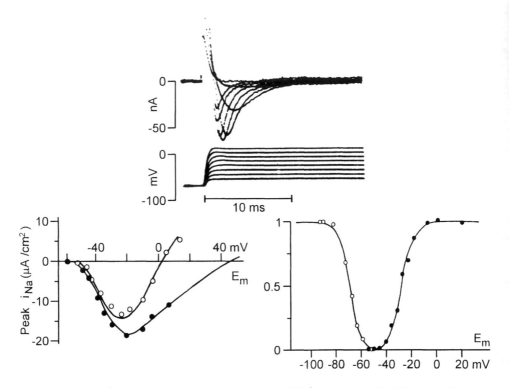

Figure IV.1. Na$^+$ current. Upper panel: time course of Na$^+$ currents in rabbit Purkinje fibres at different membrane potentials. Modified from [195]. Lower left: current-voltage relation in 155 (filled symbols) and 20 mM [Na$^+$]$_e$ (open symbols). Lower right: steady-state activation and inactivation curve. Modified from [196].

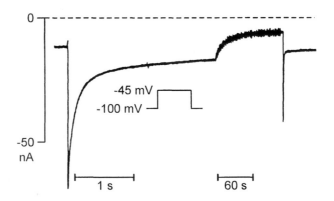

Figure IV.2. Time course of the tetrodotoxin-sensitive sodium current in rabbit Purkinje fibres, showing the presence of a very slowly inactivating component (note the change in time scale). Modified from [139].

In a limited range of potentials, where activation and inactivation overlap, a small steady-state Na$^+$ current, the so-called window current, can be recorded [37,372,848]. Also a small component of slowly inactivating Na$^+$ current (Fig. IV.2) can be recorded over a broad range of potentials in many types of cardiac cells of different species, including expressed human cardiac Na$^+$ channels [169,918,1215]. Recovery from inactivation is normally very fast (1-10 ms), with rates increasing upon hyperpolarisation. Following long depolarisations recovery can become very slow (order of seconds) [139,1004].

1.1.1.1.3   Ion permeation
The channel is highly selective for Na$^+$. The single channel conductance is 20-25 pS in the presence of 150 mM Na^+_e [1012].

1.1.1.1.4   Modulation
Na$^+$ channels are phosphorylated by PKA, but increase as well as decrease of Na$^+$ current have been described (see Chapter V) [for review see 991]. An increase in [Ca^{2+}]$_e$ results in a shift of voltage-dependence of the kinetics in depolarising direction, while lower [Ca^{2+}]$_e$ has the opposite effect. Extracellular as well as intracellular acidification reduces the current. 3-n polyunsaturated fatty acids block i$_{Na}$ and shift its activation to more positive potentials and its inactivation to more negative potentials [633].

Na$^+$ currents are the target of Class I antiarrhythmic drugs (local anaesthetics), which cause a use-dependent block, and cardiac Na$^+$ currents are more sensitive to local anaesthetics than their brain or skeletal muscle counterparts. While some local anaesthetics are activated state blockers, some (e.g. lidocaine) have been described as inactivation state blockers (see Chapters I and V) [for review see 148]. However more recently evidence was obtained that the so-called inactivation state block is not due to preferential binding of these drugs to the channel in the inactivation state, but to binding to transition states along the activation pathway [418,1199] and/or to the slow inactivated state [814].

The LQT3 form of congenital Long QT syndrome (LQT) and the Brugada syndrome have been related to defects of the cardiac Na$^+$ channel α-subunit (see Chapter VIII) [for review see 89]. LQT3 is caused by a gain of function mutation resulting in slow or incomplete inactivation of the channel, causing a small but persistent Na$^+$ current during the plateau of the action potential [76]. The Brugada syndrome on the other hand is associated with loss of function mutations [170,291] or defective surface localisation of i$_{Na}$ [52], causing reduction of i$_{Na}$. While LQT3 and Brugada syndrome are respectively gain of function and loss of function mutations, the two syndromes can coexist in the same patient [1204]. Recently Na$^+$ channel

mutations have also been shown to be a cause of cardiac conduction defects
[989,1127].

1.1.1.1.5 Structure

At the molecular level the channel consists of an α-subunit and two β–subunits [for review
see 47,377]. The gene (*SCN5A*) coding for the human cardiac α–subunit ($Na_v1.5$) is
located on chromosome 3 (3p21-24), while the β-subunit (β1) is encoded by a single gene
located on chromosome 19 [695]. While cardiac Na^+ channels are specifically blocked by
TTX, they belong to a subfamily of voltage-dependent Na^+ channels that require higher
TTX doses than e.g. neuronal Na^+ channels, and that is often referred to as the TTX-
resistant Na^+ channel subfamily.

The α-subunit, which is sufficient for channel activity, is composed of 6 transmembrane
segments repeated 4 times in a tetrameric structure. The channel appears to be a bell-
shaped molecule with several cavities [976]. The permeation process is dependent on a
hydrophilic part of the α-subunit between transmembrane segments S5 and S6. The S4
segment contains a high density of positive charges and acts as the voltage sensor for
activation gating. The short intracellular segment between domain III and IV has been
identified as the fast inactivation gate. All four domains play a role in inactivation:
domains D3 and D4 and the D3-D4 linker are important for fast inactivation while D1 and
D2 are most important for slow inactivation [831].

The two β-subunits exert a modulatory role; they speed up the kinetics of activation and
inactivation and decrease block by local anaesthetics [608,693].

1.1.1.2   Sustained inward current i_{st}

A sustained inward current i_{st} was recently found in spontaneously active
SAN and AVN cells in different mammalian species (Fig. IV.3) [for review
see 748]. It is activated by depolarisation in the range of potentials of slow
diastolic depolarisation (activation range between –70 and –40 mV), and
shows only weak inactivation. The current is largely carried by Na^+ ions and
is not decreased by reducing $[Ca^{2+}]_e$. The channel has a single channel
conductance of 13 pS. The current is blocked by dihydropyridines and heavy
metal ions and is enhanced by β-adrenergic stimulation. The current is
thought to contribute to spontaneous activity in nodal tissue.

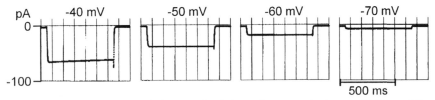
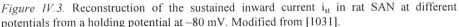

Figure IV.3. Reconstruction of the sustained inward current i_{st} in rat SAN at different
potentials from a holding potential at –80 mV. Modified from [1031].

1.1.2   Ca^{2+} channels

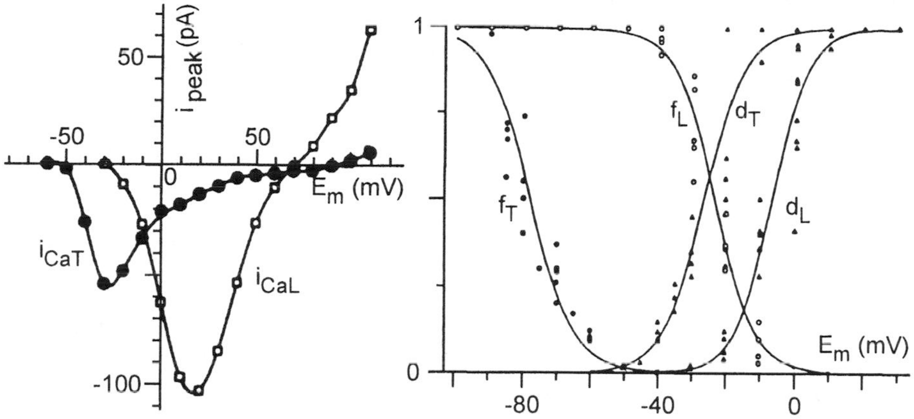

Figure IV.4. Two types of Ca^{2+} current (i$_{CaL}$ and i$_{CaT}$) in cardiac tissue. Left panel: current-voltage relation of i$_{CaL}$ and i$_{CaT}$ in canine atrial cells. Modified from [66]. Right panel: steady-state activation (d$_L$) and inactivation (f$_L$) curves of i$_{CaL}$ and of i$_{CaT}$ (d$_T$ and f$_T$) in rabbit SAN. Modified from [408].

Different types of Ca^{2+} permeable channels have been described in the plasma membrane of heart cells: the L- and T-type channels (i$_{CaL}$ and i$_{CaT}$), both voltage-activated, and a background channel [see 83,153,614,726,788,1034]. They can be differentiated on the basis of their electrophysiological and pharmacological characteristics (Fig. IV.4). The density of the T- and L-type channels differs between species and in different sections of the heart: the ratio of T-type over L-type channel is highest in Purkinje and SAN cells, where it reaches of 0.2 to 0.6; in atrial and ventricular cells the ratio is very small [66]. Under Na$^+$-free conditions a TTX-sensitive Ca^{2+} current i$_{Ca.TTX}$ was found in human single atrial cells [634], and also coexists in guinea pig ventricular myocytes with i$_{CaT}$ [443]. Whether the current reflects Ca^{2+} current through cardiac Na$^+$ channels in Na$^+$-free conditions [400] is still controversial.

1.1.2.1   L-type Ca^{2+} channel
Ca^{2+} influx through the L-type Ca^{2+} channel (i$_{CaL}$) also called dihydropyridine receptor (DHPR) (Fig. IV.5) is responsible for the upstroke of the action potential in SAN and AVN and plays an important role in determining the plateau and eventual spike - dome appearance of the action potential in other cardiac cells [for review 463,726,1109]. It is also responsible for the coupling between excitation and contraction, by inducing release of Ca^{2+} from the sarcoplasmic reticulum.

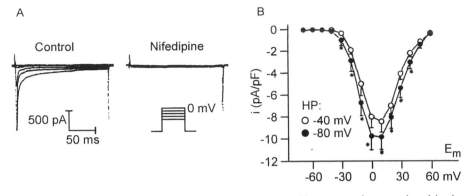

Figure IV.5. i_{CaL} in human right ventricular myocytes. A: Time course in control and in the presence of nifedipine at different potentials. B: Current-voltage relation measured from holding potential of –40 and –80 mV. Modified from [650].

1.1.2.1.1 Kinetics

Relatively large depolarisations are needed to activate the channel. The threshold for activation is around -25 mV and half-maximum activation is attained at about -15 mV for most cells [see 726] (Fig. IV.6) and at more positive potentials (-3 mV) in the AVN [419].

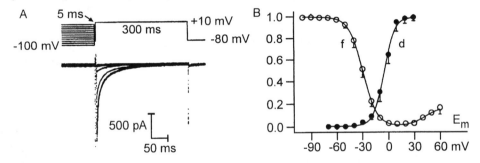

Figure IV.6. i_{CaL} in human right ventricular myocytes. A: Currents recorded from different holding potentials. B: Steady-state activation and inactivation curves of i_{CaL} (B). Modified from [650].

At the single channel level three modes of activity have been distinguished. In mode 1 the channel shows repetitive short (<1 ms) openings and closures (0.2 and 2 ms), forming a burst of activity separated from other bursts by longer closures. Mode 2 occurs in the presence of dihydropyridine (DHP) agonists [442] or following β-receptor stimulation [155,864], and is characterised by much longer open times. A third mode is characterised by the complete absence of openings or presence of only rare short openings, and its probability increases with preceding depolarisations. This mode corresponds to the inactivated state of the channel.

Activation and inactivation show a pronounced overlapping (window current) [452,1035]. Half-maximum steady-state inactivation occurs at −20 to -30 mV. The inactivation curve shows a minimum at about 0 mV and increases again at more positive potentials, and this dip in the curve is absent when intracellular Ca^{2+} is well buffered, while also the decay of the current during a pulse is much slower. A large variety of experiments have demonstrated that this type of behaviour is due to the presence of two types of inactivation: inactivation is dependent on voltage as well as on intracellular Ca^{2+} concentration. The Ca^{2+}-induced inactivation is the faster process, while the voltage-induced inactivation is rather slow. The Ca^{2+} concentration that controls the Ca^{2+}-induced inactivation of the channel is obviously the subplasmalemmal Ca^{2+} concentration, which may strongly deviate from the bulk cytosolic $[Ca^{2+}]$. The concentration seen by the channel may be much higher, especially during the first 50 ms of a depolarisation [657]. It is especially the Ca^{2+} originating from the sarcoplasmic reticulum (SR) which is responsible for the inactivation process during the first 50 ms of depolarisation [893,1047,1113]. The Ca^{2+}-induced inactivation acts as a negative feedback process: a large increase of intracellular Ca^{2+} enhances the rate of inactivation, thereby limiting further Ca^{2+} influx and preventing Ca^{2+} overload of the cell.

Experiments under conditions where a rise of $[Ca^{2+}]_i$ is excluded demonstrated the presence of a slow voltage-dependent inactivation [see 726].

Recovery from inactivation upon hyperpolarisation is also dependent on voltage as well as on $[Ca^{2+}]_i$. For the voltage-induced inactivation the rate and the degree of recovery is greater the more hyperpolarised the membrane, with time constants in the order of 300 ms at -50 mV and 100 ms or shorter at -80 mV. A much slower component (seconds) is seen following long depolarisations, indicating the presence of slow inactivation [109,990]. This slow inactivation may play a role in overdrive suppression [1257]. Recovery from Ca^{2+}-induced inactivation as such is voltage-independent [1047,1048] but indirectly it is modulated by voltage, since the fall in $[Ca^{2+}]_i$ is dependent in part on the extrusion of Ca^{2+} from the cell by the Na^+/Ca^{2+} exchanger, which is faster the more negative the membrane potential.

At negative holding potentials recovery from inactivation may show an overshoot, i.e. the Ca^{2+} current transiently becomes larger than in steady-state. Such facilitation also can occur during high frequency stimulation, and requires a moderate increase in intracellular Ca^{2+} concentration [62,649,699,872,1154].

1.1.2.1.2   Permeation and selectivity

The channel is 500 to 1000 times more permeable to divalent cations than to monovalent cations. The exclusion of monovalent ions depends on the presence of a minimum concentration of divalent ions [see review 1161]. Despite the low permeability of the channel for K^+ ions, K^+ is responsible for a substantial current through the channel, because the intracellular K^+ concentration is very high compared to the free Ca^{2+} concentration in the cell. The contribution of K^+ to the net current flow through the channel also explains why the reversal potential of the Ca^{2+} current is much less positive than expected from the equilibrium potential for Ca^{2+} ions, and it was demonstrated that net influx of Ca^{2+} occurs at potentials where the net current through the channel is outward [1351].

The conductance of the channel for divalent ions increases with the concentration and shows saturation. The single channel conductance at the physiological Ca^{2+} concentrations is about 5 to 7 pS [402,1334].

The permeation and selectivity properties of the channel have been explained by assuming the presence of multiple ion binding sites within the channel pore. While several ions may be simultaneously present in the channel, they can only pass through the channel in a single file. This multi-ion occupancy of a single file channel can explain the high conductance and at the same time the high selectivity. High selectivity is conditioned by high affinity of the ion binding sites within the pore; high conductance is due to electrostatic repulsion between the ions simultaneously occupying the channel at different binding sites [1161]. However more recently this hypothesis has been questioned, and ion permeation was explained on the basis of electrostatic screening and volume exclusion between ions and carboxylate groups of four glutamate residues (EEEE locus) in the pore that appear essential for high Ca^{2+} specificity [812].

1.1.2.1.3   Modulation

L-type Ca^{2+} currents are blocked in a use-dependent way by phenylalkylamines (such as verapamil), benzothiazepines (e.g. diltiazem) and dihydropyridines (like nifedipine), and are major targets for therapeutic drug action [for review see 148,459].

Channel activity is enhanced by β-adrenergic stimulation via PKA [1159]. The effect is mainly due to β1 stimulation, but also β2-receptor stimulation increases i_{CaL} in certain myocardial preparations [1095] [see 1302]. The effect of α-receptor activation and PKC is complex, with both stimulation and inhibition of i_{CaL} being observed [474,545,1294]. Rate-dependent facilitation of the channel is enhanced by isoproterenol [872] and is impaired in human failing hearts [54].

NO as well as cGMP can produce stimulatory and inhibitory effects on i_{CaL} [357,1187]. The effects in human atrial myocytes are mediated via opposite action of cGMP on the phosphodiesterases PDE2 and PDE3 [1187].

Extracellular as well as intracellular acidification cause inhibition of the channel. The channel can act as an oxygen sensor. It is inhibited in hypoxia, and the human cardiac L-type channel was found to be modulated by redox agents. SH-oxidising agents cause a decrease of the current [321,322,613], while also a marked transient stimulatory effect has been described [1307]. Hypoxia also affects the response of the channel to α- or β-adrenergic modulation [470].

Aldosterone upregulates Ca^{2+} current in adult rat cardiomyocytes; the effect may be important in cardiac remodeling [73].

1.1.2.1.4 Structure

The cardiac L-type Ca^{2+} channel consists of 4 subunits: two α-subunits, $Ca_v1.2$ (α1C) and an α2, a β-, and a δ-subunit (a γ-subunit is exclusively expressed in skeletal muscle). The human $Ca_v1.2$-subunit is encoded by the *CACLN1A1* gene on chromosome 12p13.3. The $Ca_v1.2$-subunit is sufficient to express channel activity. It resembles the Na^+ channel, with 4 repeats each with 6 transmembrane segments, a highly charged S4 segment which probably acts as the voltage sensor for activation and a P region between S5 and S6.

The highly conserved glutamate residues located in the pore region of all four repeats (the EEEE locus) are involved in high-affinity binding of divalent cations, providing high Ca^{2+} selectivity as well as high rates of permeation of Ca^{2+} through the channel [1322]. Ca^{2+}-dependent inactivation as well as facilitation is due to Ca^{2+}-dependent binding of calmodulin to consensus calmodulin binding sequence (the IQ motif) present at the C terminus, but not all determinants involved reside on the C terminus. The proximal C terminus is also involved in voltage-dependent inactivation [1360,1361] [see 440].

The function of the α-subunit is markedly modulated by the β-subunit. Co-expression of the two subunits results in a marked increase of peak current [535,793,852,1263], and the β-subunit appears to be required for facilitation of the channel [546].

1.1.2.2   T-type Ca^{2+} channel

A so-called T-type Ca^{2+} current (i_{CaT}) [66,801] of short duration is activated at potentials more negative than the threshold for the L-type Ca^{2+} current (Fig. IV.4) [for review 788,1196]. Fig. IV.7 shows single channel currents and ensemble average currents of i_{CaT} in guinea pig ventricular myocytes at different membrane potentials. i_{CaT} was described in all types of cardiac cells, but in most species the expression of this current in adult atria or ventricle is low and the current was not found in adult human atrium or ventricle [85,312,649,917]. The current is well represented in neonatal myocytes: the T-type Ca^{2+} channel was identified in mid-gestational fetal myocardium of developing mouse heart [224], but declines with maturation. The channel has been proposed to play a role in pacemaking.

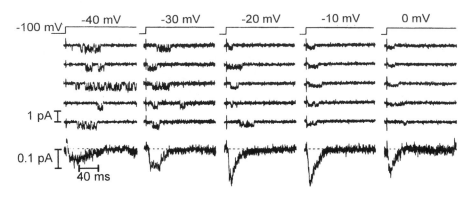

Figure IV.7. Single channel current of the T-type Ca^{2+} channel (i_{CaT}) in guinea pig ventricular myocytes at different membrane potentials. The lower panels show the corresponding ensemble average from a large number of repeated measurements. Modified from [278].

1.1.2.2.1   Kinetics

Threshold for activation is around -70 mV to -50 mV and maximum activation is seen at –30 mV to -10 mV [see 1196]. Inactivation is rapid and complete, with time constants of 30 ms at -50 mV, becoming shorter at more depolarised levels. Steady-state inactivation extends from -85 mV to -40 mV with half-maximum around -60 mV and slope of 5.5 mV. Repriming is voltage-dependent and with time constants of the order of the order of 100 ms. It is slower the longer the preceding depolarisation, suggesting the existence of slow inactivation.

1.1.2.2.2   Permeation

In 100 mM [Ca^{2+}] the single channel conductance is about 7 pS, [278] compared to 20 pS for the L-type. Extracellular protons inhibit the channel with greater efficiency than the L-type current, while intracellular protons have no effect [1165]. Extracellular Mg^{2+} ions reduce the current and shift the activation and inactivation curves in the positive direction [1298].

1.1.2.2.3   Modulation

T-type Ca^{2+} currents are blocked by mibefradil [310,741]. However mibefradil also blocks tetrodotoxin-sensitive Ca^{2+} current, which was shown to coexist with i_{CaT} in guinea- pig ventricular myocytes [443], and at higher concentrations also i_{CaL} and other currents. The channel is insensitive to β-adrenergic stimulation [1166]. The expression of T-type Ca^{2+} channel in myocardium is modulated by arachidonic acid [1349]. The myocardial expression declines with maturation [1304], but is reactivated in some disease models [191]. Inhibition of the channels by mibefradil was found to protect against atrial remodeling caused by atrial tachycardia [318].

1.1.2.2.4 Structure

$Ca_v3.1$ ($\alpha 1G$) and $Ca_v3.2$ ($\alpha 1H$) [854] are T-type Ca^{2+} channel isoforms found in cardiovascular tissue [101,223]. $Ca_v3.2$ was cloned and expressed from human heart, it has properties similar (but not identical) to the cardiac i_{CaT} [851]. $Ca_v3.2$ is coded by the *CACNA1H* gene mapped to human chromosome 16p13.3. $Ca_v3.1$ is coded by *CACNA1G* on chromosome 17q22. $Ca_v3.1$ is present in neonatal rat hart and in mouse midgestational myocardium and may contribute to excitability [224,635]. The gene is reexpressed in rat ventricular myocytes during remodeling after myocardial infarction [475].}.

1.1.2.3 Background Ca^{2+} channels

Two types of Ca^{2+} permeable channels which do not require voltage steps for activation and are insensitive to dihydropyridines have been identified in single channels studies [216,936]. Activity of one of these channels is enhanced by exposure to oxygen free radicals and metabolic inhibition [1244].

1.1.3 K^+ channels

Cardiac cells show a large variety of K^+ channels [see 239,796,925,1058]. Functionally, distinction can be made between voltage-activated channels (i_{to}, i_{Kur}, i_{Kss}, i_{Kr} and i_{Ks}), ligand-activated channels ($i_{K.ACh}$, $i_{K.ATP}$, $i_{K.Na}$ and $i_{K.AA}$) and a channel (the inward rectifier i_{K1}) that is not gated by voltage or extracellular ligands and can be called a background current. Structurally the $i_{K.ACh}$, $i_{K.ATP}$ and i_{K1} channels belong to the same family (Kir) of inward-rectifying K^+ channels (Fig. IV.8).

Since the membrane potential at rest and during cardiac activity is less negative than the equilibrium potential of K^+ ions, net K^+ current is outward, repolarising the membrane during the action potential or stabilising the membrane at a hyperpolarised level. Under physiological circumstances the voltage-activated K^+ currents and $i_{K.ACh}$ and i_{K1} play an important role for the diastolic potential and in shaping the normal action potential. Under ischaemic conditions, ligand-activated currents, especially $i_{K.ATP}$ and $i_{K.AA}$ become dominant, while some of the "physiological" K^+ currents are inhibited.

The amino-acid sequence and topology of many K^+ channels is known [see 36,193] and the molecular structure of the pore has been elucidated from x-ray analysis of the crystallised molecule [276] [see 95]. The voltage-gated K^+ channels show a remarkable homology with the Na^+ and Ca^{2+} channels. However, whereas Na^+ and Ca^{2+} channels consist of four tandemly-linked domains of six transmembrane segments which are connected in one long strand, only one domain with six transmembrane segments is found for the K^+ channel. The S4 segments act as the voltage sensor. Two types of inactivation have been described in expressed channels [902]. In N-type inactivation the negatively charged N-terminal acts as a ball that can block the open channel. In C-type inactivation conformational changes on the extracellular side close to the pore result in some kind of constriction. C-type inactivation is sensitive to drug binding and extracellular K^+ [for review see 796].

The inward-rectifying channels have a simpler structure and contain only two transmembrane segments separated by a pore region. To this family belong the strong inward rectifiers (IRK), The G protein coupled, weakly inward-rectifying K^+ channels (K_G), the ATP-sensitive K^+ channels (K_{ATP}) and some K^+ transporters (Fig. IV.8 right panel).

A tetrameric structure for all these K^+ channels is highly likely. The pore in K^+ channels is formed by a stretch of 19 amino-acids in the linker between S5 and S6 in the four subunits. The motif GYG (or GFG) in the P-region is the signature of K^+ selectivity but other residues also participate in determining K^+ selectivity.

Recently a new family of K^+ channels with two pore segments in tandem and four transmembrane segments have been described [for review see 380,845]. They are called two-pore domain K^+ channels or 2P/4TM. Several subfamilies such as TASK, TREK, TWIK, TALK etc., have been identified, and a few of its members have been identified in cardiac cells.

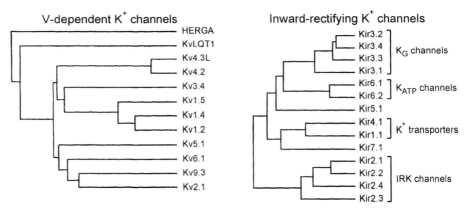

Figure IV.8. Families of voltage-gated and inward-rectifier K^+ channels.

1.1.3.1   Voltage-dependent channels

Voltage-gated K^+ channels can be subdivided in a number of families: K_v1 (*Shaker*), K_v2 (*Shab*), K_v3 (*Shaw*), K_v4 (*Shal*), K_v5-9 (eag family, with subfamilies *eag*, *elk* and *erg*) and the KvLQT1 family. A large variety of voltage-gated K^+ channels are expressed in cardiac cells (see Table IV.1 and Fig. IV.8 left panel) [for review see 796,925,1058,1107]. The main voltage-dependent K^+ currents in the heart are the transient outward K^+ currents i_{to} and the delayed outward currents i_{Kr}, i_{Ks} and i_{Kur} (Fig.IV.9). Each of these currents exists in a number of variants, while in some cardiac cells additional components are present, such as i_{Kss}, which is non-inactivating and is also called background current. These currents play a major role in shaping the action potential and adapting its duration to changes in frequency.

Table IV.1. Voltage-gated K^+ currents / channels in mammalian heart. Modified from [796].

Current	Activation	Inactiv.	Blocker	Tissue	Species
i_{to}					
$\quad i_{to,f}$	Fast	Fast	mM 4-AP	Atrium	Dog, human, mouse, rat
			Flecainide	Ventricle	Cat, dog, ferret
			HaTX, HpTX		human, mouse, rat
$\quad i_{to,s}$	Fast	Slow	mM 4-AP	Atrium	Rabbit
				Ventricle	Ferret, human,
					mouse, rabbit, rat
				Node	Rabbit
i_K					
$\quad i_{Kr}$	Moderate	Fast	E-4031	Atrium	Dog, guinea pig,
			Dofetilide		human, rat
				Ventricle	Cat, dog, guinea pig, rat
					human, mouse, rabbit
			Lanthanum	Node	Rabbit
$\quad i_{Ks}$	Very slow	No	NE-10064	Atrium	Dog, guinea pig, human
			NE-10133	Ventricle	Dog, guinea pig, human
				Node	Guinea pig, rabbit
$\quad i_{Kur}$	Fast	No	μM 4-AP	Atrium	Dog, human, rat
$\quad i_{Kp}$	Fast	No	Ba^{2+}	Ventricle	Guinea pig
$\quad i_K$	Slow	Slow	mM TEA	Ventricle	Rat
$\quad i_{K,slow}$	Fast	Slow	μM 4-AP	Atrium	Mouse
			mM TEA	Ventricle	Mouse
$\quad i_{K,slow}$	Fast	Very slow	mM 4-AP	Atrium	Human, rat
$\quad (i_{K,DTX})$			DTX		
$\quad i_{ss}$	Slow	No	mM TEA	Atrium	Mouse, rat
			mM 4-AP	Ventricle	Dog, human, mouse, rat

4-AP = 4-aminopyridine; HaTX = hanatoxin; HpTX = heteropodatoxin;
TEA = tetraethylammonium; DTX = dendrotoxin.

1.1.3.1.1   Transient outward current i_{to}

The transient outward current consists of several components. i_{to}, also called i_{to1}, is carried by K^+, while a Ca^{2+}-activated Cl^- current also results in a transient outward current, which is often called i_{to2} (this current will be discussed in section 1.1.4.3) [208,1157]. i_{to} is a transient outward K^+ current, which is rapidly activated and is also inactivated during depolarising steps. It can be blocked by millimolar concentrations of 4-AP. Its properties are similar to the A-type current in neurons. i_{to} was found to be present in all cardiac cell types [see 796] including SAN [632] and AVN [744]. The major effects of i_{to} are found phase 1 repolarisation of the action potential in atria and in ventricular subepicardial cells.

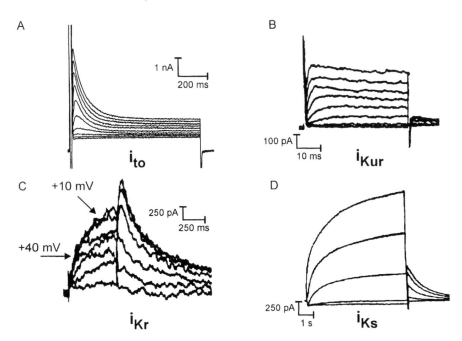

Figure IV.9. Time course of the most important voltage-dependent K^+ channels in cardiac cells. A: i_{to} in human ventricular myocytes. Modified from [1100], B: i_{Kur} cloned from human heart [325] C: i_{Kr} from mouse ventricular myocytes [1238] D: i_{Ks} in guinea pig ventricular myocytes [970].

Based on kinetics, two transient outward K^+ current types can be distinguished: a fast component i_{tof} and a slow component i_{tos}. [111,1157] both of which are present in human heart [772,1270]. The distribution of the two components is species-dependent and it also varies in different parts of the heart [for a recent review see 796].

In human atrial cells only i_{tof} has been identified [327,1249], while in ventricular myocardium both components have been described [772,1270].

The density of i_{to} varies between different parts of the heart. Differences in expression of i_{to} are present between right and left ventricle: density of i_{tof}

expression is higher in right versus left ventricular midmyocardial M cellslumenal [1221]. Also transmural differences in density of i_{to} have been described (see also Chapter VI). In the ventricle from different species, including humans, density of i_{tot} is higher in subepicardial and midmyocardial cells than in subendocardial cells [647,665]. In the subendocardial cells, inactivation and recovery of i_{to} is slower, and these properties are similar to those of i_{tos} in other species [772,1270]. The differences in expression of i_{to} across the ventricular wall result in important transmural differences in shape of the action potential (see also Chapters I, III and VI). Also in atrial cells i_{to} is more expressed in subepicardial than in subendocardial cells [1253].

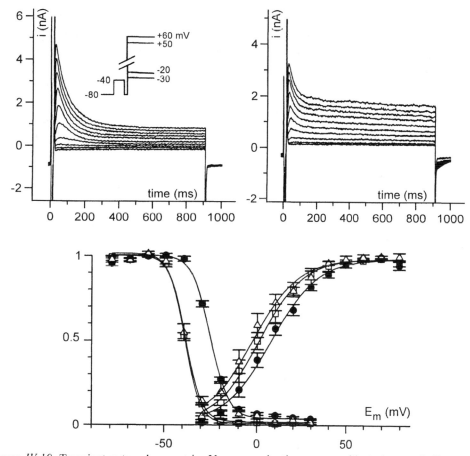

Figure IV.10. Transient outward current i_{to}. Upper panels: time course of i_{to} in human (left) and rat (right) ventricular myocytes. Lower panel: Steady-state activation and inactivation curves of i_{to} in rat ventricular myocytes in control (squares), at pH_e 6.0 (filled circles), and upon return to normal pH (triangles). Extracellular acidification shifts both curves in depolarising direction. Modified from [1100].

i_{to} is also present in Purkinje fibres, but its properties (e.g. sensitivity to block by tetraethylammonium (TEA)) appear to be different than those that have been reported in cardiac i_{to} of atrial or ventricular myocytes or from cloned K^+ channel subunits known to participate in cardiac i_{to} [416].

1.1.3.1.1.1 Kinetics

The i_{to} current is activated upon depolarisation. Midpoint voltage values for steady-state activation vary between -10 to +20 mV (Fig. IV.10) [135,324].

i_{tof} has fast activation, inactivation and recovery from inactivation. The time course of inactivation has been described as mono-exponential or bi-exponential. Time constants also vary but are in the order of 25 to 75 ms and are voltage-independent. Steady-state inactivation shows half-maximum potentials between -50 and -15 mV [see 134]. Recovery from inactivation is very sensitive to voltage, being faster the more hyperpolarised the membrane. Actual time constants for recovery vary with species. In most species, including human atrial cells [18,338,395] and ventricular epicardium, recovery is fast, with time constants in the order of 20 to 60 ms at -80 mV; frequency-dependence is small.

In other cell types [see 134] including human subendocardial fibres [772] i_{to} is due to i_{tos} and recovery is slow to very slow (time constants of 1 to 6 s). In these latter preparations the current is markedly reduced [327] and shortening of the action potential markedly less at elevated frequencies [559].

1.1.3.1.1.2 Permeation

The i_{to} current is carried by K^+ ions. The single channel current-voltage relation of the two types of channels is linear, and single channel conductances in 145 mM $[K^+]_e$ are respectively in the order of 10 pS and 30 pS [75,186,785].

1.1.3.1.1.3 Modulation and block

i_{to} is blocked by 4-aminopyridine, and the components can be separated by different sensitivity to drugs and toxins [450] [see 796].

i_{to} expression is affected by humoral status and changes during development. It is reduced by α- and $\beta 1$-receptor activation (see Chapter V). The density of i_{to} in the heart increases after birth [314,525,701,1239], while also changes in kinetics have been reported [966]. Calcitonin gene-related peptide has been shown to suppress i_{to} [1099]. Angiotensin II alters i_{to} in subepicardial cells to resemble unincubated subendocardial cells, but did not alter mRNA levels of $K_v4.3$ or $K_v1.4$; the effect could be due to accessory subunits [1330].

Recent evidence indicates that the channel is modulated by the redox state of the cell via oxidation - reduction of specific thiol groups [1033].

The transient outward current is altered in a number of pathological situations and remodeling. i_{to} density is reduced in patients with terminal heart failure [86] and in long-term cardiac memory by long term pacing of ventricular myocytes [1331]. In human atrial myocytes of patients with heart failure i_{to} density was increased and kinetics was altered, which can contribute to the shorter duration of the action potential [992]. i_{to} density is reduced in dilated human atria [623] and chronic atrial fibrillation [386,1337] [see 1184].

1.1.3.1.1.4 Structure

$K_v1.4$, $K_v4.2$ and $K_v4.3$ reveal rapidly activating and inactivating 4-AP-sensitive K^+ current resembling cardiac transient outward K^+ current, and they are present in cardiac cells, but like the functionally described i_{to}, their distribution varies with species and cell type. As molecular substrates for i_{tof}, $K_v4.2$ and $K_v4.3$ have been proposed. However in dog and human $K_v4.3$ appears to be responsible for i_{tof} in atrial [1249] and ventricular cells [538], and Kv4.3 is down-regulated in remodeling human atrial fibrillation [386]. $K_v1.4$, which was also detected in human ventricle [538], seems be at the origin of i_{tos} in ventricular subendocardial cells [860,1249].

$K_v4.2$ and to a lesser extent also $K_v4.3$ interact with a small protein MiRP1 (MinK-related peptide 1) encoded by *KCNE2* on chromosome 21q22.12. The presence of MiRP1 changes the kinetics of the channels [1348]. β subunits called K_v channel-interacting proteins (KChIPs) have also been identified for the K_v4 family of ions channels [19,1348]. Although not yet described in cardiac cells, the eventual presence of accessory subunits could partly explain the variability of the properties of i_{to}. Also hetero-oligomerisation may be at the origin of the large diversity in properties.

1.1.3.1.2 Delayed K^+ currents

On the basis of kinetics, rectification, sensitivity to blockers and modulation by intracellular messengers, three delayed K^+ currents i_{Ks} (slow delayed K^+ current), i_{Kr} (rapid delayed K^+ current) and i_{Kur} (ultrarapid delayed rectifier K^+ current) can be distinguished [178,746,792,796,971]. i_{Kr} shows activation and inactivation, i_{Ks} only activation, while i_{Kur} activates very rapidly and shows no or very slow inactivation. Delayed rectifiers are important for regulating the duration of the action potential and also play a role in SAN automaticity.

The currents have been recorded from all cardiac cell types, but density of i_{Kr} and i_{Ks} varies with species and cell type [824]. Despite contrary reports, i_{Kr} and i_{Ks} have both been found in human atrium and ventricle, although in human ventricle the amplitude of the delayed rectifying K^+ current is small (Fig. IV.11) [86,105,494,594,615,646,1203,1251]. In human heart i_{Kur} has only be clearly identified in atrial cells. Differences in channel density are also found between apex and base of the ventricle and in different transmural layers (see also Chapter VI): expression of both currents is smaller in rabbit apical than in basal myocytes [175], and i_{Ks} is smaller in canine ventricular mid-myocardium than in epicardium [664]. These findings partially explain the differences in action potential duration (APD) between these cells.

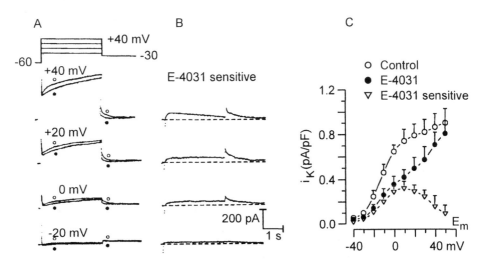

Figure IV.11. The delayed outward current in human ventricle contains i_{Ks} and i_{Kr}. A: Time course of the current in control (open symbols) and in the presence of E-4031 (a blocker of i_{Kr}). The time-dependent current in the presence of E-4031 represents i_{Ks}. B: The E-4031-sensitive current (=i_{Kr}). C: Voltage-dependence of the amplitude of the delayed rectifying current in control, and i_{Ks} (current in the presence of E-4031) and i_{Kr} (E-4031-sensitive current). Modified from [648].

1.1.3.1.2.1 The slowly activated delayed K$^+$ current i_{Ks}

1.1.3.1.2.1.1 Kinetics

The i_{Ks} current only shows activation and no inactivation. Activation occurs over a broad range of depolarising potentials (Fig. IV.12). Half-maximum values vary considerably from -13 mV to +26 mV [48,648,721]. Kinetics are slow and the time course of the activation is sigmoidal. Time constants reported vary with species. In human ventricle the time course was fitted by two exponentials with time constants of about 350 ms and 8.5 s [648]. Deactivation time course also varies largely with species: deactivation is slow in the guinea pig but relatively fast in the dog and human [371,494,1192].

1.1.3.1.2.1.2 Permeation

The i_{Ks} current is largely carried by K^+, although the channel is less selective than i_{Kr} [721]. The fully activated current-voltage relation approaches linearity. Single channel conductance is relatively low with estimations of 3 to 5.4 pS in mammalian ventricular or atrial cells [48,472]. Extracellular K^+ ions have no direct effect on the conductance. A rise in $[Na^+]_i$ or $[Ca^{2+}]_i$ enhances i_{Ks} [802,1149].

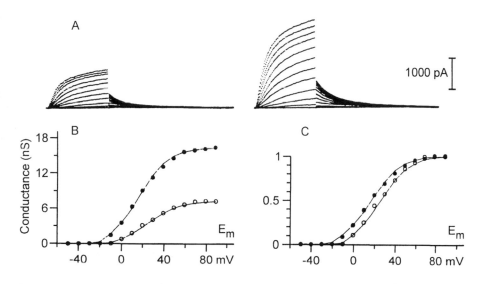

Figure IV.12. Stimulation of PKA by isoproterenol increases the amplitude of i_{Ks} in guinea pig ventricle. Panels A show i_{Ks} current in control (left) and in the presence of adrenaline (right). Lower panels: Amplitude of the tail currents (B) and the steady-state activation curve (C) in control (open symbols) and in the presence of adrenaline (filled symbols). Modified from [1232].

1.1.3.1.2.1.3 Modulation and block

β-adrenergic stimulation increases i_{Ks}, causes a negative shift of its activation curve and slows deactivation (Fig. IV.12) [884,1160,1232]. Also α-adrenergic stimulation [1231], PKC activation or a rise in $[Ca^{2+}]_i$ [1149] result in an increase of i_{Ks}. Chronic amiodarone as well as hypothyroidism decreases i_{Ks} [106,107,543]. In a dog with chronic complete atrioventricular block and biventricular hypertrophy i_{Ks} densities of left and right ventricle were significantly lower than in control [1224].

1.1.3.1.2.1.4 Molecular structure

Cardiac i_{Ks} is due to coexpression of *KCNQ1* (originally named K_v.LQT1) and a small peptide minK (I_{sK}) (Fig. IV.13) [51,968]. The *KCNQ* family of K^+ channel proteins has the classical constitution of voltage-activated K^+ channels, but lacks the tetramerisation domain that mediates subunit association of the K_v channel family. The minK protein, coded by gene *KCNE1* on chromosome 21q22.12, consists of a single putative transmembrane domain. It does not show channel properties, but modulates the activity of the pore forming subunit. Coexpression of *KCNE1* (minK) reversed pH regulation of *KCNQ1* from inhibition to activation by acidic pH_i. In addition, *KCNE1* altered the pharmacological properties of *KCNQ1* [1170]. The most common form of Long QT syndrome, LQT1 is linked to defects on chromosome 11p15.5, resulting from mutations in *KCNQ1* [1242]. Mutations in minK give rise to LQT5 [290,1088].

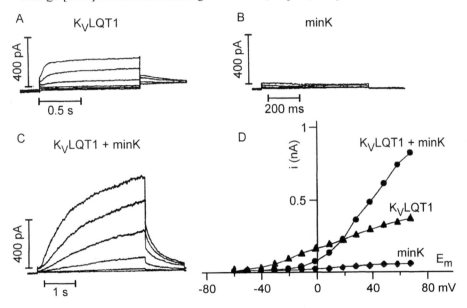

Figure IV.13. Coexpression of K_vLQT1 (= *KCNQ1*) with minK subunit results in the typical appearance of i_{Ks} in cardiac cells. Panels A to C show the time course of the currents, while in panel D the amplitudes of the steady-state currents are plotted as function of potential. Modified from [36].

1.1.3.1.2.2 The rapid delayed K$^+$ current i_{Kr}

The rapid delayed K$^+$ current plays a important role for the APD.

1.1.3.1.2.2.1 Kinetics

i_{Kr} activates rapidly for depolarisations positive to –40 mV, with a mid-point voltage between -20 and -5 mV (Fig. IV.14); this value is independent of $[K^+]_e$ [1016]. Time constants of activation and deactivation vary among species and are dependent on the membrane potential. Activation time constants range from less than 100 ms up to 500 ms [141,971]. Values of about 100 and 200 ms were reported in human ventricular myocytes [648,1202,1203]. These time constants are shorter than the time constants of

i_{Ks}. Time constants of deactivation of i_{Kr} in human and dog ventricle were reported to be slower than deactivation of i_{Ks} [371,494,1192].

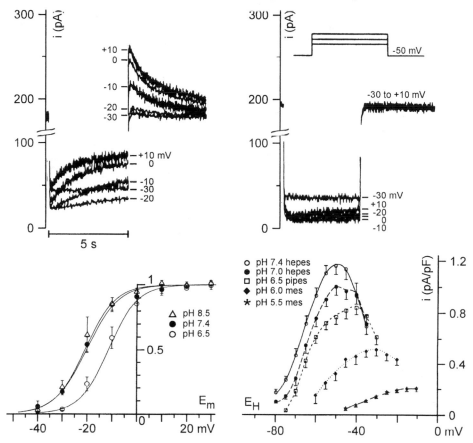

Figure IV.14. Rapid delayed rectifying K$^+$ current i_{Kr} in rabbit ventricular myocytes. Upper panels: time course of i_{Kr} during different voltage steps in control (left); the time-dependent current is blocked by the class III antiarrhythmic drug dofetilide (right panel). Modified from [141]. Lower panels: steady-state activation curve (left panel) and current-voltage relation of the "fully activated current" (right) at different external pH. Modified from [1207].

In whole cell recordings the time course of the macroscopic current shows saturation with no apparent sign of inactivation. The amplitude of the steady-state current as a function of voltage shows a maximum near 0 mV, and declines with stronger depolarisation, so that the current-voltage relation shows pronounced inward rectification (Fig. IV.14). Experiments by Shibasaki [1016] demonstrated that the inward rectification of the channel is due to a very rapid inactivation process preceding the activation [971]. Similar results were obtained in expressed *hERG* channels [969], which have been shown to be responsible for the i_{Kr} current.

1.1.3.1.2.2.2 Permeation

Although preferentially permeable to K^+, the K^+ selectivity of i_{Kr} is less pronounced than in i_{K1}. In 150 mM $[K^+]_e$, the single channel conductance is around 10 pS in human ventricular cells [1203] and other cell types. A value of less than 2 pS can be extrapolated for physiological conditions.

1.1.3.1.2.2.3 Modulation and block

While it was originally thought that i_{Kr} is insensitive to β-adrenergic stimulation, more recent experiments provided evidence that stimuli that elevate cAMP exert multiple effects on the channel. cAMP reduces the current in expressed channels by direct binding to the channel and through PKA-mediated phosphorylation [227,228,565]. It was also found that β–adrenergic stimulation can markedly enhance i_{Kr} by reducing the inward rectification of the channel. The effect is not due to PKA-induced phosphorylation of the channel, but to activation of PKC, which results from elevation of cytosolic Ca^{2+} following β-adrenergic stimulation [434].

The channel is selectively blocked by methanesulfonanilide class III antiarrhythmics (such as sotalol, dofetilide and E-4031) and by almokalant. However it is also blocked by a large number of drugs which block other channels or receptors, such as Na^+ channel blockers (quinidine, flecainide disopyramide, amiodarone), antihistamines (terfenadine and cetirizine) and drugs with multiple actions (clofilium, tedisamil) [see 148]. Methanesulfon-anilides block the channel in the activated open state, and trapping occurs upon repolarisation. The relatively slow kinetics of block development and recovery is responsible for the existence of use-dependent block; but because of the very slow recovery, block hardly varies with frequency. Short-term application of amiodarone significantly reduces i_{Kr} [543]; unlike the effect of this drug on i_{Ks} the effect on i_{Kr} is not due to hypothyroidism [106].

Decreasing K^+ leads to a decrease of the i_{Kr} current [972,1318] and enhances the sensitivity of the channel to block by dofetilide or quinidine [1317]. External divalent cations reduce the amplitude of i_{Kr} by blocking the channel [455,456,970,1062]. The current is also reduced by external acidification, which increases the rate of deactivation and causes a shift of the voltage-dependence of activation [1207].

The density of delayed rectifier channels changes during development and maturation [see 1325]. E.g. in mouse foetal cells i_{Kr} dominates i_K; in early neonates i_{Ks} becomes dominant, while in adult mouse neither i_{Kr} nor i_{Ks} is observed [1241].

In a dog with chronic complete atrioventricular block and biventricular hypertrophy i_{Kr} density was smaller in right ventricular myocytes than in control, while no difference was seen in the left ventricle [1224]

1.1.3.1.2.2.4 Structure

The i_{Kr} channel belongs to the *erg* subfamily (erg1) of the eag family of voltage-gated K$^+$ channels. The *hERG* gene [1254], located on chromosome 7q35-36, is responsible for i_{Kr} expression in the human heart [969,1086]. A small protein MiRP1 (MinK-related peptide 1) [2], coded by *KCNE2* on chromosome 21q22.12, coassembles with *hERG* and alters its kinetics and current density [724]. Mutations in the *hERG* gene are at the basis of a form (LQT2) of congenital Long QT syndrome [229], while mutations in MirP1 are responsible for LQT6 [see 177].

1.1.3.1.2.3 The ultrarapid delayed rectifier i_{Kur}

A rapidly activated K$^+$ current, with no or very slow inactivation is present in different heart preparations [see 145,792,796,992], including human atria (Fig. IV.15).

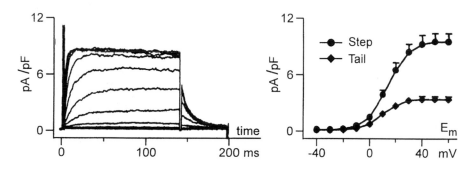

Figure IV.15. i_{Kur} in dog atria. Left panel: time course during depolarising steps. Right panel: amplitude of the current during the step, and amplitude of the tail current upon repolarisation as a function of potential. Modified from [1338].

i_{Kur} is considered an ultrarapid delayed rectifier; however in many publications this current has been described as a non-inactivating component of i_{to}. The kinetics and pharmacological properties vary largely with species and tissue. It appears that various i_{Kur} are due to different molecules, although different subunits may also be involved. In human atria a highly 4AP-sensitive i_{Kur} is present, while no such current can be seen in human ventricle (Fig. IV.16) [648].

The current is rapidly activated (almost instantaneously compared to i_{Kr} and i_{Ks}) and either does not decay or shows very slow inactivation. In human atrium half-maximum activation occurs at about 0 mV. Very slow inactivation occurs with time constants of several seconds. Midpoint inactivation potential is variable and values of -7 to -20 mV were reported in human atrium [338,1017,1250]. Recovery of inactivation is slow, and the current is markedly reduced at elevated stimulation frequencies [31,327,338,1017].

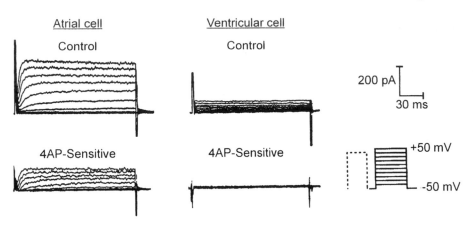

Figure IV.16. A i_{Kur} which is highly sensitive to a 4-aminopyridine (4AP) is present in human atria, but absent in the ventricle. Modified from [648].

Single channel conductance in 5.4 mM $[K^+]_e$ is in the order of $14 - 20$ pS [1336], and is sensitive to $[K^+]_e$. Fully activated current-voltage relations show outward rectification [430,1250].

In human atria the current is blocked by 4-aminopyridine and by quinidine, and is modulated by sympathetic stimulation; while β-adrenergic agonists increase i_{Kur}, α-adrenergic stimulation results in inhibition [646]. The current is downregulated in atrial fibrillation [1186].

> The $K_v1.5$ protein, coded by *KCNA5* on 12p13, is a possible molecular candidate for the i_{Kur} current in the human atrium [325,1059,1186,1250]. The protein is present in the human atrium and ventricle and is highly concentrated in the intercalated discs [723]. $K_v3.1$, $K_v1.2$ and $K_v2.1$ appear to be responsible for i_{Kur} in a number of other preparations; e.g. in dog atria i_{Kur} seems to be due to $K_v3.1$ [1338].

1.1.3.2   The inward rectifier i_{K1}

A strong inwardly rectifying K^+ channel i_{K1} belonging to the IRK group (Fig. IV.8) is present in the heart. The inward-rectifier channels can carry substantial currents at negative membrane potentials, while outward current during depolarisations to potentials more positive than about −40 mV are very small. Its current-voltage relation has a region of negative slope (Fig. IV.17) [see 150]. The inward rectification of the channel enables the channel to keep the cell at a stable negative resting potential without providing excessive repolarising current during the plateau of the action potential, thereby enabling a long plateau. The channel also plays an important role during the final rapid repolarisation of the cardiac action potential [1026] [see 1131]. The density of the i_{K1} is highest in the Purkinje and ventricular system [479], less in atrium [437]; in the SAN the i_{K1} current is absent [495] [but see 1031]. A substantial increase of the current occurs during development from the fetal stage to the neonatal and adult stage [780,1227].

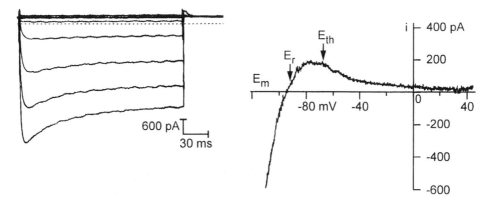

Figure IV.17. Inward-rectifying K^+ current i_{K1}. Left panel: i_{K1} during hyperpolarising and depolarising steps in guinea pig ventricular myocytes. Modified from [1226]. Right panel: current-voltage relation of i_{K1} in ventricular myocyte. Modified from [1340]. E_r = resting potential, E_{th} = action potential threshold.

1.1.3.2.1.1 Kinetics and rectification

The i_{K1} current, the first K^+ current to be characterised in cardiac cells, was considered initially to be a time-independent background current. Later it became clear that i_{K1} showed time-dependent changes, which are generated by a voltage- and time-dependent block-unblock (see Chapter II) by intracellular Mg^{2+} [717,1188] and polyamines, such as putrescine^{2+}, spermidine^{3+} and spermine^{4+} [676].

1.1.3.2.1.2 Permeation

The i_{K1} channel is very selective for K^+ ions [542,850,964]. Reported single channel conductance values in 150 mM K^+-containing solution differ appreciably, ranging from 9 to 45 pS [353,504,542,609,716,725,965,1274].

In guinea pig ventricular myocytes the channel shows a fully open state and three or four lower conductance substates [715,716,725].

1.1.3.2.1.3 Modulation and block

Many different factors are known to affect the activity of inward-rectifier K^+ channels [for review see 950]. The conductance of i_{K1} increases with $[K^+]_e$ [850,965]. i_{K1} is blocked by intracellular but not by extracellular acidification [504] and by Cs^+, and Ba^{2+}.

It is inhibited by quinidine [1015] and a number of antiarrhythmics. Amiodarone significantly reduced i_{K1}. Unlike the effect of this drug on i_{Ks} the effect on i_{K1} is not due to hypothyroidism [106].

Lysophosphatidylcholine [979] and oxidative stress decrease i_{K1} [722,784].

i_{K1} in human ventricular myocytes can be inhibited via β-adrenergic stimulation by a PKA-mediated phosphorylation and the modulation is significantly reduced in ventricular myocytes from the failing heart [598]. The effect of α-adrenergic stimulation appears to be cell type and species-dependent; human atrial i_{K1} can be inhibited by α1-adrenergic stimulation via PKC-dependent pathways [978].

The inward-rectifier K^+ current was significantly reduced in isolated human ventricular [86] and atrial [597] myocytes from patients with heart failure. In different animal models of cardiac hypertrophy increase, decrease or lack of change of i_{K1} has been described.

In rat ventricular myocytes i_{K1} current density largely increases in the late phase of the fetal period, accompanied by a marked hyperpolarisation of the resting potential [774].

1.1.3.2.1.4 Molecular structure

i_{K1} channels from cardiac cells of different species including human have been cloned and expressed [for review see 908]. Kir2.1 (IRK) is the leading candidate for the cardiac i_{K1} protein [1339]. It is encoded by gene *KCNJ2* on 17q23.1-q24.2. It belongs to the class of inward-rectifying K^+ channels (IRK) which also contains the G protein coupled inward rectifiers (GIRK) such as $i_{K.ATP}$ and $i_{K.ACh}$. The IRK class of channel are tetramers of subunits consisting of only two transmembrane segments with a pore loop sequence in between. A dramatic increase in expression of Kir2.2 rather than expression of Kir2.1 mRNA causes the hyperpolarisation in the late fetal period of rat heart [774].

1.1.3.3   Ligand-activated K^+ channels
1.1.3.3.1   ACh-sensitive K^+ channel $i_{K.ACh}$

Slowing of the heart beat can be caused by activation of specific a K^+ channel $i_{K.ACh}$ in the SAN belonging to the group of G protein coupled weakly inward-rectifying K^+ channels (K_G) (Fig. IV.8) [see review 1277]. In mammalian, the current is also expressed in atrial cells, AVN and Purkinje cells, and to a lesser extent in a number but not all mammalian ventricular cells [599]. The channel is present in human atria [436,437] Activation of the channel by ACh results in an weakly inward-rectifying K^+ current (Fig. IV.18). The channel is a major effector of vagal modulation of SAN, AVN and atrial cells. It contributes to the atrial resting potential and affects the duration of the action potential.

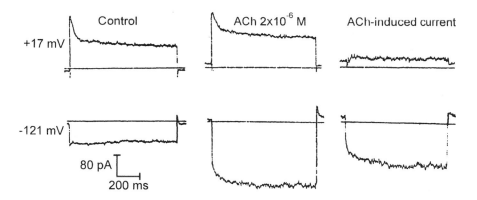

Figure IV.18. ACh-sensitive K^+ current ($i_{K,ACh}$) in human atrial cells. Net ionic current is shown during a depolarising (upper panels) and during a hyperpolarising step (lower panels), in control condition (left) and in the presence of ACh (middle). The right panels show the ACh-sensitive current measured as the difference of the current in presence and absence of ACh. Modified from [436].

1.1.3.3.1.1 Activation

Activation of $i_{K,ACh}$ normally occurs upon binding of ACh to the M2 muscarinic receptor. The receptor is coupled to the K^+ channel via G_i, a guanine nucleotide binding protein (G protein), characteristically inhibited by pertussis toxin. The presence of an agonist however is not absolutely necessary, and background openings of the channel have been observed in different situations. Open probability in human atria is very variable, from 0.03 to 0.3 in the presence of 10^{-5} M ACh [437].

Channel activity evoked by application of agonists shows fade (desensitisation): the current through the channel decreases in the continued presence of the agonist. Upon washout of the agonist the response to a second exposure remains temporarily depressed. Desensitisation occurs in up to three phases: a rapid phase (up to 30 s) is due to the channel or G protein level; in a slower phase (up to a few minutes) the receptor is phosphorylated by a receptor kinase; a third phase of fade occurs when cells have been exposed to the agonist for many hours and appears to be due to internalisation.

1.1.3.3.1.2 Permeation and rectification

The channel is very selective for K^+ ions. The conductance is highly sensitive to extracellular K^+ concentration. In symmetric conditions (150 mM $[K^+]$) the single channel conductance is 40-44 pS. At the whole cell level the current is characterised by inward rectification, but inward rectification is weaker than for i_{K1}. The current activates on hyperpolarisation and deactivates incompletely on depolarisation [810].

Similar to the i_{K1} current, rectification is explained by block of the open channel by intracellular Mg^{2+} and polyamines.

1.1.3.3.1.3 Modulation and block

G protein mediated activation of $i_{K.ACh}$ can occur by a number of agonists acting on several receptors: adenosine (P1-receptors), external ATP (P2Y-receptors) [for review see 1195], somatostatin, calcitonin gene regulated protein, endothelin. Channel activity can also be modulated by PKA, PIP2, and by arachidonic acid [see 674].

Like i_{K1}, the $i_{K.ACh}$ current can be blocked by Cs^+ or Ba^{2+}. However tetraethylammonium potentiates the activity of muscarinic potassium channels in guinea pig atrial myocytes [1233].

1.1.3.3.1.4 Molecular structure

$i_{K.ACh}$ is composed of two inward-rectifier K^+ channel subunits Kir 3.1 (GIRK1) coded by *KCNJ3* gene on chromosome 2q24.1, and Kir 3.4 (GIRK4) coded by *KCNJ5* gene on chromosome 11q24 [162,602,604].

Activation of the channel is due to binding of the βγ-subunits of G_i to the C-terminal of the channel. A defective β3-subunit (C825T polymorfism) was found to increase $i_{K.ACh}$ and to reduce the response to carbachol, suggesting that it results in constitutive activity of $i_{K.ACh}$ [267]. βγ-subunits activate GIRK channels by stabilising interactions between PIP2 and the K^+ channel [476]}..

1.1.3.3.2   ATP-inhibited K^+ channel $i_{K.ATP}$

The $i_{K.ATP}$ channel was first described in heart cells [805]. It belongs to the inward-rectifying K^+ channel family (Fig. IV.8). It is present in many other cell types [see 502,1000], e.g. in pancreatic β cells, where it plays an essential role in insulin secretion. An ATP-sensitive channel exists also in inner mitochondrial membranes; it has different ATP sensitivity and pharmacological properties. In heart the plasmalemmal K_{ATP} channel is expressed in ventricular, atrial as well as nodal cells from different species, including the human heart [42]. The channel appears to exert a protective role during an ischaemic insult: by shortening of the action potential, generation of inexcitability and shifting the membrane potential closer to the equilibrium potential for K^+ ions, excessive loss of K^+ is avoided. Activation of the mitochondrial channel also seems responsible for preconditioning or protection against a second insult.

1.1.3.3.2.1 Kinetics and regulation

In inside-out patches a K^+ channel with a high conductance is activated when the cytoplasmic [ATP] is decreased below a critical concentration (Fig. IV.19). ATP normally decreases the open probability. The K_d is around 0.1 mM [799,805]. However K_d values measured for individual channels may differ by as much as 3 orders of magnitude and range from 9 to 580 µM [335]. Hill coefficients vary between 1.0 and 5.0.

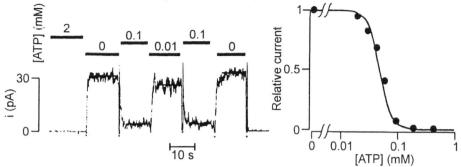

Figure IV.19. $i_{K,ATP}$ at different intracellular ATP concentrations, and dose response curve of $i_{K,ATP}$ in rat ventricular myocytes. Modified from [626].

Since the K_d value is much lower than the normal [ATP] of 5 mM or more, the question arises how the channel can cause important electrophysiological effects, as have been described to occur during ischaemia or hypoxia. Three considerations should be made:

1. The subsarcolemmal [ATP] is much lower than the bulk value when the Na^+/K^+ ATPase [888,1162] or adenylyl cyclase [473,982] are activated, or when anaerobic glycolysis is blocked [1266].

2. The sensitivity to block by ATP is strongly dependent on many different cellular parameters (see section 1.1.3.3.2.3), and the K_d values determined may not reflect the values in pathophysiological conditions.

3. The maximal current that can be obtained is very large, due to a high single channel conductance and high channel density. Therefore activation of a very small fraction of the channels will have marked effects on the action potential configuration.

1.1.3.3.2.2 Permeation

The ATP-dependent channel shows a high conductance of 80 pS in symmetrical $[K^+]$ conditions [539,805]. It is very selective for K^+. At physiological $[K^+]_e$ the conductance is about 25 pS [334]. While in the presence of high $[K^+]_e$ the channel shows inward rectification, at normal physiological $[K^+]_e$ however, the current shows no rectification or even outward rectification up to 0 mV [798,1091]. Outward rectification is also characteristic for the current generated during metabolic inhibition [499], hypoxia [74] and in the presence of potassium channel openers.

1.1.3.3.2.3 Modulation and block

The sensitivity to block by ATP is strongly dependent on many different cellular parameters [for references see 145], such as long chain fatty acids

(LCAC) and their acyl-CoA esters [666], intracellular pH [63], lactate, MgADP, PIP2 [819], which all increase open probability of the channel at a given $[ATP]_i$. Activation is also facilitated by PKC–dependent phosphorylation and via G proteins coupled to P2 or M2-receptors [912].

K^+ channels openers, such as cromakalim, pinacidil and nicorandil, activate the K_{ATP} channel in the heart [see 352], while diazoxide activates pancreatic K_{ATP} channels, but has little effect on native cardiac plasmalemmal K_{ATP} channels, except when ADP concentration is raised [245]. Opening of the K_{ATP} channel may result in cardioprotective as well as proarrhythmic effects [see 1281]. Sulfonylurea drugs such as tolbutamide, glibenclamide and HMR 1883 are inhibitors of K_{ATP} channels [see 376].

1.1.3.3.2.4 Molecular structure

The cardiac K_{ATP} channel is of heteromultimeric nature [491,1000], composed of a protein (Kir6.2) from the "inward-rectifying" Kir family, and a sulfonylurea-receptor (SUR2A), which belongs to the group of ATP binding cassette proteins [8]. The channel forming protein Kir6.2 is encoded by gene *KCNJ11* on 11p15.1 [491], while the SUR2 gene is found on chromosome 12p12.1 [181]. ATP inhibits the channel by binding to the Kir6.2 subunit [389]. The SUR subunits are characterised by multiple membrane spanning domains and two nucleotide binding folds (NBD). They act as receptors for sulfonylurea drugs and potassium channel openers.

1.1.3.3.3 Na$^+$-activated K$^+$ channel

The Na$^+$-activated K$^+$ channel belongs to the ligand-activated channels and is activated by intracellular Na$^+$. The $i_{K.Na}$ channel is highly selective for K^+ ions, and it shows a very high conductance with values up to 200 pS [541,685,967,1252]. The channel is selectively activated by $[Na^+]_i$; however the sensitivity to $[Na^+]_i$ is variable: while it was reported that very high concentrations of $[Na^+]_i$, are required (K_d 66 mM) [541,928], inhibition of the Na$^+$/K$^+$ ATPase for a few min already revealed the Na$^+$-activated K$^+$ current in guinea pig ventricular myocytes [621].

1.1.3.3.4 K$^+$ channel activated by fatty acids and amphiphiles

Arachidonic acid (AA), unsaturated fatty acids and phospholipids activate K$^+$ selective channels in rat atrial and ventricular cells [571,572]. Activation occurs upon addition of fatty acids (FA) to either side of the membrane but is more efficient if applied from the cytosolic side. Available evidence suggests that unsaturated fatty acids with two double bonds are required for efficient activation. Arachidonic acid activates the channel directly and not via one of its metabolites. Once activated by FAs, activity can be increased by low pH and pressure [569]. A channel with slightly different rectification characteristics is activated by phospholipids [1230].

The channel is rather selective for K^+ ions. The channel activated by AA shows outward rectification; the channel activated by phospholipids has a linear current-voltage relation [571,1230]. The single channel conductance is 94 pS in 140 mM K^+ symmetrical conditions. As possible molecular substrate a 2-P (two-pore) forming K^+ channel has been proposed [336,573].

1.1.3.4   Background K^+ channels

A family of two-pore domain K^+ channels, or 2P/4TM, belonging to the *KCNK* gene family, has been described [for review see 380,845], and several subfamilies such as TASK, TREK, TWIK and TALK have been identified.

TREK-1-like currents, which are activated by extracellular ATP, have been found in rat ventricular myocytes [10]. TASK-1 channels encoded by *KCNK3* are expressed in murine [574,677] and human heart [293]. In mouse they are expressed throughout the heart, but expression is more prominent in the ventricles [677]. TASK-1 channels act as background channels. They are open pore rectifiers with linear current-voltage relation in symmetrical K^+ conditions, but outward rectifying at physiological K^+ concentrations. The channels are blocked by external pH [677], and are opened by halothane. The channel influences the amplitude and duration of the plateau of the action potential.

1.1.4   Cl⁻ channels

Cl⁻ channels belong to a large family [for review see 355,426,453,478,526,1068] Several members of the anion channel family have been cloned and expressed, such as the cystic fibrosis transmembrane regulator or CFTR channel, responsible for the PKA-stimulated channel, and the large ClC family [see 1229], several members of which have been shown to be expressed in mammalian heart.

Table IV.2. Properties of functionally identified sarcolemmal Cl⁻ channels in cardiac cells [for review see 478].

Current	Activation	γ (pS)	I-V ([Cl⁻]$_e$ > [Cl⁻]$_i$	I-V ([Cl⁻]$_e$ = [Cl⁻]$_i$	Gene
$i_{Cl.PKA}$	PKA	7–13	Outward rectification	Linear	CFTR
$i_{Cl.Ca}$	Ca^{2+}_i	2	Outward rectification	Linear	CLCA1?
$i_{Cl.vol}$	Cell swelling Basally active	30-60	Outward rectification	Outward rectification	ClC-3?
$i_{Cl.ir}$	Cell swelling Basally active	3-7	Inward rectification	Inward rectification	CLC-2?

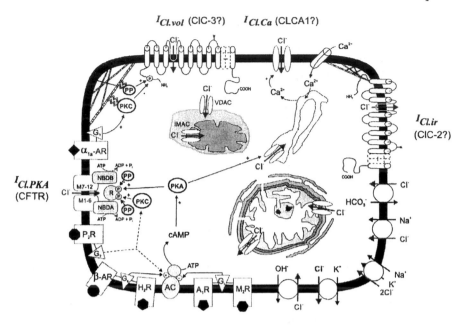

Figure IV.20. Cardiac anion transport pathways. Modified from [478].

Initially six types of sarcolemmal Cl⁻ currents were functionally identified in cardiac cells. However more recent evidence indicates that some of these currents may be mediated by the same channel. Functional and molecular studies indicate that four different types of Cl⁻ channels are present in cardiac cells [for review see 426,478,1068]: (1) a channel activated by PKA-dependent phosphorylation (2) a $[Ca^{2+}]_i$-activated channel, (3) an outwardly rectifying channel activated by cell swelling $i_{Cl.vol}$ and (4) an inwardly rectifying channel activated by cell swelling $i_{Cl.ir}$. Most Cl⁻ channels (except the PKA-induced Cl⁻ channel and $i_{Cl.ir}$), can be blocked by disulphonic stilbene compounds (DIDS and SITS).

Since the E_{Cl} is positive to the resting potential activation of Cl⁻ current causes depolarisation of the resting potential but accelerates repolarisation early during the action potential [282]. The physiological role of Cl⁻ currents however cannot strictly be delineated: the expression and density of the currents depends on cell type and species, and their expression in different human cardiac cells is far from clear. Furthermore conditions to activate some of the currents may only be present in pathophysiological situations. In addition to Cl⁻ channels, a large number of Cl⁻ transporting proteins are present in the plasma membrane. Furthermore several Cl⁻ channel and transporters have been described in membranes of intracellular compartments (e.g. IMAC, VDAC in mitochondria) (Fig. IV.20).

1.1.4.1 PKA-dependent Cl⁻ current

The PKA-activated Cl⁻ channel [for review 355,356,478] has been described in cardiac cells from different species, but is typically more present in the ventricle than in the atrium. However electrophysiological evidence for functional expression in human heart is weak.

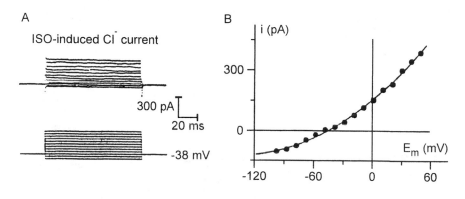

Figure IV.21. PKA-activated Cl⁻ current in guinea pig ventricular myocytes. A: Cl⁻ current induced by application of isoproterenol at different membrane potentials. B: Current-voltage relation of PKA-activated Cl⁻ current shows outward rectification in physiological condition with $Cl_e > Cl_i$. Modified from [425].

The PKA-dependent channel is activated following activation of β-receptors (Fig. IV.21) [355] or histamine H2-receptors [425,485]. These receptors are positively coupled to adenylate cyclase and PKA. Negative coupling occurs via M2 [1133], and angiotensin-II (Ang II) AT1 receptors [817] and endothelin-A (ETA) receptors. PKA-dependent phosphorylation results in activation of the channels [301] and modulation of their kinetics [486] (see Fig. V.23).

In guinea pig ventricular myocytes, acute activation of endogenous PKC alone did not activate PKA-dependent Cl⁻ channels, but potentiated PKA-dependent responses [736]. AT1 receptors [817] ETA receptors are coupled to PLC, activating PKC (see Fig. V.23).

The single channel conductance of the PKA-activated Cl⁻ channel is between 7 and 14 pS [777]. The current-voltage relation is linear in symmetric Cl⁻ concentrations, but the current shows outward rectification when $Cl_e > Cl_i$. It has been suggested that the channel acts as a permeation pathway for ATP and could be responsible for the release of ATP during ischaemia, but this point is still controversial.

The PKA-dependent Cl⁻ channel corresponds to the CFTR (cystic fibrosis transmembrane conductance regulator), the gene of which has been cloned by Riordan et al. [919]. It belongs to the family of ATP binding cassette (ABC) transporters. The CFTR protein is a monomer, consisting of two homologous membrane domains each consisting of 6 transmembrane segments, and two cytoplasmic nucleotide binding domains (NBD) and one cytoplasmic regulatory domain. The biochemical pathway for activation involves phosphorylation of the regulatory domain of the CFTR protein. The gating is coupled to ATP hydrolysis at the nucleotide binding domain (for reviews see [355] and Physiological Reviews 1999 vol 79, which was fully devoted to the CFTR channel).

While molecular evidence strongly indicate that CFTR is expressed in human atrial and ventricular cells, the role of PKA-activated Cl⁻ currents is still unclear, and electro-physiological evidence for functional expression of CFTR in human heart is weak [1068].

1.1.4.2   Volume-activated Cl⁻ current

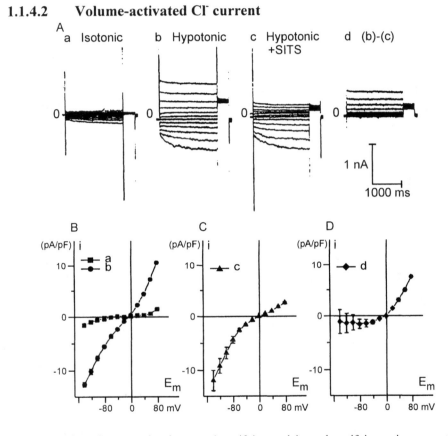

Figure IV.22. Volume-regulated outward-rectifying and inward-rectifying anion current in guinea pig ventricular myocytes can be separated by application of SITS, which blocks outward-rectifying channels, while the inward rectifiers are largely insensitive to SITS. Upper panels show the currents in isotonic condition (a), and in hypotonic condition in the presence (c) or absence (b) of SITS, and the SITS-sensitive current in hypotonic condition (d). Lower panels show the corresponding current-voltage relations. Modified from [284].

Volume-activated Cl⁻ channels were found in nearly every cardiac cell type examined. They are present in human atrial cells and possibly also in human ventricle. These channels can be activated by cell swelling or membrane stretch, and some of the channels are active in basal conditions. Outward- as well as inward-rectifying anion channels have been identified in the heart (Fig. IV.22) [113] [for references see 478].

1.1.4.2.1   Outward-rectifying volume-sensitive Cl⁻ current

Evidence for volume-activated currents in cardiac cells was first obtained in canine atria and ventricles [1067,1155]. Activation occurs by exposure of cells to hypotonic solutions, and can be experimentally evoked by procedures causing membrane deformation. Under isotonic conditions the channel is active in a small percentage of cells [for review see 478,618]. The primary physiological role of the channel appears to be cell volume homeostasis. Cell swelling-induced depolarisation and shortening of the cardiac action potential could be attributed to the outward-rectifying volume-activated Cl⁻ channel [1189,1190].

This volume-activated channel is outwardly rectifying, with a conductance of about 30 pS at the reversal potential and 50-60 pS at positive potentials. Taurine and inositol efflux that occurs upon cell swelling probably passes via this pathway [508]. cAMP causes inhibition of the channel [773]. The channel can be blocked by stilbene derivatives such as SITS.

Expression from ClC-3, which was cloned from guinea pig ventricle, provided evidence that the outward-rectifying volume-sensitive Cl⁻ current in the heart is carried by ClC-3, while dialysis of guinea pig cardiac myocytes with anti-ClC-3 antibodies abolishes native volume-sensitive Cl⁻ currents [113,283,285,773]. However the view that ClC-3 is a swelling-activated channel was questioned by other authors and it was reported that expression of ClC-3 is essentially absent from heart [1271].

1.1.4.2.2   Inward-rectifying Cl⁻ current $i_{Cl,ir}$

An inwardly rectifying anion channel has been identified in mouse and guinea pig atrial and ventricular myocytes. In isotonic conditions it is activated by hyperpolarisation at potentials negative to −40 mV. Cell swelling by exposure of the cells to hypotonic solutions increases the amplitude of the current [284]. The role of the channel remains unclear. It could play a role in the regulation of resting membrane potentials, but may become important in some pathological conditions, like ischaemia. Its biophysical and pharmacological properties show a number of similarities with ClC-2 [1140].

1.1.4.3   Ca²⁺ᵢ-activated Cl⁻ current

A transient Ca^{2+}_i-dependent outward current, $i_{Cl,Ca}$ often called i_{to2}, carried by Cl⁻ ions has been demonstrated in atrial and ventricular myocytes and Purkinje cells [944,1211] [for references see also 426,478,1068]. Its presence in human heart is still uncertain: while a Ca^{2+}-activated transient outward current has been reported in human atria [313], Li et al. [645] were unable to confirm its presence.

The channel is impermeable to large organic anions [560]. The current-voltage relation has been described as outward-rectifying [1363] or linear in symmetric conditions [1046]. In canine ventricular cells [199] the channel has a small single channel conductance of 1.5-2 pS and it shows long openings.

During the cardiac action potential this Cl^- current is activated by Ca^{2+} ions released from the SR, subsequent to entry of Ca^{2+} via L-type Ca^{2+} channel. The apparent K_d for intracellular Ca^{2+} is rather high 150 μM; however, the $[Ca^{2+}]$ seen by the channel can be very different from the bulk concentration. The finding that the Cl^- current decays much faster than the Ca^{2+} transient [1046,1153] is likely to be due to the high K_d value which causes the channel to be open only during the short time during which the local subsarcolemmal Ca^{2+} concentration reaches very high levels. It contributes to the notch of the ventricular action potential and thereby affects the plateau of the action potential and may serve as a negative feedback mechanism to limit Ca^{2+} entry. The channel can also be active at negative potentials, contributing to the transient inward current that causes delayed afterdepolarisations   (DAD)   in   conditions   of Ca^{2+} overload [417,1048,1211,1362], and may thus play a role in the genesis of arrhythmias.

While Ca^{2+}-activated Cl^- currents, belonging to the CLCA family, are ubiquitous across different tissues, molecular identification of the cardiac channels has not yet been made.

1.1.5   Pacemaker current i_f

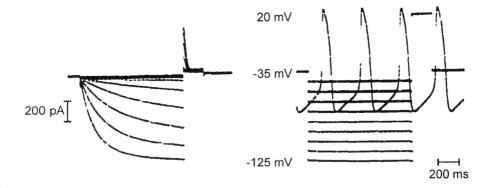

Figure IV.23. i_f current in rabbit SAN (left) during different hyperpolarising voltage steps (right) in the range of SAN diastolic and more negative potentials. Modified from [243].

The normal heartbeat is initiated by pacemaking of the SAN, resulting from a diastolic depolarisation. Many currents contribute to pacemaking [806]. One of the important currents is i_f (funny current), which is the equivalent to i_h, the hyperpolarisation-activated current found in neurons [for review see 254,259,558]. The channel is activated by hyperpolarisation during the final repolarisation phase of the action potential and generates an inward current (Fig. IV.23). The i_f current has been described primarily in SAN, AVN, and Purkinje cells [255]. It is also present in atrial [297,883,1145] and ventricular myocardium [157,1329], although in the adult it does not appear to play a role in these cells in physiological conditions.

1.1.5.1   Activation

Upon hyperpolarisation of the SAN membrane from -40 mV to more negative levels an inward current (i_f) is activated that slowly increases to a steady level [see 806] (Fig. IV.23). The current is rapidly deactivated upon return to depolarised levels. In SAN cells the steady-state activation curve extends from about -45 mV down to -100 mV. Reported half-maximum values show large variability. In Purkinje cells activation of i_f occurs at more negative potentials than in the SAN [132,1328]. In normal adult ventricular cells the activation range of i_f is more negative than the resting potential, so that it plays no role in normal electrical activity in these cells.

Time course of activation is of the order of seconds at depolarised levels but becomes shorter with hyperpolarisation. The kinetics of the channel can not be described by Hodgkin-Huxley kinetics, and allosteric opening and closing transitions and modulation by cAMP have been proposed [17].

1.1.5.2   Permeation

The fully activated current-voltage relation is linear and reverses at -10 to -20 mV. The channel is a non-selective cation channel, which passes K^+ and Na^+ ions [252,454]. In the range of diastolic potential the current is inward and mainly carried by Na^+ ions. The amplitude of the fully activated current is enhanced by increasing $[K^+]_e$ [252,343,708]. The current is inhibited in a voltage-dependent way by millimolar concentrations of external Cs^+ ions, which is used as a tool to study the properties of this channel [252,343,454,496]. At the single channel level small currents have been recorded revealing a conductance of only 1 pS [253].

1.1.5.3   Modulation

β-adrenergic stimulation shifts the steady-state activation of the pacemaker current towards less negative potentials (Fig. IV.24) via direct binding of cAMP to the channel [4,258,261]. This results in increased inward current at a given level of negative membrane potential. In the presence of β-adrenergic stimulation, ACh and adenosine cause a shift of the activation curves towards more negative values by inhibiting adenylate cyclase activity [5,262,1343]. External K^+ was found to increase the Na^+ conductance of the channel in rabbit SAN [343].

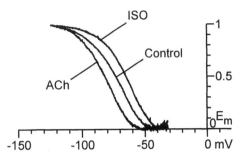

Figure IV.24. Effect of isoproterenol and acetylcholine on the pacemaker current in rabbit SAN. Modified from [6].

The i_f channel in Purkinje cells as well as in SAN is blocked by UL-FS related bradycardic agents in a potential and use-dependent way. Block requires open channels but hyperpolarisation disfavours block [374,1030].

i_f is under strong developmental control. Channel density and voltage-dependence changes during development from newborn to the adult stage [6,319,921,1015]. In rabbit SAN the current density decreases with age corresponding with a decrease in rate of spontaneous beating [6,56]. In newborn rat ventricle the activation threshold is around −70 mV [161,921], while in adult ventricle it is close to −90 mV [1328], so that the activation range is more negative than the normal resting potential (Fig. IV.25). Sympathetic innervation during development induces a negative shift of activation of i_f in rat ventricle via a combined action at α1B-adrenergic and NPY Y2 receptors [896].

In adult ventricular cells the current may become important in pathological conditions as a consequence of the shift in the activation curve, secondary to catecholamine secretion or to dedifferentiation [319]. When shifted to more positive potentials i_f could play a role in ischaemia-induced ventricular arrhythmias [921,1328]. In spontaneous hypertensive rats and failing human heart a large i_f activating at physiological potentials is observed [157,159,160].

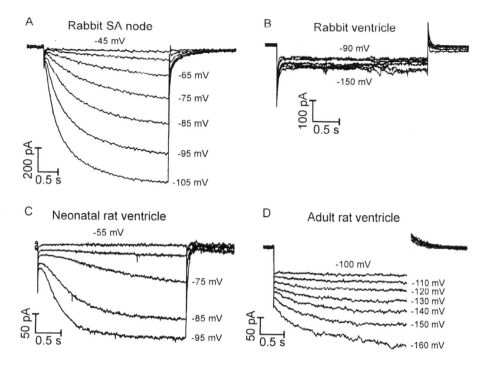

Figure IV.25. The i_f current is present in SAN. It is also present in the neonatal ventricle. In adult rat ventricular cells its activation curve is shifted towards very negative potentials out of the normal physiological voltage range. The current is absent in adult rabbit ventricle. Modified from [1015].

1.1.5.4 Structure

Recently channels responsible for i_f have been cloned and expressed [366,501,682,683,761,975,999] [for review see 92,558,681].

The i_f channels are related to the superfamily of cyclic nucleotide-gated (CNG) channels (such as the photoreceptors and olfactory receptors), and to the superfamily of voltage-gated K^+ channels. The channels are activated by hyperpolarisation. According to the current channel nomenclature, i_f channels are named hyperpolarisation-activated cyclic nucleotide-gated channels (HCN). Four different *HCN* genes have been identified. The cytoplasmic C terminus contains a cyclic nucleotide binding domain (CNBD) and regulates voltage-and cAMP-dependent gating [1216,1228]. Like the K_v family, the HCN channel protein has six transmembrane segments; it contains a typical S4 domain, and the pore region is thought to be located between transmembrane domains 5 and 6. The channel subunits are thought to form tetramers. Coexpression of different subunits [171] or tandem heteromultimers [1167] can result in the formation of functional channels. MiRP1, which was found to be expressed at significant levels in rabbit SAN, could act as a β–subunit for HCN channels (in addition to regulating i_{Kr}): MiRP1 enhances expression of HCN1 and HCN2 current and protein, and accelerates the activation of expressed HCN channels [1332]. The *hHCN2* gene maps to chromosome 19p13.3 [1173] and *hHCN4* to 15q24-q25.

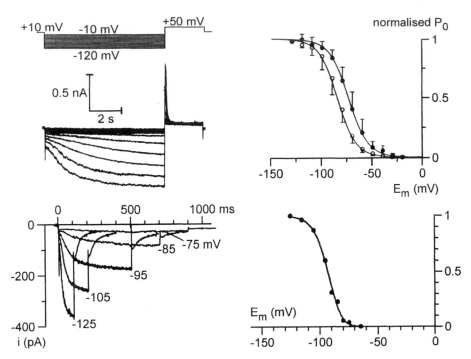

Figure IV.26. Expressed current from human HCN channels. Upper panels: Time course of expressed hHCN4 channels (left panel) and steady-state activation curve in the absence (open symbols) and in the presence of cAMP (filled symbols). Modified from [999]. Lower panels: currents during different hyperpolarising steps (left), and steady-state activation curve (right) of expressed hHCN2 channels. Modified from [761].

Expression of the different isoforms (HCN1, HCN2, HCN4) varies with species and cell type and all three are present in the heart, but the identity of the human cardiac i_f channels is still uncertain. Sinus node and Purkinje fibres contain mainly HCN4 and HCN1 [1015]. The HCN2 and HCN4 channels are prominently expressed in human ventricle and atrium [683], and expression of these channels (Fig. IV.26) resulted in hyperpolarisation-activated cation currents that are sensitive to cAMP, but have slow kinetics. *HCN1* has faster kinetics, but is insensitive to cAMP. In the rabbit and murine SAN, the dominant HCN transcript is HCN4 [501,753,1015], whereas HCN2 is the dominant isoform in rabbit ventricle. HCN2 and HCN4 are expressed in neonatal or adult rat and mouse ventricle, and the relative contribution of HCN4 markedly declines during development, paralleling the negative shift of the activation curve [1015,1320], but voltage-dependence of HCN2 also changes with stage of development [895].

1.1.6   Non-selective cation channels

In heart a number of non-selective cation channels (NSC) are activated by stimuli that also activate Cl$^-$ currents, such as a rise in $[Ca^{2+}]_i$, [204,302,446], an increase in extracellular [ATP] [350] or stretch [570,1346,1350] [see 592]. Others are activated by oxygen radicals

[506,722,1008,1134] or by amphiphiles [131,689]. Finally a NSC current has been described with no known activation mechanism and which can be regarded as a background current [226,409,581,1208,1248]. All these channels differ in permeability and block characteristics.

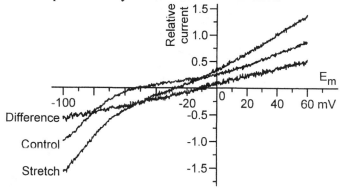

Figure IV.27. Current-voltage relation of the stretch-activated non-selective cation current in rat atrial myocytes. Modified from [1350].

Most of these NSC currents seem only to be activated in pathological conditions (increase in $[Ca^{2+}]_i$, $[ATP]_e$, stretch, radicals, amphiphiles). Since these currents carry inward current at negative membrane potentials (Fig. IV.27), they cause the resting potential to be more positive than E_K and thus favour K^+ loss through K^+ channels, of which the conductance is increased in ischaemic conditions. In situations of Ca^{2+} overload of the cells, the Ca^{2+}-activated NSC can give rise to a transient inward current and delayed afterdepolarisations and arrhythmias (Fig. IV.28) (see Chapter VIII). Stretch- or swelling-activated NSC currents potentially play a role in generating Ca^{2+} overload and triggering ANF secretion.

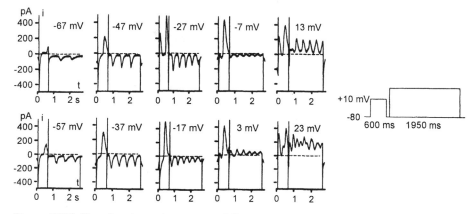

Figure IV.28. Transient inward current at different potentials after a depolarising step to −10 mV in rabbit ventricular myocytes shows a reversal potential near 0 mV (right panel). Voltage protocol (left). Modified from [1299].

Channels responsible for the cardiac NSC have not yet been identified. TRPC3, TRPC6 and TRPC7, are non-selective cation channels expressed in the heart. They belong to the transient receptor potential (TRP) family of channels, which are channels that are activated or modulated by phosphatidylinositol signal transduction pathways, and bring Ca^{2+} in the cell at hyperpolarised membrane potentials. The channels could be candidates for NSC channels described in the literature [see 184].

1.2   Pumps and exchangers

1.2.1 Na^+/Ca^{2+} exchanger

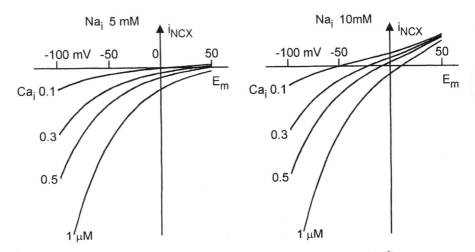

Figure IV.29. Computer simulation of current-voltage relation of the Na^+/Ca^{2+} exchange current at different $[Ca^{2+}]_i$ in 5 and 10 mM $[Na^+]_i$. Modified from [575].

The Na^+/Ca^{2+} exchanger [for review see 98,300,575,862,1019] is present in all cardiac plasma membranes. It plays an important role in the regulation of $[Ca^{2+}]_i$, in the excitation-contraction coupling process (increase of tension as well as relaxation), in determining the time course of the action potential and of the electrical restitution following a stimulus. The primary role of the Na^+/Ca^{2+} exchanger in cardiac cells is to extrude Ca^{2+} from the cell, and it was demonstrated that the largest part of Ca^{2+} entering the cell is extruded by the Na^+/Ca^{2+} exchanger [179], while a smaller part may be extruded by the plasmalemmal Ca^{2+} ATPase.

Energy for extrusion of Ca^{2+} from the cell against the electrochemical gradient is provided by the Na^+ concentration gradient across the cell membrane. The Ca^{2+} gradient across the cell membrane, which is of the order of 10000, is however much larger than the Na^+ gradient (of the order of 20). Therefore, in order to transport Ca^{2+} against such a large gradient downhill movement of at least 3 Na^+ ions is required for translocation of 1

Ca^{2+} against the electrochemical gradient. A stoichiometry of 3 to 1 has been shown experimentally for the cardiac Na^+/Ca^{2+} exchanger (however a recent report using guinea pig ventricular myocytes questions this stoichiometry, and suggests that the stoichiometry would be 4 Na^+ for 1 Ca^{2+} or variable depending on $[Na^+]_i$ and $[Ca^{2+}]_i$ [351]). Either stoichiometry implies that the exchange mechanism is electrogenic and can be characterised by a reversal potential, which is

$E_{Na,Ca} = (nE_{Na} - 2 E_{Ca}) / (n-2)$,

which in case of 3 to 1 stoichiometry amounts to

$E_{Na,Ca} = 3E_{Na} - 2E_{Ca}$

Under normal resting conditions the reversal potential is between –10 and –50 mV (Fig. IV.29). Negative to this potential the exchanger is moving Na^+ in and Ca^{2+} out of the cell (forward mode) and inward current is generated. Positive to the reversal potential Ca^{2+} is moved into the cell and Na^+ extruded (reverse mode) resulting in outward current (Fig. IV.30).

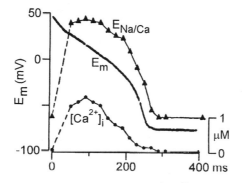

Figure IV.30. Change in reversal potential of the Na^+/Ca^{2+} exchanger during the action potential in guinea pig ventricular cells. Modified from [299].

During the initial part of the action potential the membrane potential exceeds the reversal potential of the exchanger. Therefore the carrier moves Ca^{2+} inwards, contributing to the rise of the intracellular Ca^{2+} concentration and, because of its electrogenicity, it translocates one positive charge out of the cell and thereby favours repolarisation. As Ca^{2+} is released from the SR the reversal potential of the carrier changes, becoming more positive than the plateau potential [see 84], so that the transporter reverses, resulting again in Ca^{2+} extrusion and causing slowing of repolarisation.

By regulating intracellular Ca^{2+}, the Na^+/Ca^{2+} exchanger can modulate many processes:

- Although it was suggested that Na^+/Ca^{2+} exchange might contribute to triggering Ca^{2+} release from the sarcoplasmic reticulum (SR) [625] by Ca^{2+}-induced Ca^{2+} release (CICR), more recent evidence indicates that the efficiency of reverse mode Na^+/Ca^{2+} exchange is very limited in normal conditions [315,1050]. However it may become important when $[Na^+]_i$ is elevated, i_{Ca} is depressed or expression of the Na^+/Ca^{2+} exchanger is enhanced [82].

– The exchanger plays a crucial role in the inotropic effects of cardiac steroids. The inhibition of the Na^+/K^+ pump leads to a slight rise in $[Na^+]_i$. The resulting decrease in Na^+ gradient causes a reduction in the driving force of the Na^+/Ca^{2+} exchanger, resulting in a rise of $[Ca^{2+}]_i$, which causes an increase in Ca^{2+} uptake by the sarcoplasmic reticulum (SR). As a consequence the Ca^{2+} content of the SR is enhanced. This leads to a larger release and enhanced strength of contraction during stimulation.

– The Na^+/Ca^{2+} exchanger is largely responsible for the transient inward current and delayed afterdepolarisations (DAD) which are present in conditions that cause calcium overload of the cells [984]. It can also contribute to early afterdepolarisations (EAD).

– Na^+/Ca^{2+} exchange-mediated Ca^{2+} entry has also been invoked to explain the rise in $[Ca^{2+}]_i$ during reperfusion after a period of hypoxia or ischaemia. However the role of the exchanger is still not clarified.

The modulation of the transporter has not been fully clarified. While the electrochemical gradients of Na^+ and Ca^{2+} across the cell membrane directly influence direction and size of the Na^+/Ca^{2+} exchange, the rate of transport is allosterically regulated by $[Ca^{2+}]_i$ [1262]. Negatively charged phospholipids also stimulate the activity of the transporter. The cardiac muscle Na^+/Ca^{2+} exchanger appears to be modulated by PKC- and PKA- activation dependent pathway.

While no selective inhibitors of the Na^+/Ca^{2+} exchanger are known, KB-R7943, an isothioureamethanesulfonate, inhibits the Na^+/Ca^{2+} exchanger at micromolar concentrations, but it also inhibits a number of other currents [1259,1260]. Many different substances, such as amiloride, several anti-arrhythmics, various local and general anaesthetics and Ca^{2+} entry blockers have an inhibitory effect. The exchanger is also blocked by lanthanides, Ni^{2+} and other divalent cations. A synthetic peptide XIP (exchanger inhibitory peptide) specifically binds to an intracellular loop and inhibits the exchanger.

The expression of the exchanger is enhanced after 24 hrs of α-adrenergic stimulation [909] or after thyroid hormone exposure [464] and in conditions of increased $[Na^+]_i$, e.g. following ouabain. It is also larger in infarcted hearts [661], in acute pressure overloaded hearts [563], in failing hearts [428,429,457,834,881] and in compensated ventricular hypertrophy [1052].

Overexpression of the Na^+/Ca^{2+} exchanger such as is the case in heart failure or hypertrophy can reduce Ca^{2+} transients and contractile function

[882]. However it can also improve contractility by increasing Ca^{2+} release [1052], or by increasing the rate of relaxation via enhanced Ca^{2+} extrusion [1136]. Since the Na^+/Ca^{2+} exchanger in its forward mode competes with the sarcoplasmic reticulum Ca^{2+} pump for removal of Ca^{2+} from the cytoplasm, enhanced expression of the Na^+/Ca^{2+} exchanger could result in improved diastolic function, but also in depletion of the SR resulting in systolic dysfunction. However the Na^+/Ca^{2+} exchanger acting in reverse mode could also contribute to Ca^{2+} loading during the latter part of the action potential in failing hearts [265] [see 82,304,497,579,1045]. The effect of enhanced expression of the exchanger therefore will be affected by many different factors. It depends on the Na^+ and Ca^{2+} concentrations in the cell, which are affected by heart rate and action potential waveform, and by Ca^{2+} entry through Ca^{2+} channels. It also depends on the uptake of Ca^{2+} in the sarcoplasmic reticulum (SR) by the SR Ca^{2+} ATPase, which is known to be impaired in heart failure [32,427,734,767]. Overexpression of the Na^+/Ca^{2+} exchanger by adenoviral gene transfer without change in other Ca^{2+} handling proteins was shown to depress systolic function [983].

The enhanced Na^+/Ca^{2+} exchange activity in failing hearts or in hypertrophy, can also facilitate arrhythmias [882,1052].

The human cardiac Na^+/Ca^{2+} exchanger is coded by gene *NCX1* on chromosome 2p21-p23 [600,1018] [for review see 862]. While originally it was proposed that the exchanger has 11 transmembrane segments, more recently its topology was reinterpreted to have only nine TM segments. A large hydrophilic linker between transmembrane segment 5 and 6 contains the Ca^{2+} regulatory site and the XIP binding site and contains an EF Ca^{2+} binding site and the sites for Na^+ ion binding. A section of this regulatory link acts as an inhibitor.

1.2.2 Na^+/K^+ pump

A Na^+/K^+ ATPase present in the plasma membrane transports Na^+ to the outside and K^+ to the inside of the cell, which is in the direction opposite to the electrochemical gradients of these ions, and acts to maintain these gradients. This process therefore is an active transport requiring energy. Experiments have demonstrated that the active transport of Na^+ and K^+ ions is coupled. For each ATP molecule hydrolysed 3 Na^+ ions and 2 K^+ ions are transported [for review see 30,341,1103]. Therefore, the transport process is electrogenic: the pump generates current and thereby has a direct effect on the membrane potential, while the transport is also sensitive to the existing membrane potential. Activation of the pump hyperpolarises the resting membrane potential or exerts a repolarising effect during the action potential.

The density of the pump sites per μm^2 varies from 1200 in the guinea pig ventricle [781] to 2500 in the rat ventricle [1104]. The density is larger in the ventricle than in the atria [1237] and in the ventricle it is greater in the subepicardial than in subendocardial cells. The turnover rate is about 75-100/s [781,1104]. The K_d value for $[K^+]_e$ is around 1 mM, so that the pump is maximally stimulated at physiological $[K^+]_e$. The K_d for $[Na^+]_i$ is around 10 mM; since $[Na^+]_i$ is normally around this value, the pump is mainly regulated by $[Na^+]_i$. (Fig. IV.31) [93,751,782,1104].

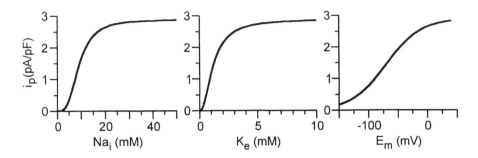

Figure IV.31. $[Na^+]_i$-, $[K^+]_i$- and potential-sensitivity of the Na^+/K^+ pump current. Modified from [1103].

The fact that the activity of the pump depends on $[Na^+]_i$, explains the sensitivity of the pump rate to frequency of stimulation. A marked increase in frequency will cause a rise of $[Na^+]_i$, resulting in enhanced outward pump current, which will cause a hyperpolarisation of the cell. In spontaneously active cells like SAN and Purkinje cells, this hyperpolarising effect counteracts the spontaneous diastolic depolarisation, acting as a negative feedback on the rate of firing, a phenomenon which is known as overdrive suppression [1193] [for references see 1288].

The amount of energy required to move 3 Na^+ ions out and 2 K^+ ions is dependent on the membrane potential and on the Na^+ and K^+ gradients across the membrane, and increases with hyperpolarisation. When the energy required for active Na^+/K^+ transport equals the energy obtained on hydrolysis of ATP, the pump will stop. The free energy of ATP hydrolysis depends on the [ATP], [ADP] and $[P_i]$. During ischaemia these concentrations can change, resulting in a reduction of pump rate.

The pump is blocked by digitalis but sensitivity is species-dependent [94,921]; the rat is very insensitive with a K_d of 2.4 x 10^{-3} M for dihydrouabain (DHO) compared to 1.4 x10^{-5} M in the guinea pig. The sensitivity to digitalis decreases with increase of $[K^+]_e$ and the opposite effect is seen when $[Na^+]_i$ is elevated [1105]. The interaction is however not competitive: DHO and K^+ do not bind at the same site. An increase in $[K^+]_e$ increases the cycling of the enzyme between different states and decreases the time that the external site is available for DHO binding; an increase in $[Na^+]_i$ has the opposite effect [94,1105].

Inhibition of the Na^+ pump (e.g. by digitalis glycoside) will result in a rise of $[Na^+]_i$, which will cause decrease of the activity of the Na^+/Ca^{2+} exchanger, leading to enhanced $[Ca^{2+}]_i$ and contraction. It was recently demonstrated in mouse ventricular myocytes that inhibition of the Na^+ pump can affect the subplasmalemmal Na^+ concentration within the time course of a single beat. As a consequence it enhances the reverse mode activity of the Na^+/Ca^{2+} exchanger and the intracellular Ca^{2+} transient and contraction during the same beat [1110].

The Na^+/K^+ pump is stimulated by β- [359] and α-receptor stimulation [361], via activation of PKA, respectively PKC.

The Na^+/K^+ ATPase protein belongs to P type ATPase superfamily [for review 40,752]. It consists of one α- and one β-subunit and is probably present as a dimer. Both have been cloned. The α-subunit is a large protein spanning the whole cell membrane: it carries the ATP binding site and a phosphorylation site at the intracellular portion, and the digitalis binding site at the extracellular face. Three isoforms exist, of which the α-1 shows low affinity and α-2 and α-3 high affinity for ouabain [1237]. The three-dimensional of the Na^+/K^+ ATPase protein has recently been clarified and shown to bear remarkable resemblance to the structure of the sarcoplasmic reticulum Ca^{2+} ATPase [916].

2. OTHER TRANSPORT MECHANISMS IN CARDIAC CELLS

2.1 Water channels in the plasma membrane

Water channels, also called aquaporins (AQP) have been found in most types of cells including cardiac cells [for review see 104,205,298,500,1182]}. Although they do not directly contribute to ionic currents, water channels play a role in cell volume regulation. By diluting or concentrating ions in the cytoplasm, net water movement may affect ionic gradients, and thereby influence ionic currents.

AQPs have been found in caveolae of atrial and ventricular myocytes [838]. The caveolae transiently function as osmometers, monitoring and reacting to net water flow from or into the subcaveolar cytosol of the myocytes. They may play an important role in situations of metabolic inhibition such as ischaemia, which can result in cell swelling.

APQ belong to the large family (more than 150 members) of MIP (Major Intrinsic Proteins of lens fibre). More than 10 different types have thus far be identified. Some of the aquaporins are selective for water, while others (the aquaglyceroporins are also permeable for glycerol and small non-electrolytes. They consist of 6 transmembrane domains. The loops connecting the second and the third transmembrane domain and between the fifth and the sixth transmembrane domain, fold back into the membrane and are thought to form the pore boundary. AQPs are thought to be formed as tetramers with four pores [173].

2.2 Intercellular channels: gap junctions

Gap junctions are responsible for the syncytial nature of cardiac tissue [for reviews see 247,394,533,957,1089,1090,1273]. They consist of arrays of intercellular channels, connecting adjacent cells. The gap junction channels are formed as multimers of connexins (Cx), which belong to a large family of proteins, at least 13 of which have been found in mammals. Their high conductance and permeability allow for fast conduction of the action potential (electrical coupling) and for an efficient flow from cell to cell of molecules or metabolites with a molecular weight up to 1.2 kD (K^+, Na^+, Ca^{2+}, cAMP, cGMP, IP3) (metabolic coupling). In the canine heart each ventricular cell is connected to about 10 other cells by way of gap junctions. Different values for the conductance between cells have been published going from 250 to 2500 nS per cell. For a normal conduction of the action potential between a pair of cells about 20 connexin channels seem to be sufficient. Since the single channel conductance is of the order of 100 pS (see section 2.2.2) there appears to be large redundancy. This contrasts with the finding that mice heterozygous for Cx43 null mutation show a 45% reduction in conduction velocity of the action potential [401] and with simulations of safety factor. However in the heart many cells contribute to the sink excitatory current.

The distribution of gap junctions in the normal adult heart is non-uniform or anisotropic [see 859]: gap channels are found almost exclusively in the intercalated disks. Large intercalated disks exist at the end of the cells, smaller along the length. A small number is present at the SAN-atrium junction and the Purkinje-muscle junction. These observations explain why conduction in the transverse direction or between the SAN and the atrium or between the Purkinje system and the ventricular muscle can be critically reduced.

Gap junctions are present in all types of cardiac cells, and three connexins, Cx40, Cx43 and Cx45, are expressed in most mammalian cardiac cells (Table IV.3), but the exact isoform of connexin present in the gap junction is dependent on species, cell type and development [for recent reviews see 247,533,1044,1090]. Junctional communication can be mediated by homogeneous or heterogeneous gap junction channels [305], and formation of heterotypic gap junction channels by Cx40 and Cx43 has been described [1175].

Table IV.3. Distribution of connexins in cardiac cells

	Cx43	Cx40	Cx45
SAN	+	++	+
Atrium	++	+++	-
AVN	-/+	++	+
His - Purkinje	+?	+++	+
Ventricle	+++	-/+	-

− Cx43 ($\alpha1$ connexin) is the most widely distributed connexin in the heart. It is the dominant connexin in the atrial and ventricular myocardium.

− Cx40 ($\alpha5$ connexin) is most important in the atria and conduction system; it is expressed in the His bundle Purkinje system, atria and SAN. Cx40 knockout mice have slower conduction in AVN and His bundle, particularly in the right bundle. Heterotypic Cx40-Cx43 channels may be present at the junctions between Purkinje fibres and ventricular muscle.

− Cx45 (human $\alpha7$ connexin) is still controversial. It was found to be present in the AVN, in the His bundle, and in the SAN. Its distribution therefore seems to be limited to nodal tissues and the His bundle [207]. The channel seems to be the first to appear during embryogenesis, but is strongly downregulated during development [13].

− Cx46 is present in rabbit SAN [1210], but does not appear to be present in human.

− Cx37 is expressed in vascular endothelial cells.

Different distribution of connexins have been reported within different regions of the SAN, and differential expression of connexins could create regions within the SAN with different conduction properties, thereby contributing to the non-uniform conduction properties seen in this tissue [612]. It was found that the primary pacemaker region of the guinea pig SAN is virtually Cx43-negative, but that more peripherally strands of Cx43-containing atrial cells invaginate the mass of SAN cells in a mosaic pattern, with only very sparse lateral connections between the two cell types, except near the end of the atrial strands [1135].

A number of authors have published results from connexin knockout studies. Heterozygous Cx43$^{+/-}$ mice revealed no significant changes in conduction velocity, or activation of the ventricular myocardium [530,578,760] [see 673]. Cx40$^{-/-}$ reduced propagation in the right branch of the His bundle without apparent delay in the left bundle branch [1126]. Double heterozygous Cx43$^{+/-}$/Cx40$^{+/-}$ knockout mice showed a small increase in QRS and QT interval [578].

2.2.1   Kinetics

The gap junction channel is gated via two important mechanisms called chemical and voltage gating, and the two processes may be interrelated [122,399].

2.2.1.1   Chemical gating

Protons cause slow and complete closing of the gap junctional channel [see 123], but the pH sensitivity of gap junctions varies with type of connexin, and may depend on the phosphorylation state. Most gap junctions containing Cx45 are closed by acidification to pH 6.7, and the pH-dependence is steep. The pKa for Cx43 appears to be at pH 6.5, while pH sensitivity of Cx40 is less. Coexpressed Cx40 and Cx43 are more susceptible to acidification-induced uncoupling than those cells expressing only one connexin isotype [399].

An increase in $[Ca^{2+}]$ also reduces the total junction conductance. Whether Ca^{2+} or pH are more important in regulating the gap junctional conductance of cardiac cells under physiological conditions is still a matter of controversy. While a rise in $[Ca^{2+}]$ can result in closure of the gap junctions, and contributes healing-over by uncoupling healthy cells from damaged cells, it appears that relatively high $[Ca^{2+}]_i$ is required.

The effects of pH and Ca^{2+} seem however to be synergistic [127,1272], and simultaneous changes in the concentrations of these two ions occur frequently e.g. during ischaemia. A decrease of pH_i to 6.0 combined to an elevation of $[Ca^{2+}]_i$ to 425 nM fully blocks the transjunctional conductance.

2.2.1.2   Voltage gating

While the instantaneous current-voltage relation of fully-open gap junction channels is linear, gap junction channels are sensitive to transjunctional voltage [756,1236]. Application of a transjunctional potential causes fast closing of the channels to a non-zero conductance state. In homotypic channels the current-voltage relation is symmetric and S-shaped, a process which can be compared to inactivation (Fig. IV.32) [1236]. Cx43 gap junction channels possess more than one mechanism of voltage gating: a slow and complete closing and a fast incomplete closing gate [50], and voltage gating may be asymmetric [49]. It was suggested that chemical gating and slow voltage gating share common structural elements [122].

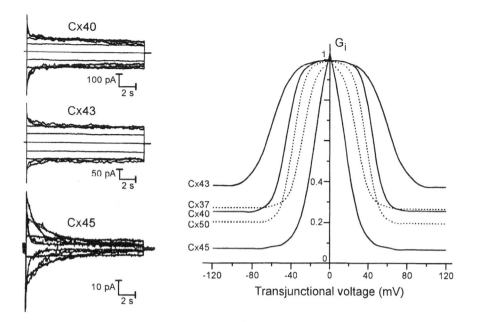

Figure IV.32. Gap junctions. Left panels: Currents at different transjunctional potentials by different connexins. Right panel: Corresponding conductance-voltage relation. Modified from [1090].

Voltage gating accelerates uncoupling during ischaemia. The transjunctional voltage-dependence, together with the effects of Ca^{2+} or pH may explain the sealing phenomenon that occurs when part of the heart tissue is injured, especially since voltage-dependent inactivation is enhanced at low pH$_i$ [399]. During ischaemia this process is useful in isolating ischaemic cells from viable functional cells. However at the same time it may be arrhythmogenic.

2.2.2   Permeation

The gap junction shows a high permeability and passes substances with a molecular weight up to 1.2 kD, including IP3 and cAMP [1201].The limiting pore diameter has been estimated at about 12 Å. Discrimination between anions and cations is limited or absent. Ca^{2+} ions easily permeate, but propagation of spontaneous Ca^{2+} waves, occurring under conditions of Ca^{2+} overload, is rather rare with a probability of 0.15 [617].

Gap junctions channels exhibit several conductance states. Values for the single channel conductance of the main state vary (45 – 100 pS for Cx43; 120 – 160 pS for Cx40; 30 pS for Cx45) and this variability may be related to the relative expression of the three connexins, the state of phosphorylation and the voltage [128,755,1124,1200].

2.2.3 Modulation

The extent of coupling of cardiac cells is determined by many factors and is regulated by diverse processes of synthesis, trafficking and degradation. Connexins have been shown to have a very large turn-over. Cx43 and Cx45 have a half-life of about 2 hrs in cultured neonatal rat heart cells [see 957]. Gap junctional communication is affected by many factors in addition to voltage gating and chemical gating by pH and Ca^{2+} [for review see 247,394,957]. Hypotonic media, phorbol esters, arachidonic acid have all been shown to decrease gap junction conductance. Pulsatile stretch increases expression of Cx43 [1355].

Phosphorylation by PKA, PKC, tyrosine kinase have been reported to affect the permeation properties of connexins as well as the trafficking of connexins between intracellular pools and the plasma membrane. However the effects of protein kinases on cardiac gap junctional intercellular communication (GJIC) depend on type of connexin and cell type [611]. Cx43, which is the main connexin in atrial an ventricular myocardium, is a phosphoprotein, and is targeted by several protein kinases that regulate myocardial cell-cell coupling. While PKC [266], mitogen-activated protein kinase (MAPK), or tyrosine kinase were reported to decrease GJIC, PKA [230] was reported to stimulate Cx43-mediated GJIC. The phosphorylation state may affect the properties of the gap junctions or the trafficking of Cx43 between the plasma membrane and intracellular pools. Uncoupling during ischaemia is associated with dephosphorylation of Cx43 [67]. Macroscopic conductance and permeability of human Cx40 gap junction channels are strongly increased by cAMP [1183].

Pharmacological blockage of gap junctions can be obtained by long chain alcohols such as heptanol or by halothane. Block by halothane is least for Cx40, more for Cx43, and most for heteromeric channels [433].

Changes in gap junction structure [596] and expression of different connexins during development and dedifferentiation have been reported [20]. Changes in gap junctional communication can play an important role in pathological conditions [see 533]. Metabolic inhibition such as occurs in acute hypoxia or ischaemia can cause intra- and extracellular acidification and an important increase in $[Ca^{2+}]_i$. These changes can result in an increase in gap junctional resistance, causing hampered intercellular communication. GJIC can also be altered during remodeling. Decreased Cx43 expression and altered distribution have been described in ischaemic and infarcted myocardium [720,859,955,956]. In healing infarction redistribution of gap junctions is observed, with dispersion of small gap junctions over the whole membrane. In healed regions bordering canine infarction a reduction of number of gap junctions as well as the size was found, with a larger reduction in the number of side-to-side connections. In ventricular hypertrophy Cx43 showed pronounced dispersion over the entire cell surface [1172]. During the progression of cardiac dysfunction in cardiomyopathic hamsters, which mirror many aspects of heart failure, gap junctional communication is reduced via c-Src-mediated tyrosine kinase phosphorylation of Cx43 [235,1152]. Pacing-induced atrial fibrillation gave rise to inhomogeneities in the distribution pattern of Cx40 [1176].

2.2.4   Formation and structure of gap junctions

Channels responsible for the large conductance of the gap junction membrane consist of two hemi-channels or connexons in two apposing cells [see 1323]. Each hemi-channel is composed of six subunits or connexins. Each subunit or connexin consists of 4 transmembrane segments, M1 to M4, two extracellular loops and one intracellular loop. In the formation of gap junctions, hemi-channels act as ligands for each other. Six cysteines in the extracellular loop of the connexin molecule are involved in docking and/or opening of channels. M3 is amphiphatic and probably part of the pore structure. Amino-acids at or near the N terminus and the M1/E1 border form part of a charged complex and may act as a voltage sensor. The C-terminal together with the intracellular loop between M2 and M3 form the so-called proton gate. The mechanism whereby protons close the gap junctions is proposed to be a ball-receptor inactivation process: protons increase the positive charge of the receptor site and allow the negatively charged ball of the C-terminal to bind and to occlude the channel pore. The cytoplasmic loop between M2 and M3 probably acts as the receptor site of the Cx43 gap junction.
Human Cx43 is coded by gene *GJA1* localized on 6q21-6q23.2, Cx40 by *GJA5* on 1q21.1, and Cx45 by *GJA7* on chromosome 17.

2.3   Ion channels in intracellular organelles

Different channels are present in intracellular compartments, and their activity regulates Ca^{2+} signaling and cellular activity. The main Ca^{2+} compartments involved are the sarcoplasmic reticulum (SR) and the mitochondria, but also the nucleus and the Golgi compartment contribute to intracellular Ca^{2+} signaling. Although intracellular channels do not directly contribute to electrical activity of the plasma membrane, they have a number of indirect effects. E.g. the Ca^{2+} released from the SR can affect the activity of plasmalemmal ion channels and transporters. Ca^{2+} release affects the normal electrical activity by causing inactivation of i_{CaL}. The rise in cytoplasmic $[Ca^{2+}]_i$ also modulates the Na^+/Ca^{2+} exchange current during the action potential. In Ca^{2+} overload Ca^{2+} release can also occur during or after the final repolarisation of the action potential. This will cause stimulation of the Na^+/Ca^{2+} exchanger and activation of non-selective cation channels and Ca^{2+}-sensitive Cl^- channels, which may all participate in the genesis of early and delayed afterdepolarisations. In conditions of Ca^{2+} overload the RyR channel thus plays an indirect but important role in generating triggered activity. Ca^{2+} release induced by i_{CaT} can also contribute to automaticity in pacemaker cells by causing local Ca^{2+} release from the SR, resulting in activation of the electrogenic Na^+/Ca^{2+} exchanger [99,484].

2.3.1   Sarcoplasmic reticulum channels

The SR membrane is a leaky membrane with a high conductance for K^+ and Cl^- [for review see 731]. The only important gradient is that of Ca^{2+} ions, while K^+ and Cl^- ions seem to be equally distributed across the membrane. The free Ca^{2+} concentration in the SR has been estimated to be 700 µM. With a cytoplasmic concentration of about 0.1 µM the estimated Ca^{2+} equilibrium potential is thus larger than 200 mV, while the SR potential is estimated to be 0 mV. This implies the existence of a large electrochemical gradient for Ca^{2+} from lumen to cytoplasm, and a low Ca^{2+} permeability of the SR membrane under basal conditions. The Ca^{2+} permeability strongly rises during electrical activity, causing Ca^{2+} to be released from the SR. During this Ca^{2+} release the SR interior becomes negative by at most a few mV, because of passive movement of K^+ and H^+ into the SR and movement of Cl^- in the opposite direction.

Two Ca^{2+} release channels have been described: the ryanodine receptor (RyR) channel and the inositol 1,4,5-trisphosphate receptor (IP3R) channel [for review see 705].

2.3.1.1 Ca^{2+} release channels
2.3.1.1.1   Ryanodine receptor RyR

In mammalian cardiac cells the SR represents the store from which Ca^{2+} is released during the action potential. In this process a Ca^{2+} permeable channel in the SR, which can be specifically blocked by ryanodine and therefore has been called the ryanodine receptor or RyR, plays an important role. The RyRs are clustered in the SR at the narrow (12 nm) dyad or triad junctions between the SR and plasmalemma, or T tubular membrane, or in SR not associated with plasma membrane (corbular SR). They play a crucial role in excitation-contraction coupling in normal and failing hearts [for recent reviews see 82,83,304,706,1278].

2.3.1.1.1.1 Kinetics
The cardiac RyR is a Ca^{2+}-gated channel, and the trigger for activation of the RyR is the rise in $[Ca^{2+}]_i$ consequent to Ca^{2+} influx during the cardiac

action potential [317]. This process is called Ca^{2+}-induced Ca^{2+} release (CICR) (Fig. IV.33). The mechanism in cardiac cells is different from the Ca^{2+} release in skeletal muscle, which is voltage-dependent Ca^{2+} release. A voltage-sensitive Ca^{2+} release mechanism, which was recently proposed also to exist in cardiac muscle [for review see 331], is very controversial [863].

The kinetics of the RyR is very complex, with multiple gating modes (spontaneous activity changes due to transitions between periods of high and low levels of activity and inactive periods), and Ca^{2+}-dependent inactivation at high Ca^{2+} concentrations. The channel was also reported to show adaptation [407]: upon application of a constant step in $[Ca^{2+}]$, activation decreases with time, but the channel is not inactivated, since Ca^{2+} release can occur again upon a second application of Ca^{2+}. However the existence of adaptation is still controversial [616,959,1053]. Several 'modal gating' schemes and other models have been proposed to explain the complex gating behaviour of the RyR [333,959,1102].

2.3.1.1.1.2 Permeation

The RyR behaves as a high conductance but poorly selective cation channel. It is permeable to divalent and monovalent cations. The P_{Ca}/P_K ratio is 6. The conductance is large; it is about 100-150 pS in the presence of 50 mM $[Ca^{2+}]$ at the lumenal side [167,168,1147,1163].

2.3.1.1.1.3 Role in excitation-contraction coupling.

Excitation-contraction coupling in cardiac cells is due to Ca^{2+}-induced Ca^{2+} release. Calcium entering through plasmalemmal Ca^{2+} channels results in a rise in cytosolic Ca^{2+} concentration. Ca^{2+} binding to the RyR causes opening of the RyR Ca^{2+} channels. Due to high Ca^{2+} concentration in the lumen of the SR, Ca^{2+} passively leaks from the SR to the cytoplasm (Fig. IV.33). The stimulus for Ca^{2+} release during a contraction is provided by Ca^{2+} entering the cell via L-type Ca^{2+} channels. Although release can also occur upon Ca^{2+} entry via T-type channels [1049,1352] or via reversed Na^+/Ca^{2+} exchange [1050] or via a TTX blockable Ca^{2+} current (i_{CaTTX}) [7,974], these triggers are less important.

The amount of Ca^{2+} released by the SR is roughly ten times larger than the amount of Ca^{2+} entering through the plasmalemma. The rise in cytoplasmic Ca^{2+} concentration causes contraction by binding to troponine C (TnC) on the myofibrils. Relaxation is caused by a fall in $[Ca^{2+}]_i$; Ca^{2+} is taken up by the Ca^{2+} ATPase in the SR, and also partially extruded through the plasma membrane by the Na^+/Ca^{2+} exchanger and to some extent by the Ca^{2+}ATPase in the plasma membrane. Also the mitochondria can be involved in Ca^{2+} uptake.

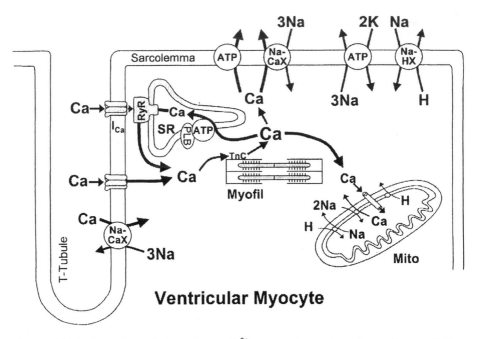

Figure IV.33. Overview of the role of Ca^{2+} transport processes in cardiac excitation-contraction coupling. Modified from [82].

   The Ca^{2+} release by the SR is graded: the rate and amount of calcium released from the SR depends on the Ca^{2+} current flowing through the L-type Ca^{2+} current in the plasma membrane. Such graded control is paradoxical: since the released Ca^{2+} is roughly ten times larger in amount than the trigger, the released Ca^{2+} would be expected to stimulate further CICR, acting as a positive feedback and resulting in a regenerative release. In recent years it has however become clear that the Ca^{2+} concentration regulating the CICR is not the bulk cytoplasmic Ca^{2+} concentration. Rather than global cytosolic $[Ca^{2+}]$, the stimulus evoking Ca^{2+} release from RyRs are local nanodomains of $[Ca^{2+}]$, as was proposed by Stern [1101] in the "local control" hypothesis [see 1102]. According to this hypothesis a variable number of individual functional "release units" can be recruited via a local control mechanism. Such a release unit consists of a single i_{CaL} channel interacting with a limited number of RyR channels through a functionally local subspace. Although Ca^{2+} released in each unit is much larger than the trigger, there is no propagation to other units. The non-regenerative aspect of Ca^{2+} release, and the local activation have been confirmed by analysing the behaviour of "Ca^{2+} sparks".

   Microscopic Ca^{2+} release events called "Ca^{2+} sparks" [174] have been detected using confocal microscopy with Ca^{2+}-sensitive fluorescent dyes [for review see 800,1278]. They consist of small local rises in $[Ca^{2+}]$, which decay within about 100 ms. Such a spark occurs when an SR release unit is activated, resulting in a small Ca^{2+} flux from the lumen of the SR to the cytosol. Sparks can occur spontaneously in quiescent heart cells or can be evoked by limited activation of the plasmalemmal Ca^{2+} current. Individual release sparks result from the independent opening of multiple Ca^{2+} release channels clustered within discrete SR junctional regions [97,188]. Very small events "quarks" with estimated Ca^{2+} release fluxes 20-40 times smaller than those calculated for a typical Ca^{2+} spark were also resolved. These events appear to arise from the opening of a more limited number of RyRs [658]. Recent evidence indicates that unitary Ca^{2+} current through a single RyR under physiological conditions should be about 0.35 - 0.6 pA [733]. Using a combination of patch clamp and confocal Ca^{2+} imaging, it was demonstrated that a "Ca^{2+} sparklet", which is the local Ca^{2+} signal produced by a single opening of a single L-type Ca^{2+} channel, can trigger about $4 - 6$ ryanodine receptors to generate a Ca^{2+} spark [1243]. The experiments indicated that the spark duration is relatively independent of the trigger, and gave evidence for use-dependent inactivation or adaptation.

The Ca^{2+} transient is thought to result from spatial and temporal summation of Ca^{2+} sparks, each triggered locally by the flow of current through a single Ca^{2+} channel. Mobilization of a variable number of Ca^{2+} sparks enables cardiac cells to show graded cellular Ca^{2+} transients [658]. Under normal conditions, Ca^{2+} release is not propagated, but the action potential is responsible for the propagation.

The amount of Ca^{2+} released depends not only on the Ca^{2+} influx through the plasma membrane, but also on the amount of Ca^{2+} present in the SR. The relationship is not linear. Higher lumenal Ca^{2+} concentrations result in a larger fraction of the SR Ca^{2+} being released at a given Ca^{2+} concentration at the cytosolic side of the RyR. Under conditions of high lumenal and low cytosolic $[Ca^{2+}]$, Ca^{2+} may be released spontaneously from the SR and this release may propagate along the cell, causing the occurrence of Ca^{2+} waves. Increasing the Ca^{2+} load enhances the frequency of the spontaneous release events. Spontaneous Ca^{2+} release from the SR in conditions of Ca^{2+} overload are at the basis of transient inward current and DADs [553], mainly by activating Na^+/Ca^{2+} exchange [984].

For the heart to be in a steady-state exactly the same amount of Ca^{2+} that had entered from the outside has to be extruded, while there also has to be an exact balance between the amount of Ca^{2+} released and the amount taken up again by the SR. Several processes act as negative feedbacks, causing autoregulation. E.g. more Ca^{2+} entering the cell, or a higher Ca^{2+} load of the SR, will cause more Ca^{2+} release, resulting in higher cytosolic Ca^{2+} concentration. This will however have many effects: e.g. stronger Ca^{2+}-induced Ca^{2+} inactivation of the L-type Ca^{2+} channel, higher rate of Ca^{2+} extrusion by the Na^+/Ca^{2+} exchanger, and secondarily reduced residual SR Ca^{2+} content. These autoregulatory mechanisms provide a simple way to control the Ca^{2+} content of the SR [see 304].

β-adrenergic stimulation enhances the magnitude of the Ca^{2+} release and increases the contraction and the rate of relaxation by PKA-dependent phosphorylation of target proteins such as DHPR, phospholamban and the RyR. It increases the fidelity of the coupling between DHPR and RyR [1213] and enhances synchronization of SR Ca^{2+} release at the onset of depolarisation [1063]. PKA-dependent hyperphosphorylation of the RYR can however result in heart failure (see next section).

2.3.1.1.1.4 Modulation

Among the substances that increase the open probability of the channel are caffeine and cADP-ribose. Ryanodine at low concentrations increases the open probability by stabilising the channel in a substate; at high concentrations it blocks the channel [941]. Open probability also can be decreased by local anaesthetics such as tetracaine [147, see 731].

Ca^{2+} release is modulated by the presence of nucleotides and by phosphorylation. ATP as well as phosphorylation increase the Ca^{2+}-sensitivity of the RyR [846]; ADP and H^+ result in an opposite shift [1303].

The RyR is associated with the FK506 binding protein (FKBP12.6). Binding of FKBP12.6 stabilises the RyRs [886]. Dissociation of this protein from the RyR results in increased Ca^{2+} sensitivity of the RyR. The binding is decreased by PKA-dependent phosphorylation and immunophilins [711].

In cardiac hypertrophy and failure the coupling may become deficient [382]. The enhanced expression of the Na^+/Ca^{2+} exchanger and the reduction of the SR Ca^{2+} pump is accompanied by a downregulation of RyR levels. Also defective coupling between RyR and L-type Ca^{2+} channel has been reported. In failing human hearts, RyR is PKA-hyperphosphorylated, causing dissociation of FKBP12.6 from the calcium release channel, resulting in increased sensitivity to Ca^{2+}-induced activation [711]. An abnormal Ca^{2+} leak through the RyR [742,826,1319] could cause enhanced diastolic Ca^{2+} release. Enhanced diastolic release of Ca^{2+} from the SR would decrease the SR Ca^{2+} load, resulting in a decreased Ca^{2+} transient and contraction, and could also trigger arrhythmias. Recently it was observed that in an animal model of heart failure after myocardial infarction Ca^{2+} sparks showed large temporal and spatial heterogeneity. The poorly coordinated production of Ca^{2+} sparks is likely to contribute to the diminished and slowed macroscopic Ca^{2+} transients [662]. Recently missense mutations in the cardiac RyR were detected in four independent families with arrhythmogenic right ventricular dysplasia type 2 (ARVD2), an autosomal dominant cardiomyopathy causing effort-induced arrhythmias and sudden death [1148].

2.3.1.1.1.5 Molecular structure.

Vertebrates have three genes encoding the RyR [for review see 1069]. In mammals RyR2 (coded by *RYR2* on 1q42.1-q43) represents the cardiac muscle isoform [778,835,1164]. The RyR channel has a homotetrameric structure with a fourfold symmetry and with a large cytoplasmic domain, giving it a mushroom-like appearance; each domain is thought to contain six putative transmembrane segments [899,1164,1225]. The protein contains a central channel which branches into four radial channels. The N-terminal and the shorter C-terminal protrude in the cytoplasm and form the foot structure seen in electron microscope studies [see 81,710].

2.3.1.1.2 Inositol trisphosphate receptor IP3R

Both atrial and ventricular myocytes express IP3Rs, with approximately six-fold higher levels of InsP3Rs in atrial cells [567,656,763,853]. Expression is larger in Purkinje fibres than in other cells [384]. The IP3Rs are arranged in the subsarcolemmal space, where they largely co-localise with the junctional RyRs.

While the role of IP3-receptors is well established in smooth muscle and non-excitable cells [80] their role in heart is much less understood. However IP3 is released from the plasma membrane following activation of different receptors (M2, M1, P2, ET) [435,878,1096,1214], and IP3 can cause Ca^{2+} release, indicating that these channels could modulate EC coupling [88,369,656,1220,1354]. Like the RyR, the IP3R may become regeneratively active in conditions of Ca^{2+}-overload [421,564].

2.3.1.1.2.1 Modulation

IP3 and Ca^{2+} interact in the activation of the channel. The IP3 affinity is about 27 nM. In the presence of 100 nM IP3 a rise of Ca^{2+} in the concentration range from 10^{-8} to 10^{-7} M increases the open probability of the IP3-receptor [901]. In addition to IP3 and Ca^{2+}, a large number of factors influence the function of IP3Rs [see 488,534,739]. IP3Rs are modulated by PKC, PKA, Ca-CaM kinase II and tyrosine kinases, ATP-Mg and pH. The positive inotropic effect [878] as well as the proarrhythmic effect [1014] of α-receptor stimulation has been related to IP3 production.

During end-stage human heart failure, IP3R1 mRNA and protein are upregulated whereas RyR2 mRNA and protein are downregulated [705].

2.3.1.1.2.2 Permeation

The single channel conductance of the IP3R is smaller (70 pS) than that of the RyR, but the permeability series of divalent ions is the same with a permeability ratio of divalent over monovalent cations around 6 [901].

2.3.1.1.2.3 Structure

In vertebrates three different IP3R isoforms are present encoded by three different genes [see 847,1069]. Both atrial and ventricular myocytes express mainly type 2 IP3Rs, but small amounts of the other types are present [238,656,853]. The type 2 IP3R shares considerable homologies with type 1 and with the RyR, and can be divided in three domains: a large cytoplasmic N-terminal containing the IP3 receptor, a hydrophobic channel domain with six transmembrane segments, and a short cytoplasmic tail [1111].

2.3.1.2   Other sarcoplasmic reticulum channels

K^+ channels [940], Cl^- channels [561,939] and possibly H^+ channels [640,732] constitute high conductance pathways in the sarcoplasmic reticulum membrane, which keeps the potential across the membrane of the SR at about zero potential. Ca^{2+} movement across the SR membrane does therefore not result in building up of electrical gradients which would oppose further Ca^{2+} movement. The flux of K^+, H^+ or Cl^- as counter ions facilitates the passive release as well as the active uptake of large amounts of Ca^{2+}.

2.3.2   Mitochondrial channels

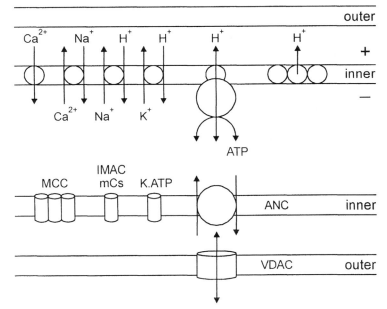

Figure IV.34. Ion transporters in inner and outer mitochondrial membranes.

In the mitochondria energy is transferred from different substrates to ATP by way of oxidation. Since one of the key reactions serves to build up a proton gradient, the inner membrane of the mitochondrion was supposed to be relatively impermeable. The outer mitochondrion membrane, on the other hand has long been considered to act as a sieve. This view has changed dramatically during recent years (see topical reviews J Physiol 2000, 529).

2.3.2.1 Outer mitochondrial membrane

The most important channel in the outer membrane is a voltage-dependent anion channel called VDAC (Fig. IV.34). Together with the adenine nucleotide carrier in the inner membrane VDAC plays an important role in the traffic of ATP and ADP between the cytoplasm and the mitochondrial matrix [700].

2.3.2.1.1 Voltage-dependent anion channel VDAC

Isolated in lipid bilayers, VDAC shows a maximum open probability at zero membrane potential which falls off at either positive or negative voltages [200]. The importance of this voltage gating remains unclear since the voltage gradient over the outer membrane is of unknown amplitude.

The VDAC is permeable for molecules up to 1 kD (650 pS at 0 mV) and is slightly more permeable to anions than to cations (ratio of 2/1). It allows passage of ATP and ADP. The flux of ATP is high (10^6 molecules ATP per second) [937]. Permeability is modulated by the NADH concentration. It is estimated that fluctuations of NADH can result in a six fold change of the permeability to adenine nucleotides with consequent changes in the intensity of respiration [667]. The VDAC should thus be considered a sensor of glycolysis since cytoplasmic NADH is mainly determined by glycolysis. The VDAC channel has been crystallised [1143] and forms groups of six transmembrane pores, each pore consisting of a single 30-35 kD VDAC subunit [96].

2.3.2.2 Inner mitochondrial membrane

Under physiological conditions the permeability of the inner membrane is low [577]. In ischaemic conditions however this permeability barrier can be weakened or completely vanish by opening of large channels. A number of channels have been described (Fig. IV.34) of which the three most important are: a multiple conductance channel (MCC) or mega channel permeable to large cations and anions, an ATP-dependent K^+ channel, and a 107 pS slightly anion-selective channel, known as the mCS channel (mitochondrial centopicosiemens) or IMAC (inner membrane anion channel). The molecular nature of these channels is unknown. From drug sensitivity studies the K.ATP channel structure can be supposed to be similar but not identical to that of the plasma membrane K.ATP channel.

2.3.2.2.1   Multiple conductance channel MCC

A combination of elevated, μmolar intramitochondrial $[Ca^{2+}]$ with low [ATP] activates the channel [225,288,1117]. Activation is facilitated by the presence of long-chain acyl-coA [873], pro-oxidants and dithiol-oxidatives; it is inhibited by H^+, Mg^{2+} and the immune suppressive drug cyclosporin [1118]. Since intramitochondrial Ca^{2+} concentrations are normally low and matrix [ATP] high, the MCC is not expected to be activated under normal conditions. In ischaemia or Ca^{2+} overload conditions, and especially upon reperfusion with high O_2 tension, the channel may be activated and is probably responsible for the permeability transition. Pore opening uncouples oxidative phosphorylation (comparable to the effect of the uncoupling protein in brown fat cells) and acts as a drain for glycolytic ATP. Activation is accompanied by depolarisation and release of the mitochondrial content, especially Ca^{2+} itself. This release of Ca^{2+} may trigger a Ca^{2+} wave from one mitochondrion to the other [487]. The effect is reversible when activation is transient. However, if activation is steady, the cell will die [288,1118].

The mega channel has a variable conductance between 40 and 1000 pS and is unselective to cations or anions. Large anions such as ADP and ATP can permeate.

2.3.2.2.2   ATP-dependent K^+ channel

The ATP-dependent K^+ channel [492] has the same conductance and the same activation pattern of K.ATP channels in the plasma membrane, but a different pharmacological profile. It opens by reduction of the [ATP] below a critical concentration and this process is facilitated by PKC-dependent phosphorylation [980]. It is blocked by glibenclamide and activated by pinacidil; in comparison with the plasma membrane channel, it is more sensitive to block by hydroxydecanoate and to activation by diazoxide [833].

It plays an important role in volume regulation and in preconditioning (see remodeling). The concentration of K^+ ions in the matrix is supposed to be close to the concentration in the cytoplasm, implying that the continuous passive influx through the channel (because of the negative matrix potential) has to be compensated by an efflux through the K^+/H^+ exchanger at the expense of the proton gradient [362]. Activation of the channel results in an enhanced K^+ influx and has the following consequences:

– When activation is accompanied by an important anion influx through the IMAC channel, the influx of salt will lead to a concomitant water transport and swelling of the matrix. This osmotic challenge has been shown on isolated mitochondria to lead to activation of fatty acid oxidation and increased ATP synthesis [363,412].
– When K^+ influx is not accompanied by an enhanced anion influx it will cause depolarisation. This in turn leads to a reduction of Ca^{2+} influx and

limits the Ca^{2+} load, avoiding activation of the mega channel and preventing irreversible loss of the cell [225,287].

The volume regulatory role is functionally important for ATP synthesis. Both volume regulation as well as restriction of Ca^{2+} overload have been proposed to play a role in preconditioning. With respect to preconditioning a third process, caused by K.ATP channel opening, has been proposed, nl. an increased production of radicals and secondary activation of kinases [839].

2.3.2.2.3 Anion-selective pathway (IMAC; mCS)

Initially distinction has been made between an anion-selective pathway described in osmotic challenge experiments (IMAC) [364] and an anion-selective channel analysed in electrophysiological experiments (mCS) [1066]. More recent evidence favours the hypothesis of a single unit [see 833]. The process of activation is far from solved. In patch clamp experiments the channel was activated under alkaline conditions and low divalent ion concentrations; it was predominantly closed at negative matrix potentials [1066]. For these reasons it is difficult to imagine how this channel may be functional under metabolic stress conditions. However, more recent data obtained with inhibitors suggest activation under ischaemic conditions [833].

3. ACTION POTENTIAL MORPHOLOGY AND IONIC CURRENTS

Cardiac cells are coupled by gap junctions, and thereby form a functional syncytium. Therefore, contractility of the heart cannot be regulated by recruitment. While in skeletal muscle the action potential is only a trigger for the Ca^{2+} release that causes the contraction, cardiac excitation-contraction coupling is controlled by regulating Ca^{2+} influx and release from intracellular stores via modulation of ionic currents during the action potential. Large differences exist in shape of the action potentials between different cardiac cell types. Differences are seen in upstroke of the action potential between nodal cells and myocardial cells, in diastolic potentials between pacemakers and myocardial cells, and in the shape of the plateau phase throughout the heart. These differences are governed by cell-dependent expression of a large variety of ionic currents (see section 1), which makes it possible to modulate the shape of the action potential. Of special importance is the duration of the cardiac action potential: the long duration ensures a long refractory period, while the fraction of time spent at depolarised potentials determines to a large extent balance between Ca^{2+} influx and efflux, and hence the contractility. However the large variety of

modulatory influences also makes the action potential vulnerable to
pathological effects, although it also provides for important redundancy of
regulatory mechanisms.

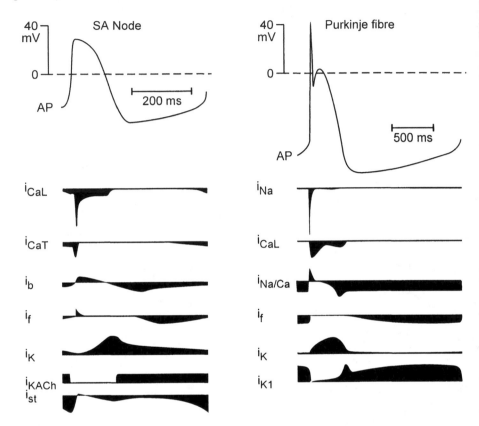

Figure IV.35. Schematic overview of the time course of the main ionic currents involved
during the action potential and diastolic depolarisation in SAN (left) and Purkinje fibres
(right). Larger thickness of the current trace is intended to approximately indicate the phase of
the cycle in which the current is important. The scale of the different currents is not the same.

At each moment during the cardiac cycle, the rate of change of the
membrane potential is directly proportional to the net ionic current flowing
through the membrane at that moment ($C_m.dE_m/dt = i_{net}$). Since many
currents contribute to the net ionic current, the time course of the action
potential or the contribution of different ionic currents to the net ionic
current during the action potential is difficult to predict, since both depend
on a large number of equations and parameters. Several models simulating
ionic currents and action potentials in different cardiac cells types have been
published in the literature for Purkinje fibres [260], ventricle [688,887,1285]
(Heart program from Oxsoft Ltd, Oxford U.K.), SAN [241,1283] and atria

[217,296,445,816]. Although none of the models is able to simulate all aspects of electrical activity, they attempt to summarise the available knowledge on ionic currents at the time of publication of the model and are a great help for understanding possible influence of physiological, pathological or pharmacological effects on electrical activity. Fig. IV.35 and Fig. IV.36 give a schematic overview of the time course of the most important currents during the cardiac cycle on the basis of experimental results and simulations. The next sections will discuss the different phases of the action potentials in relation to the contribution of the most important ionic currents in normal conditions. Further chapters will discuss how cardiac electrical activity is affected by different factors in normal and pathological conditions.

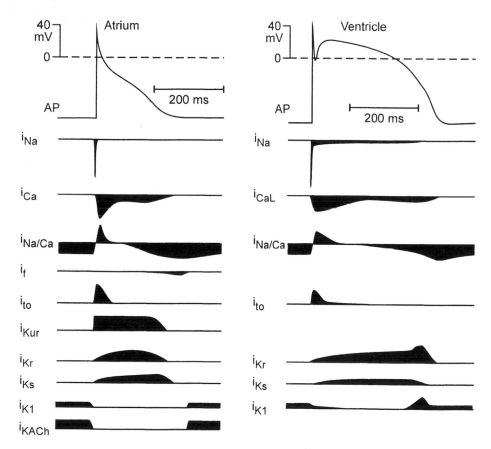

Figure IV.36. Schematic overview of the main ionic currents involved during the action potential in atria (left) and ventricle (right). Like in previous figure, a large size of a current only indicates the phase where the size of the current is large.

3.1   Upstroke

3.1.1   Fast response cells

In fast response cells (atria, His bundle, Purkinje and ventricular myocardium), phase 0 of the action potential is governed by the tetrodotoxin-sensitive Na^+ current. In these cells the Na^+ channel density is very large. Stimulation to potentials above threshold leads to activation of enough Na^+ channels to overcome the outward K^+ current; hence the net current will be inward, causing further depolarisation and opening of more Na^+ channels, leading to a regenerative depolarisation (see Chapter III). Since the kinetics of the Na^+ channel is fast, this leads to a very rapid activation of a large number of Na^+ channels, causing a fast and large rise of i_{Na}. Especially in the His bundle and the Purkinje system, the Na^+ current is very large, resulting in a fast depolarisation (up to 800 V/s) and fast conduction of the action potential (see Chapter III). The current during phase 0 of the action potential reaches a peak at a potential of about –20 mV within about 1 ms.

During the fast depolarisation the Na^+ current is much larger than the other currents; the upstroke velocity (which is proportional to the net ionic current) is therefore almost exclusively determined by i_{Na}, especially since the K^+ conductance of the cell shows a very fast drop, due to the inward rectification of i_{K1}. After rising to a peak, the Na^+ current rapidly declines. This is due a decrease of the driving force (the membrane potential becomes closer to the E_{Na}), and to inactivation of the channel. However, since the net current is still inward, the declining Na^+ current causes further depolarisation of the cell. The membrane potential becomes positive and reaches a peak at potentials near the Na^+ equilibrium potential within a few ms. At that moment the action potential shows an overshoot of about +40 mV, but the potential does not reach E_{Na}, because of the presence of outward currents (K^+ e.g. is now far from equilibrium, and i_{to} activation is fast enough to contribute to outward current during the final portion of phase 0) and also because of the inactivation of the Na^+ channel. At the peak of the action potential the net current is zero.

In pathological situations, such as ischaemia, depolarisation of the cell can result in inactivation of Na^+ channels, and eventually failure of excitation and conduction can occur. Also large activation delays, due to increased intercellular coupling resistance, can cause inhibition of the Na^+ current, by a process called accommodation: the slow depolarisation of the cell during the foot of the action potential (before the threshold is reached) enables channel inactivation to occur concomitant with activation, so that no channel opening occurs. Under such conditions i_{CaL} can be activated, especially in the presence of catecholamines, and cause slow conduction [929].

3.1.2   Slow response cells

In SAN and AVN (the so-called slow response cells) the upstroke of the action potential is not carried by Na^+ current but by the L-type Ca^{2+} current. While Na^+ channels appear to be present in the SAN, the low value of the diastolic potentials results in complete inactivation of the channels. The diastolic depolarisation however leads to activation of T-type Ca^{2+} channels, which contribute to the current during the final diastole and the initial phase 0. When the threshold is reached, i_{CaL} becomes the dominant inward current. The Ca^{2+} current is however much smaller, and is also slower than the Na^+ current in the fast response cells. The Ca^{2+}-dependent action potentials therefore have a low upstroke velocity, which is of the order of 10 V/s, and conduction is also slow. The Ca^{2+} current depolarises the cells to positive potentials of about +30 to +40 mV. This peak potential is much lower than the Ca^{2+} equilibrium potential (which for a cell at rest is of the order of +150 mV). The large difference between the peak potential and this E_{Ca} is due to several causes: first, the finite permeability of the channel for K^+ ions allows important efflux of K^+ ions through the channel (intracellular K^+ ion concentration is five to six orders of magnitude larger than the intracellular Ca^{2+} concentration); second, the large rise in intracellular Ca^{2+} concentration, especially near the cell membrane, causes a reduction of E_{Ca}; third, Ca^{2+} current is small so that the contribution of outward current to the net current during the upstroke of slow response cells is more important than in fast response cells; finally, the slow time course of phase 0 (which is due to i_{Ca} being small and slow) also allows activation of outward currents to be relatively important at the time of the peak of the action potential.

3.2   Initial repolarisation

After the peak of the action potential the cells start to repolarise. The final repolarisation to diastolic potentials is however delayed by about 100 to about 400 ms, depending on the cell type and frequency. Between the initial depolarisation (phase 0) and the final repolarisation (phase 3), cardiac cells have a plateau phase (phase 2). This plateau can be distinct, as is especially the case in ventricular cells, or shorter and less pronounced, gradually evolving in a final repolarisation, as is the case in atria and SAN. The plateau phase can be preceded by a marked initial early repolarisation (phase 1), as is seen in atria, Purkinje cells and ventricular subepicardial and midmyocardial M cells. In atria, in ventricular epicardium and M cells and in some Purkinje cells a small secondary depolarisation can follow the initial repolarisation phase and lead to the plateau, resulting in a so-called notch, which gives the action potential a spike - dome appearance (see also Chapter VI). No such clear distinction between phase 1 and 2 can be made in SAN, AVN and atrial and ventricular subendocardial cells. In SAN, AVN and ventricular subendocardial cells the plateau of the action potential starts from the peak of phase 0, without a pronounced phase 1. In atrial cells the action potentials have a short duration and most, but not all, action potentials have a more or less triangular shape so that the transition between phases 1, 2 and 3 is gradual and the distinction between these phases is less clear.

The initial fast repolarisation following phase 0 of the action potential is largely due to the inactivation of i_{Na} and the rapid activation of the transient outward current. The transient outward current is mainly carried by i_{to} (i_{to1}), but a Ca^{2+}-activated Cl^- current $i_{Ca,Cl}$ (i_{to2}), which rises in parallel with intracellular Ca^{2+}, can also contribute to the outward current. In atria the ultrarapid delayed rectifier i_{Kur} is also involved. The different expression of i_{to} in different cardiac cells explains the important variation in early repolarisation and shape of the action potential. The current is large in atrial cells and in subepicardial and midmyocardial ventricular cells, but small and slower in subendocardial cells (see also Chapters I and VI).

The effect of the transient outward current on the duration of the action potential in human ventricular cells is still controversial and can be different in subepi- and subendocardial cells. Some simulations show no prolongation of the action potential upon inhibition of i_{to} [887]. Other simulations demonstrate that a mild increase of i_{to} can even result in a prolongation of the action potential by causing a deep notch between the fast upstroke and the plateau, which results in a larger driving force for Ca^{2+} and delayed secondary activation of i_{CaL}. A large increase in i_{to} can however prematurely interrupt the action potential [388].

3.3   Plateau

Cardiac action potentials have a duration that is much longer than the duration of the action potentials in nerve or skeletal muscle. The slope of the plateau phase in different cardiac cells is small to very small (it is smaller in the ventricle than in atrial cells, and within the ventricular myocardium it is smallest in midmyocardial M cells). The long plateau phase of the cardiac action potential is due to a close balance between outward and inward currents, the outward currents slightly dominating, so that the net current is small and slightly outward. The small size of the net ionic current implies that relatively small changes in any of the currents can have large effects on the net current, on the rate of repolarisation during the plateau and thus on the duration of the action potential.

3.3.1 Ventricle

An important factor for the genesis of the plateau of the ventricular action potential is the high membrane resistance during this phase of the action potential, which is due to the inward rectification of i_{K1}. The inward rectification of i_{K1} enables the channel to carry large currents at negative potentials, thereby stabilising the resting potential, while limiting the K^+ efflux during the plateau (Fig. IV.37), and thereby also decreasing the net inward current necessary to prevent the occurrence of a fast repolarisation. By reducing passive current flow during systole, the inward rectification enables the existence of a long plateau without excessive energy cost.

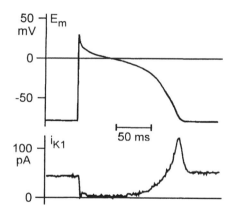

Figure IV.37. Due to the inward rectification of i_{K1} the amplitude of the K^+ current is largely decreased during the action potential in ventricular myocytes. Modified from [1340].

3.3.1.1 Inward currents

The main channel providing inward current during the plateau of the cardiac action potential is i_{CaL}. This channel is activated more slowly than i_{Na}, and the amplitude of the Ca^{2+} current is much smaller than that of the Na^+ current, so that it does not contribute to phase 0 depolarisation in fast response cells. In ventricular subepicardial and midmyocardial cells, which have an important i_{to}, the activation of i_{CaL}, concomitant with the inactivation of i_{to}, can give rise to a brief phase of secondary depolarisation after phase 1, which gives these action potentials their typical spike - dome appearance. The Ca^{2+} conductance gradually declines during the plateau, due to Ca^{2+}- and voltage–dependent inactivation. The exact time course of i_{CaL} is however difficult to predict in the absence of detailed knowledge of subplasmalemmal

Ca^{2+} concentrations. The decline of the Ca^{2+} current is partially counteracted by the effect of repolarisation, and by the decrease of $[Ca^{2+}]_i$, during the intracellular Ca^{2+} transient, which causes an increase of the electrochemical gradient for Ca^{2+} influx. As the cells more and more repolarise, the amplitude of i_{CaL} can temporarily show a small increase (Fig. IV.38 left panel) when the potential enters the range of window current. Slow and / or incomplete inactivation of i_{Na} also contribute somewhat to the inward currents.

3.3.1.2   Outward currents

A gradual rise is seen in the amplitude of the delayed rectifier K^+ currents i_{Kr} and i_{Ks} during the plateau of the ventricular action potential. The increase in outward current together with the decrease in inward current will finally terminate the plateau. The contribution of the two delayed rectifier K^+ currents however varies between cell types.

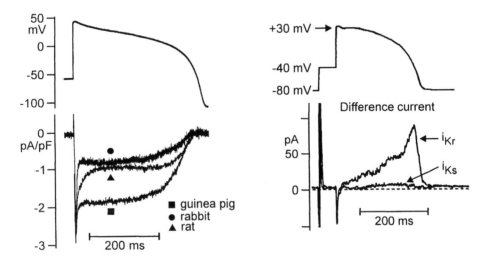

Figure IV.38. Time course of i_{CaL}, i_{Kr} and i_{Ks} during the action potential in ventricular myocytes. Left panel: Time course of i_{CaL} in guinea pig (squares), rabbit (circles) and rat (triangles) ventricular myocytes during the action potential. Modified from [654]. Right panel: Contribution of i_{Kr} and i_{Ks} to the outward current during the plateau and repolarisation of the action potential in dog ventricle. Modified from [1192]. The currents were measured in voltage clamp experiments where a command potential was imposed with the shape of the normal action potential. Repeating the experiment with the same command potential, but in condition where one current component is blocked, shows the time course of contribution of that current to the net ionic current during the normal action potential.

i_{Kr} rises faster during the plateau than i_{Ks}. Its time course of activation is fast enough to enable a large fraction of the channels to be activated during the late plateau of the ventricular action potential and deactivated during the final repolarisation and diastole. Its inward rectification limits the maximum size of the current at positive potentials. As the potential becomes gradually more negative during the plateau, the amplitude of the current can show an extra rise at the end of the plateau, since the change in membrane potential brings the channel out of the potential range of inward rectification (Fig. IV.38 right panel).

i_{Ks} activates very slowly, and at low rates of stimulation it remains small throughout the plateau of the action potential. Since studies in guinea pig ventricular myocytes had shown slow deactivation during diastole, it was proposed to contribute to the rate-dependent action potential abbreviation, by accumulating through subsequent cardiac cycles at higher frequencies. Since the channel does not show inward rectification, the size of the current is not limited by the depolarisation of the cell. Therefore, it could carry appreciable outward current at high frequency, especially in cells with elevated plateau level. β-receptor stimulation increases the size of the current, resulting in a reduction of APD. The rate-dependent reduction in the duration of the ventricular action potential is important, since it allows more rapid heart rates, while preserving a diastolic interval large enough to enable efficient filling of the ventricles. The small expression of i_{Ks} in canine midmyocardial M cells explains the long duration of the action potentials of these cells, and their vulnerability to failure of normal repolarisation resulting in early afterdepolarisations (EAD) (see Chapter VIII). The contribution of i_{Ks} to the outward currents during the action potential in human ventricular cells was questioned however, since whole cell clamp experiments show only very small i_{Ks} currents in these cells. Nevertheless, defects in the gen coding for i_{Ks} are at the basis of LQT1.

3.3.1.3   The Na^+/Ca^{2+} exchanger

The Na^+/Ca^{2+} exchanger is not only important for Ca^{2+} homeostasis, but it can also modulate the electrical activity: because of its electrogenicity (presumably with 3 Na^+ to 1 Ca^{2+} stoichiometry), the Na^+/Ca^{2+} exchanger directly contributes to the net ionic current, and by affecting $[Ca^{2+}]_i$ it can influence other ionic currents during the action potential. During diastole, the reversal potential of the exchanger is more positive than the membrane potential. Early after the upstroke of the action potential however, the large depolarisation causes reversal of the electrochemical gradient of the exchanger (Fig. IV.29), resulting in Ca^{2+} entry through the exchanger. $i_{Na/Ca}$ is outward during this phase. The rise in intracellular Ca^{2+} concentration (mainly due to Ca^{2+} release from the sarcoplasmic reticulum) causes a change in reversal potential of the Na^+/Ca^{2+} exchanger, so that within a short time the reversal potential of the exchanger becomes more positive than the plateau potential. The exact time course of current carried by the exchanger is difficult to estimate, since the Ca^{2+} concentration in the subplasmalemmal space may be very different from the bulk cytosolic Ca^{2+} concentration. During a large part of the plateau phase the net current carried by the Na^+/Ca^{2+} exchanger is presumably relatively small, since the reversal potential is not very different from the high plateau potentials of ventricular cells. At the end of the plateau, but especially during the final repolarisation, the electrochemical gradient becomes larger, and the Na^+/Ca^{2+} exchanger extrudes Ca^{2+} from the cytoplasm, causing inward current, which tends to slow the repolarisation.

3.3.2   Atria

During phase 2 of the action potential, atrial cells show a gradual repolarisation that is faster than the plateau of the ventricular action potential (implying a somewhat larger net outward current density), with a less clear transition between phase 2 and 3.

The inward rectification of the K^+ current is less pronounced in supraventricular cells, since expression of i_{K1} in atria is much smaller than in the ventricle, and $i_{K.ACh}$, which participates to the K^+ currents in atrial cells, is more weakly inward rectifying than i_{K1}.

In human atria i_{CaL} and the Na^+/Ca^{2+} exchanger are the most important carriers of inward current during the plateau of the action potential. i_{CaL} is important for the rate-dependence of the APD. The contribution of the Na^+/Ca^{2+} exchanger to the inward current is larger in atrial than in ventricular cells [803], since the low plateau potentials of atrial cells causes a larger electrochemical gradient than in ventricular cells.

In human atrial cells a fast i_{to} and i_{Kr} and i_{Ks} are present. i_{to} is important throughout a large part of the plateau [327], so that it contributes to the shorter duration of the atrial action potential as compared to ventricular cells. The ultrarapid delayed rectifier i_{Kur} also contributes to the outward currents in human atria, where its amplitude is at least as large of that of i_{to}. It was found to contribute considerably to the action potential morphology; because of its non-inactivating characteristics it is important for ending the plateau and repolarisation to the resting potential. Because of their slower time course of activation the contribution of i_{Kr} and i_{Ks} to the outward currents during the atrial action potential is less than that of i_{to}. i_{Kr} appears to be important for the rate-dependence of atrial cells. Because of its slow activation, the contribution of i_{Ks} is not important during the plateau at normal rates.

A sensitivity analysis on a mathematical model indicated that i_{to}, i_{Kur}, and i_{CaL} are the most important determinants of the action potential shape during the plateau of human atrial cells [816]. Also $i_{K.ACh}$ can contribute, while i_{K1} only participates to the final phase of the repolarisation.

In contrast to atrial cells it was described that i_{Kr} is important in rabbit AVN. In these cells i_{Kr} activates rapidly and remains elevated throughout the plateau and early repolarisation and only starts to decline rapidly during the late repolarisation [745].

3.4　　Final repolarisation

3.4.1　　Ventricle

The final repolarisation (phase 3), which follows the plateau of the action potential, is largely initiated by the inactivation of the L-type Ca^{2+} current and by the activation of the delayed rectifying K^+ current. The exact contribution of delayed outward currents to repolarisation in human ventricle is still not clear. Although i_{Kr} as well as i_{Ks} are present, the amplitude of the currents appears to be small in human ventricle. However, as can be seen from the prolongation of the ventricular action potential by methane-sulfonanilide class III antiarrhythmics, which specifically block i_{Kr}, and from the effect of LQT2, which is a defect of the channel responsible for i_{Kr}, the fast component of the delayed rectifier K^+ current is an important determinant of APD in human ventricle. Due to the gradual rise in amplitude of i_{Kr} during the plateau, the outward current finally overwhelms the inward currents, which causes an increase of the rate of repolarisation and the start of phase 3 [648]. Despite the reduction of the K^+ electrochemical gradient, the amplitude of i_{Kr} can still temporarily rise during the initial part of the final repolarisation, because of the inward rectification of i_{Kr}.

The role of i_{Ks} for the repolarisation of the ventricular action potential is still a matter of debate, and depends on the location of the cell within the ventricular wall [175], since expression of i_{Ks} varies between subendocardial, subepicardial and midmyocardial cells. Because of the slow activation kinetics of i_{Ks} as measured in voltage clamp experiments, i_{Ks} activation during normal action potentials is expected to be limited, but it could become important in conditions of prolonged APD, during β-adrenergic stimulation or at higher rates of stimulation [see e.g. 1181]. Several arguments favour a contribution of i_{Ks} to the initiation of the final repolarisation of the action potential: i) The longer APD of midmyocardial M cells as compared to subepi- or subendocardial cells was related to the low density of i_{Ks} channels in the M cells. ii) Defective i_{Ks} channels are the basis of LQT1. iii) Block of i_{Ks} was reported to result in longer APD. However action potential clamp experiments using i_{Ks} blockers in normal canine ventricular muscle (see Fig. IV.38 right panel) and Purkinje fibres showed little contribution of i_{Ks} to the ionic currents during normal action potentials over a wide range of stimulation frequencies [1192]. The slow activation and the relatively fast deactivation of i_{Ks} in human [494] and dog [371] ventricle (in contrast to the findings in guinea pig ventricular myocytes [971]) may preclude marked accumulation of i_{Ks} at higher stimulation frequency.

During the final phase of repolarisation the contribution of the delayed rectifiers to the outward current decreases because of the decreased electrochemical gradient. However the inward rectifier plays an important role in the final phase of the repolarisation, especially in the ventricular myocardium and conduction system. Because of its strong inward-rectifier characteristics (Fig. IV.17) the channel was shut off during the action potential, but as during the final repolarisation the membrane potentials becomes more negative than about −55 mV, i_{K1} becomes larger again (Fig. IV.37), despite the decrease in electrochemical gradient for K^+. The contribution of i_{K1} helps to realise a relatively fast final repolarisation. The lower expression of i_{K1} in atrial cells explains the more gradual final repolarisation of these cells.

Several inward currents still play a role during the initial phase of the final repolarisation. The decrease of the intracellular Ca^{2+} concentration following uptake of Ca^{2+} by the sarcoplasmic reticulum resulted in a negative shift of the reversal potential of the Na^+/Ca^{2+} exchanger during the plateau of the action potential. The Na^+/Ca^{2+} exchanger thus acts again in the forward mode extruding Ca^{2+}, driven by influx of Na^+. Therefore it carries inward current which is expected to counteract to some extent the outward currents. During the repolarisation the potential moves through the zones of window current of i_{CaL} and somewhat later through the window of i_{Na}, which can result in a small increase of inward current that can become important in situations of reduced outward current. The inward current carried by the Na^+/Ca^{2+} exchanger, the slowly inactivating component of i_{Na}, and the Na^+ and Ca^{2+} window currents can all be responsible for the occurrence of EADs in situations of reduced outward current.

3.4.2   Atria

In atrial cells the repolarising current during phase 3 is mainly produced by i_{to} and i_{Kur}, with only a very limited contribution of i_{Kr}. The effect of these outward currents is counteracted to some extent by the inward current of the Na^+/Ca^{2+} exchanger.

3.5 Diastole

3.5.1 Resting potential in myocardial cells

3.5.1.1 Ventricle

The diastolic potential (phase 4) in ventricular myocardium is governed by a large K^+ conductance, which is due to i_{K1}, and which develops in extra-nodal myocytes during later stages of development [698]. The large K^+ conductance ensures a resting potential close to the K^+ equilibrium potential. A small background conductance for cations results in net inflow of positive charges, primarily carried by Na^+, which is present at the highest extracellular concentration. The background current causes the membrane potential to be less negative than E_K by about 5 to 10 mV. Also the Na^+/Ca^{2+} exchanger can contribute a small inward 'background' current. The electrogenic Na^+/K^+ pump can provide a small outward current, contributing a few mV to the resting potential. Block of the pump results in a small depolarisation amounting to a few mV, while activation of the pump by high frequency stimulation causes a small hyperpolarisation.

Increasing external K^+ concentration causes depolarisation of the cell, which closely follows the Nernst equation. It also results in a higher conductance of i_{K1}. A limited decrease of $[K^+]_e$ causes a small hyperpolarisation, while a large decrease can cause a depolarisation, because lowering $[K^+]_e$ decreases the conductance of i_{K1}. The situation is similar in the His bundle Purkinje system, except that these cells show a diastolic depolarisation caused by i_f (see section 3.5.2.3).

3.5.1.2 Atria

Two different K^+ channels, i_{K1} and $i_{K.Ach}$, contribute to the normal resting potential in human atrium [437,597]. Although the size of i_{K1} in atrial cells is smaller than in the ventricle, the basal conductance in the absence of agonists in human atrial cells is largely determined by i_{K1}. The relative contribution of the two channels differs between species. In human atrial cells the K^+ conductance that can be induced by ACh is of the same order of magnitude as the basal K^+ conductance.

3.5.2 Pacemaker activity

The SAN is the primary pacemaker of the heart. However also the AVN and the His bundle Purkinje system possess automaticity, although at lower frequency. These cells are therefore called subsidiary pacemakers. Atrial and ventricular myocardial cells show no spontaneous activity in normal conditions, but they may become spontaneously active in pathological situations.

Pacemaker activity is due to a progressive slow depolarisation of the membrane potential during diastole, which finally reaches the action potential threshold. This diastolic depolarisation is caused by the flow of net inward current. Since the rate of depolarisation (which is proportional to the net current) is rather constant during a large part of the diastolic depolarisation, the net inward current remains nearly constant during this phase. However the net current is outward during the final repolarisation, to become zero at the maximum diastolic potential; the diastolic depolarisation must therefore be initiated by a time-dependent change from net outward to net inward current at the end of the action potential. This can be due to a time-dependent increase of inward currents or to a decrease of outward currents, or a combination of both.

3.5.2.1   Normal automaticity in the sinoatrial node

The frequency of pacemaker activity in the sinoatrial node varies largely with species (Fig. IV.39 upper panel). The diastolic potential in the SAN is in the range between about –65 and –40 mV, and depends on the location of the cells within the SAN (outermost cells have more negative potentials due to electrotonic interactions with atrial cells). This low membrane potential is due to the lack of i_{K1} in SAN of most species [809] [but see 1031]. A number of ion channels contribute to the net ionic current in this range of potential, and there may be important variation in the channels contributing to diastolic depolarisation among different species. Several of the channels that are active during diastole provide time-dependent currents and can thereby directly contribute to pacemaker activity in the SAN; assigning the name pacemaker current to anyone of them is therefore misleading. Other channels provide a background current or play a role in modulating pacemaker activity. The exact role of each of these channels is still a matter of debate, and modifying one current influences many other currents. Given the importance of SAN pacemaker activity for functioning of the heart, it does not appear surprising that the SAN possesses marked redundancy in pacemaker mechanisms, and it was shown that different current components can substitute for each other and thereby stabilise SAN pacemaker frequency.

Four channels carrying inward current (i_f, T- and L-type Ca^{2+} channels and the sustained inward current i_{st}) have been proposed to directly contribute to the voltage- and time-dependent currents responsible for SAN pacemaker activity [for reviews see 136,254,259,495,1340]. In addition to these voltage-dependent channels, background currents and the Na^+/Ca^{2+} exchanger contribute to the net inward current during diastole [see 659].

Also the voltage-dependent outward current (delayed rectifying K^+ current) plays an important role in SAN pacemaker activity [672,822,1194,1341].

The delayed outward current, which was activated during the action potential, deactivates during early diastole, and this deactivation contributes to the diastolic depolarisation. While an outward current like i_K cannot by itself be responsible for depolarisation, the deactivation of i_K in the presence of a background inward current will result in the net current becoming less outward and eventually more inward with time. In rabbit SAN i_{Kr} is largely responsible for i_K, while in porcine SAN i_{Ks} is functionally dominant, which may in part account for the slower heart rate of the pig [824].

The i_f current is an inward current; it is mainly carried by Na^+ ions, and is activated during hyperpolarisation, which makes it a good candidate for directly contributing to pacemaker activity. The role of the i_f current for SAN pacemaking has however been questioned because its range of activation would be too negative to contribute a significant current in the range of diastolic potentials [808,1031,1060,1194,1315]. However, despite the finding that i_f activation is small and slow (<10% of maximal activation) in the region of pacemaker potentials, the magnitude of the i_f current generated may be large enough to account for the net current during diastolic depolarisation [1180,1341]. Zaza et al. [1341] however showed that during diastole an outward current (i_{Kr}) larger than i_f, is present, which indicates that other channels besides i_f must contribute inward current during this phase. In a study on rat SAN, the absence of i_f in about half of the spontaneously active SAN cells, or the presence of spontaneous activity when i_f was only seen at very negative potentials, provided arguments to conclude that spontaneous activity was independent of i_f [1031]. Furthermore very large reductions of i_f [242] [672] result in only moderate changes in SAN cycle length, as was also found from simulation using numerical models (Heart OXSOFT 4.2, Oxsoft Ltd, Oxford U.K.). It may be that several mechanisms of automaticity interact, resulting in feedback stabilisation of automaticity as is suggested by simulations, or alternatively that i_f is not very important for normal SAN automaticity, only providing a protection in case of failure of the other mechanisms.

Two types of Ca^{2+} channels can provide time-dependent inward current contributing to the pacemaker potentials of SAN cells [270,408]. The low threshold Ca^{2+} channel (i_{CaT}) is densely expressed in nodal cells, and inhibition of this current lowers the rate of diastolic depolarisation by depressing the later portion of the diastolic depolarisation [408,1353]. Although the channels are expected to be largely inactivated in the diastolic range of potentials, they appear to carry a significant amount of inward current contributing to the later two thirds of the diastole. The L-type Ca^{2+} current, which provides the inward current for the upstroke of the SAN action potential, could also contribute to the net inward current during diastole and was reported to modulate the entire diastolic depolarisation in the SAN [807,1209], but is expected to contribute most to the final phase. Facilitation of i_{CaL} at high frequency or depolarisation is present in rabbit SAN and may provide an important regulatory mechanism of SAN automaticity [699].

A sustained inward current (i_{st}) which is activated by depolarisation within the range of diastolic potentials was found in SAN from different species (Fig. IV.39 lower panels) [for review see 748]. Since it is activated by depolarisation and provides inward current that causes more depolarisation its activation is thought to constitute a positive feedback loop driving the diastolic depolarisation

The role of the TTX-sensitive Na^+ channel in SAN cells is not clear. In adult it does not play a role in pacemaker activity, but it may contribute to the shape of the action potential of more peripherally located SAN cells [590]. It also appears to contribute to the current flowing during the diastolic depolarisation in neonatal rabbit pacemaker myocytes and may be responsible for the higher sinus rate in the neonate [57].

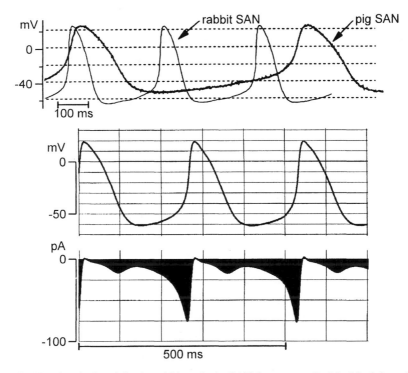

Figure IV.39. Electrical activity in rabbit and pig SAN (upper panel). Modified from [824]. Estimated contribution of i_{st} during the diastolic depolarisation and action potential in rat SAN (lower panels). Modified from [1031].

In addition to the time-dependent currents a background current mainly carried by Na^+ has been described in SAN [409]. Other currents such as the electrogenic Na^+/K^+ and the Na^+/Ca^{2+} exchanger may also affect pacemaker activity, and the activity of these electrogenic transporters is affected by electrical activity of the cell. Recently it has been proposed that Ca^{2+} entry via T-type Ca^{2+} channels may increase subsarcolemmal Ca^{2+} by triggering local release from the sarcoplasmic reticulum. The rise in subsarcolemmal Ca^{2+} could stimulate Ca^{2+} extrusion by Na^+/Ca^{2+} exchanger. The resultant net inward Na^+/Ca^{2+} exchange current, would contribute to automaticity [99,484]. This mechanism could also play a role in ectopic atrial arrhythmias.

As already mentioned the contribution of the different currents to SAN automaticity is not clear and may depend on species, developmental stage [698] and the presence of hormones, transmitters and humoral factors. In general it is thought that both Ca^{2+} currents and i_{st} provide a positive feedback loop driving diastolic depolarisation, since their activation during depolarisation will cause further depolarisation [1031,1209]. i_f en i_K and the depolarisation-induced facilitation of i_{CaL} on the other hand could provide a negative feedback loop stabilising diastolic depolarisation. The activation of i_f during hyperpolarisation would cause depolarisation which tends to turn off activation. The deactivation of i_K causes a decrease of outward current, which will tend to depolarise the cell and activate the channel, although this effect plays a minor role because activation occurs mainly during the action potential. Prolongation of the diastolic depolarisation could result in depolarisation-induced facilitation of i_{CaL}, which is expected to oppose excessive slowing of the heart rate [699].

Automaticity is modulated by the autonomic system. Sympathetic as well as parasympathetic stimulation have marked chronotropic effects. By activating adenylate cyclase β-adrenergic stimulation enhances spontaneous activity by several mechanisms. It increases the amplitude of i_{CaL} and i_{st}, enhancing inward current. It also shifts i_f activation kinetics towards less negative potentials. At a given potential in the range of diastolic depolarisation, more i_f channels are activated and also the rate of activation is enhanced [1343]. The mechanisms by which β-adrenoceptor agonists increase pacemaking rate in SAN pacemaker cells include also an increase in the rate of deactivation of i_K [631]. β-receptor stimulation is also expected to enhance inward current through the Na^+/Ca^{2+} exchanger by enhancing Ca^{2+} influx through the L-type Ca^{2+} channel, and by phosphorylation of the exchanger.

Parasympathetic activity and adenosine counteract the effect of sympathetic stimulation by its inhibitory effect on adenylate cyclase, decreasing i_{CaL} and i_{st}, and shifting i_f in the hyperpolarising direction [1343].

Furthermore ACh also activates $i_{K.ACh}$, thereby enhancing outward current, causing hyperpolarisation and a decreased net inward current resulting in a decreased rate of diastolic depolarisation and lower frequency.

3.5.2.2   Automaticity in the atrioventricular node

The AVN can be functionally divided into AN, N and NH regions. The AV nodal cells have a low diastolic potential in the region of -60 to -50 mV, but the potential is more negative in the regions bordering the His bundle (NH) or the atria (AN) by electrotonic interactions. The AVN has a slow diastolic depolarisation and the rate of spontaneous activity is slower than in SAN. It can act as a subsidiary pacemaker. The contribution of the different currents to pacemaker activity has not been clarified and it may be different in different areas of the AVN and contribute to the complex electrophysiological properties observed in the intact AV node [768]. The ionic currents contributing to AVN pacemaker activity appear to be very similar to the currents in SAN: i_{CaL}, i_{Na}, i_f, and i_{Kr} and i_{Ks} have been described, and in rabbit AVN i_{Kr} was found to dominate i_K and to play an important role in the diastolic depolarisation [183,420,593,745,977].

Like in SAN, β-adrenergic stimulation enhances the rate of diastolic depolarisation. ACh and adenosine decrease i_{CaL} and also activate $i_{K.ACh}$, causing hyperpolarisation and slowing of the rate of diastolic depolarisation [71].

3.5.2.3   Automaticity in His bundle Purkinje system

The mechanism of automaticity is more simple and much better understood than that in nodal tissue. In Purkinje fibres the diastolic depolarisation occurs at more negative potentials (around -80 mV in normal conditions) than in the SAN due to the presence of a large i_{K1}, which keeps the diastolic potential range close to the K^+ equilibrium potential (see section 3.5.1.1). The primary current responsible for the diastolic depolarisation in these cells is i_f, which is large enough to counteract i_{K1}. Like i_f in nodal cells the current is a mixture of Na^+ and K^+ current, but due to the larger electrochemical gradient for Na^+ than for K^+ in the range of diastolic potentials, the current is mainly carried by Na^+ [132,251,1328]. A small i_{CaT} is present in Purkinje cells [451], but its contribution to diastolic depolarisation has been questioned [870].

Increasing the external K^+ concentration results in depolarisation of the cell, according to the Nernst equation. An increase in $[K^+]_e$ also results in a higher conductance of i_{K1}, counteracting the effect of inward current, and thereby reducing the rate of spontaneous activity. A limited decrease of $[K^+]_e$ causes a small hyperpolarisation, while a large decrease depolarises the cell, because of the reduction of the conductance of i_{K1}. β-adrenergic stimulation enhances the rate of diastolic depolarisation by shifting the activation kinetics of i_f to less negative potentials. ACh counteracts this effect.

Higher rates of stimulation cause overdrive suppression by stimulating the electrogenic Na^+/K^+ pump, resulting in hyperpolarisation and slowing of the rate of diastolic depolarisation. This is the basis of the overdrive suppression of the spontaneous activity of the His bundle Purkinje system at normal heart rates.

Chapter V

Modulation of electrical activity

1.   MODULATION OF ACTION POTENTIAL BY RATE

1.1   Description

   In the description of the changes in action potential duration (APD) as a function of rate distinction should be made between steady-state condition, transient changes when the rate is suddenly increased or decreased, and the restitution process which refers to changes in APD for an extra stimulus applied at a variable interval following attainment of steady-state. Most information available is related to the ventricular action potential.

   For frequencies above $1s^{-1}$ the APD in steady-state is shorter the higher the frequency. At frequencies lower than $1s^{-1}$, depending on the species, the APD may tend to a steady value or become slightly shorter again. In the rat and mouse ventricle the APD barely changes with frequency [see 110,137,650]. A number of equations have been proposed to correct for differences in heart rate in comparing QT intervals in clinical electrocardiography, among which the best known is the Bazett formula [65].

   For a sudden increase in frequency three types of evolution can be distinguished, which differ mainly by the change occurring for the first action potential(s) upon acceleration or deceleration of the rate. In human ventricle an important initial shortening is followed by a slow and gradual decrease in duration, which develops over a time course of tens of seconds to a few minutes (Fig. V.1). In the cat a considerable initial shortening is succeeded by a lengthening which however is transient and finally results in a further shortening. In the rabbit ventricle the initial change is a prolongation, which is followed by a pronounced but slowly developing shortening. For a sudden decrease in frequency the opposite changes occur.

   Restitution describes the changes in APD when an extra stimulus is applied following the repolarisation process. For extra stimuli given at times shorter than the steady-state cycle the action potential usually is shortened (except e.g. in the rabbit). In many species, including human, the restitution process is described by an exponential with time constant in the order of 100 to 200 ms. In dog and cat the fast phase shows an overshoot, during which the APD temporarily lengthens above the steady-state value. For times longer than the steady-state cycle length, the action potential lengthens and the time constant of the relationship is in the order of minutes (Fig. V.2).

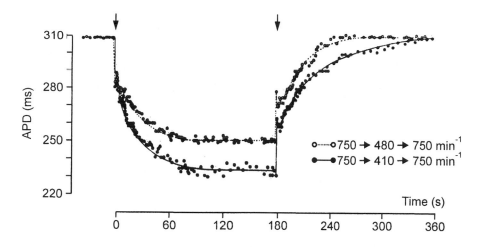

Figure V.1. Two phases in the adaptation of the human ventricular action potential duration to step changes in cycle length (see inset). A rapid initial phase is followed by some oscillatory change before continuing into a much slower phase. Modified from [346].

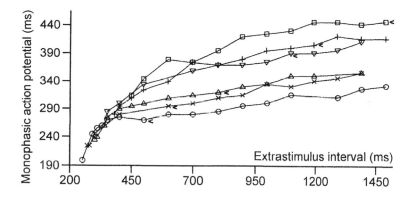

Figure V.2. Restitution of the duration of human ventricular action potential at different drive cycles. Monophasic derivations from an endocardial site in the right ventricle. Note two phases: an initial rapid phase is followed by a slower one (basic cycle length indicated by an arrow head). Modified from [757].

Restitution time course is important to understand the propensity to arrhythmias. When the slope of the fast phase as a function of cycle length is greater than one, the incidence of arrhythmias is high. A high slope means that small changes in cycle length are accompanied by larger changes in APD. Since these changes are not exactly the same in every cell, dispersion of APD is generated and conditions are fulfilled which facilitate reentry (see Chapter VIII)

1.2   Underlying mechanisms

From the description of the adaptation of the APD to acceleration or deceleration and during restitution it is evident that two phases should be considered: an initial rapid phase which is followed by a slow phase.

1.2.1   The fast initial changes

The initial fast changes in APD can be explained by the gating characteristics (activation, deactivation, inactivation, repriming) of specific currents that play a role in determining the APD. When an extra stimulus is given shortly after repolarisation, currents that undergo inactivation during an action potential are decreased in amplitude and their amplitude grows with time as inactivation is removed. This is the case for inward currents such as i_{Na} and i_{CaL}; incomplete recovery of inward current results in shortening of the APD. For outward currents such as i_{to} and i_{Kur}, incomplete recovery from inactivation results in lengthening of the APD. Other outward currents, such as i_{Kr} and i_{Ks} only undergo activation during the action potential and deactivate during diastole. Following repolarisation they remain partly activated and may thus show accumulation during an extra stimulus, with shortening of the APD as the outcome.

The immediate shortening of the APD upon increase of frequency in the human ventricle and most other species can be explained by summation of outward currents (i_{Kr}, i_{Ks}) and/or inactivation of inward currents (i_{Na}, i_{CaL}) [522,650] (Fig. V.3). In the rabbit and sheep an initial lengthening occurs, which is caused by the marked inactivation of the outward current i_{to} [559].

Rapid changes also occur in currents carried by transporters. The amplitude of the Na^+/Ca^{2+} exchange current during an extrasystole is markedly reduced [522]. The amplitude of this current depends largely on the amount of Ca^{2+} released from the SR, and this amount is smaller when an extra stimulus is applied directly after repolarisation. The reason is incomplete refilling of the SR or availability of Ca^{2+} for release. The fall in exchanger current will be translated in a shorter APD; in the ferret e.g. the change in Na^+/Ca^{2+} exchange current is the major determinant of the restitution process [522]. The impact of changes in Na^+/Ca^{2+} exchanger current is more pronounced in atria than in ventricles. In the dog atrium fast changes in APD are absent when the modulatory function of the exchanger is eliminated by blocking the release of Ca^{2+} from SR by ryanodine [424].

> Initial rapid phase
> shortening of APD:
>   repriming i_{Na}, i_{CaL} and $i_{Na/Ca}$
>   deactivation of i_{Kr}, i_{Ks}
> lengthening of APD: repriming i_{to}, i_{Kur}

Very often oscillations of the APD (alternans) are present during the initial seconds of a change in rate. They are caused by changes in diastolic interval, which is very short for the first stimulus at the elevated rate and may then show some type of long-short sequence before gradually attaining a steady-state.

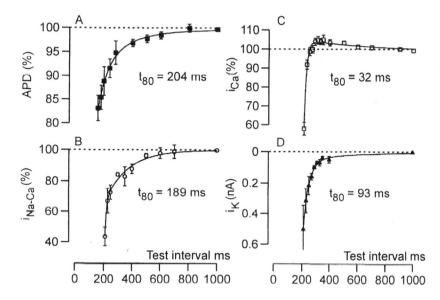

Figure V.3. Comparison of the time course of electrical restitution of the action potential duration and repriming of $i_{Na/Ca}$, i_{CaL}, and i_K. Note that the y-axis in D has been inverted to allow comparison of time course. Repriming of i_{to}, which exerts a lengthening effect, is not shown. The time to 80% recovery (t_{80}) of each curve is indicated. Preparation ferret ventricle. Modified from [522].

The effect of fast changes in current, as described above, will be different in the atria versus ventricle, in subendocardial versus subepicardial, and in base versus apex. The differences are related to the variability in the expression of certain currents and/or their kinetics. In atria the modulation of i_{to} will be more important than that of i_{Kr} or i_{Ks}, because these latter are less activated during the short atrial action potential. A change in i_{Kur} will also mainly affect the atrial action potential, because the current is less expressed in the ventricle. Also the Na^+/Ca^{2+} exchange current will play an important role in atria: due to the rather negative plateau the inward current through the exchanger is larger than in the ventricle. In ventricular subepicardial cells i_{to} is more expressed and its recovery from inactivation is faster than in subendocardial cells [772]; shortening of the APD is greater in subepicardial cells and increase in rate will be accompanied by modulation of the T wave morphology.

1.2.2   The slower changes

The slower changes in APD are more straightforward: shortening for an increase in frequency, lengthening for a decrease in frequency. The shortening can be explained by i) changes in ion concentrations $[K^+]_e$, $[Na^+]_i$ and $[Ca^{2+}]_i$, causing a change in the permeation and the gating of ionic channels and the flux through ion transporters, and by ii) modulatory effects of receptors on the same processes.

Slow phase
modulation of currents by ion concentration
        rise in $[K^+]_e$: enhancement of i_{K1} conductance
        rise in $[Na^+]_i$: stimulation of Na^+/K^+ pump
        rise in $[Ca^{2+}]_i$:faster inactivation of i_{CaL}
        stimulation of $i_{Na/Ca}$
modulation of currents by β -receptor stimulation

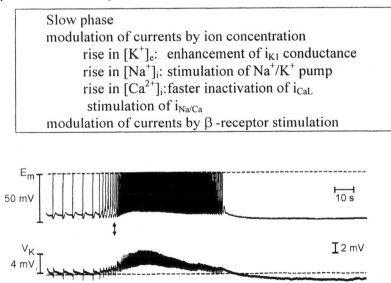

Figure V.4. Changes in membrane potential (top trace; record has been cut off) and extracellular $[K^+]_e$ (bottom trace) during triggered activity in an atrial fibre of the canine sinus coronarius. Stimulation rate was increased and led to triggered activity (arrow). Note accumulation of K^+_e which after reaching a maximum, decreased and led to subsequent K^+ depletion during the spontaneous arrest of the activity. Record by R.P.Kline. Modified from [1289].

    i) Increases in $[K^+]_e$, $[Na^+]_i$, and $[Ca^{2+}]_i$ at higher frequency have been well documented experimentally and the information has been included in theoretical models. A rise in $[K^+]_e$ increases the conductance of i_{K1} leading to shortening of the APD [138]. In multicellular tissues the increase of extracellular K^+ concentration during stimulation has been shown using ion-sensitive electrodes (actual concentrations in the T-tubules may even be higher). Simultaneous measurement of diastolic membrane potential shows depolarisation during the first minute concomitant with rise in $[K^+]_e$, followed later by hyperpolarisation, probably as a consequence of enhanced activity of the Na^+/K^+ pump and secondary reduction of $[K^+]_e$ (Fig. V.4).

The enhanced Na^+ pump activity is caused by the increased influx of Na^+ during the greater number of action potentials, with consequent rise in subsarcolemmal $[Na^+]_i$. The shortening of APD as a result of pump activation may play a larger role in subepicardial cells, since $[Na^+]_i$ has been shown to be more elevated in these cells compared to endocardial cells [206]. Although an increased pump current also reduces $[K^+]_e$ and causes a fall in current through i_{K1}, the outward current through the pump dominates. The rise in $[Na^+]_i$ also favours outward current through $i_{Na/Ca}$.

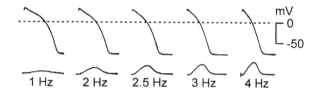

Figure V.5. Frequency-dependence of action potential duration and force of contraction in guinea pig right ventricle. Shortening of action potential duration is accompanied by a rise in contraction force. Modified from [903].

An increase in frequency is accompanied in most preparations (except rat, and in heart failure) by a rise in Ca^{2+} load and consequently by more Ca^{2+} release from the SR. As a result also contraction increases (positive Treppe phenomenon, Bowditch). The importance for the ionic processes underlying the repolarisation is evidenced by the inverse relationship which exists in many instances between APD and force of contraction (Fig. V.5). The increase in Ca^{2+} load with increase in rate is due to a shortening of the diastolic interval, disturbing the dynamic equilibrium between Ca^{2+} influx via i_{CaL} during the action potential and Ca^{2+} efflux via the Na^+/Ca^{2+} exchanger mainly during diastole. The increase in $[Ca^{2+}]_i$ has consequences for the Ca^{2+} current itself and for outward K^+ current, and will thereby affect APD: i_{Ks} is potentiated by Ca^{2+}-dependent phosphorylation [1149], and the i_{CaL} current shows faster inactivation induced by the increased Ca^{2+} release [1047]. Faster inactivation does not exclude that the peak of the Ca^{2+} current is eventually increased as a result of facilitation. Ca^{2+}-induced inactivation of

i_{CaL} may be quite important in determining APD since a gradual shortening of the action potential has been shown to accompany slow increases in tension upon increase of rate. These observations seem to imply that increased inward current carried by the Na^+/Ca^{2+} exchanger consequent to the increase in $[Ca^{2+}]_i$ may have less impact on the APD than the faster inactivation of i_{CaL}.

ii) Modulation of APD by stimulation of sympathetic activity. Increase in frequency in vivo is mostly caused by increased sympathetic activity. Stimulation of β -receptors leads to a number of reactions most of which cause shortening of the APD (Fig. V.6). Activation of adenylate cyclase activity and consequent increase in the concentration of cAMP stimulates PKA, leading to phosphorylation and stimulation of the Ca^{2+} channel, the Cl^- channel, the slow delayed K^+ channel and the RyR channel. The enhanced peak Ca^{2+} current which in itself causes more depolarisation also elevates the plateau, and consequently results in a greater activation of the two delayed outward currents.

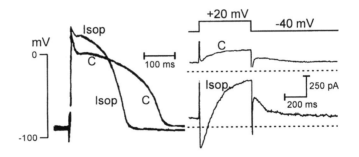

Figure V.6. Effect of isoproterenol (Isop) on the action potential (left) and i_{CaL} and i_K (right) in a canine ventricular myocyte. The plateau phase is shifted in the positive direction and shortened. In the voltage clamp records, both inward i_{CaL} and outward delayed K^+ currents are increased. Modified from [1158].

A second consequence of an enhanced Ca^{2+} current is an increased SR Ca^{2+} load and release. The enhanced systolic Ca^{2+} transient causes Ca^{2+}-induced inactivation and shortens the duration of the current, acting as a negative feedback and bringing influx and efflux in equilibrium [304]. The rise in SR Ca^{2+} load and increased systolic Ca^{2+} release also causes activation of i_{Cl}; it stimulates PKC, which may be responsible for a rise in i_{Kr} and Na^+ pump current. All these processes help to shorten the action potential duration.

1.3   Changes of the rate-dependence in pathology

In **atrial fibrillation** the normal shortening of the atrial APD at higher rates is absent or even reversed (see Chapter IX). The underlying phenomenon for this reversion is electrical remodeling of i_{CaL}. In atrial cells i_{to} and i_{CaL} play an important role in determining the APD. With development of atrial fibrillation, i_{CaL} and i_{to} are both reduced, the shortening of the APD essentially being due to the reduction in i_{CaL}. The absence of time-dependent currents showing activation-inactivation gating seems to be at the basis of the frequency-independence of APD in this condition.

The opposite change occurs in chronic **hypertrophy** and this has been shown in animal models as well as in the human [1150]: the frequency-dependence of APD of ventricular cells becomes steeper in hypertrophy, with action potential prolongation especially pronounced at low frequencies. Such prolongation results frequently in EADs and arrhythmias of the torsade de pointes type (TdP), and an increased risk of sudden death. Mechanisms responsible for this effect are reduced outward currents, i_{to} and more importantly i_{Kr} and i_{Ks}. Upregulation of the Na^+/Ca^{2+} exchanger also plays an important role and its contribution to the prolongation of the APD becomes more evident in heart failure [1052].

QT-RR relationships are also steeper in **congenital LQTs** and the heart shows a greater susceptibility to arrhythmias. In the congenital LQT1 and LQT2 syndromes changes in i_{Ks}, respectively i_{Kr} similar to hypertrophy are present. **Drug-induced LQTs** are caused by block of i_{Kr} and thus can be compared to LQT2. In LQT3 a persistent Na^+ current during the plateau is responsible for the prolongation of the APD especially at low frequencies. At higher rates, some inactivation of the "persistent" current and i_{Ks} summation will act in the opposite way on the APD.

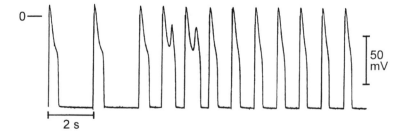

Figure V.7. Acceleration-induced early afterdepolarisation accompanied by transient prolongation of the action potential in the M region of a canine left ventricle, pretreated with E-4031, a i_{Kr} blocker. Basic cycle length was decreased from 2 s to 1 s. Modified from [124].

Sudden acceleration can cause an initial prolongation of the APD in species characterised by a pronounced i_{to} with slow recovery kinetics (e.g.

rabbit). This prolongation however is rapidly followed by a shortening. A prolongation which is present for many beats up to several seconds has been described in preparations treated with i_{Kr} blockers (Fig. V.7) [124] and in a congenital LQT3 mouse model [815] (see Chapter VIII). The prolongation of the action potential is accompanied by the generation of EADs and TdP arrhythmia. In preparations treated with i_{Kr} blockers, generation of extra Na^+/Ca^{2+} exchange current as a consequence of Ca^{2+} overload has been proposed to be responsible. In accord with this explanation it was found that the lengthening of the action potential and the accompanying EADs disappeared following treatment with ryanodine, a blocker of the Ca^{2+} release mechanism in the SR [124].

An explanation of the prolongation of the APD upon sudden acceleration in the LQT3 mouse model can be given along the same lines. The LQT3 mouse model is characterised by the existence of an increased peak Na^+ current and of a slowly inactivating Na^+ current during the plateau, which may cause a rise in $[Na^+]_i$ and consequently result in Ca^{2+} overload. Ca^{2+} overload causes extra stimulation of the Na^+/Ca^{2+} exchanger and eventually potentiation of the i_{CaL} via enhanced Ca^{2+}-dependent phosphorylation [1300]. Another explanation is some type of potentiation of the slow Na^+ current itself. The mutated channel shows an increased probability to enter a bursting mode and to stay for some time in this mode. When the stimulation rate increases, accumulation of channels in the bursting mode will enhance the slow Na^+ current, prolong the APD and promote the appearance of EADs [182].

2.   MODULATION OF ELECTRICAL ACTIVITY BY NEUROTRANSMITTERS, HUMORAL, AUTOCRINE AND PARACRINE FACTORS, HORMONES

2.1   Modulation by autonomic neurotransmitters

2.1.1   Sympathetic stimulation

Sympathetic stimulation causes release of noradrenaline (NA) and adrenaline. Acetylcholine (ACh) is the neurotransmitter of the parasympathetic system. At the prejunctional level, the sympathetic and parasympathetic neurones are interconnected, with each system exerting a negative effect on the other. It is also important to realise that activation or sensitisation of the sympathetic or parasympathetic system is possible secondary to the interaction with other neurotransmitters, autocrine and paracrine factors and hormones. Angiotensin for instance stimulates the release of NA from the sympathetic system and at the same time inhibits the secretion of ACh. Bradykinin also enhances NA release. Atrial natriuretic peptide has the opposite effects. Thyroid hormone sensitises cardiomyocytes for NA by upregulation of the number of β-receptors and the levels of G_{sa} proteins.

In this section we will describe the acute electrophysiological effects of the neurotransmitters released from the sympathetic and parasympathetic system. During recent years it has become evident that the same molecules also exert mid-term and long-term effects on ion channels, receptors and structural molecules. These processes are important during the normal development and play a role in the remodeling process that occurs in certain disease states (see Chapter IX). From clinical experience with β-receptor blockers it is evident that β-receptor stimulation exerts long-term effects. These effects consist in changes of the density of channels (e.g. gap junctions), of the receptors themselves and/or of the coupling to the effectors. α-receptor stimulation in a similar way has been implied in growth and adaptive processes in myocardial infarction. The pathways involved however are far from clarified and information remains incomplete (see Chapter IX).

In the heart noradrenaline (secreted by sympathetic nerves) and adrenaline (released by the adrenal medulla) bind to different types of receptors. One distinguishes α- and β-receptors which are further subdivided in α1A-, α1B-, α2-, β1-, β2- and β3 types [323]. About 80% of the α-receptors are of the α1B-type. In the heart of primates and man the ratio of β-/α-receptors is 2.5 and the β-effect is the most important physiological mechanism [1098]. The relative importance of the two receptor systems changes with development and in pathological situations such as ischaemia and hypertrophy.

2.1.1.1 β-receptor stimulation
2.1.1.1.1 β-receptors and transduction to effectors

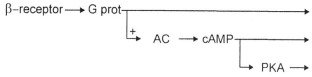

Figure V.8. Coupling between β-receptors and effectors.

For β1-receptors three types of coupling with ascending complexity have been described (Fig. V.8). In its simplest way, the receptor is coupled to the effector directly via a G_s protein (e.g. i_{CaL} [1036]), in a second type the coupling occurs via cAMP binding to the channel (e.g. i_f [261]) and in a third type the effector is phosphorylated by PKA, and probably other kinases (many channels). The most frequent coupling is via PKA-dependent phosphorylation. At the channel level, β 1-receptor activation results in stimulation of a number of currents (i_{CaL}, i_f, i_{st}, i_{Kr}, i_{Ks}, i_{Kur}, $i_{K.ATP}$, i_{Cl}, i_{gap}, $i_{Ca.RyR}$), while only a few show reduced activity (i_{to}, i_{K1}) [for references see 145].

β 2-receptors are also coupled to adenylate cyclase and PKA [1054]; however there is increasing evidence for an cAMP-independent modulation by β 2-receptors of the chronotropic and inotropic effect. Stimulation of β 2-receptors may become more important in failing and aged hearts, where β 1-receptors are downregulated and their coupling to the effectors less efficient.

2.1.1.1.2   Electrophysiological aspects of β -receptor stimulation

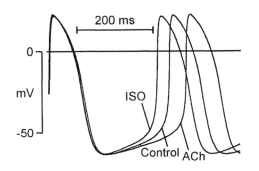

Figure V.9. Action potentials recorded from a rabbit single SAN myocyte in control solution and during perfusion with isoproterenol (ISO) (0.1 μM) or acetylcholine (ACh) (0.03 μM). Modified from [256].

Electrophysiologically the result of β-receptor stimulation is enhancement of sinus pacemaker frequency (Fig. V.9) secondary to an enhanced rate of diastolic depolarisation and a shortening of the systolic period [116], faster conduction in the AVN, elevation of the plateau level and mostly shortening of the action potential duration in atrial and ventricular cells [555] (Fig. V.10). In all cells excessive stimulation of β -receptors favours the appearance of spontaneous diastolic depolarisation and genesis of triggered activity.

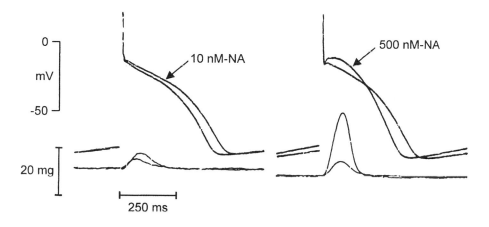

Figure V.10. Concentration-dependent actions of noradrenaline on the action potential and twitch tension of a calf Purkinje fibre. Prolongation occurs at low and shortening at high concentrations of NA. Modified from [555].

2.1.1.1.2.1 Enhanced automatism in the sinoatrial node

> Systole shortened:
> i_{Kr}, i_{Ks} increased
>
> Higher rate of diastolic depolarisation:
>   larger deactivation of i_{Kr} and i_{Ks}
>   earlier and faster activation of i_f during final repolarisation
>   larger inward current through i_{st}, i_{CaT} and i_{CaL}

The faster diastolic depolarisation in SAN cells is due to a number of changes (see box): Stimulation of the delayed K$^+$ current has two consequences: first, it causes shortening of the action potential, second, more outward current is deactivated during diastole, resulting in faster depolarisation. Deactivation of outward current (i_{Kr}) in combination with an increased sustained Na$^+$ inward current (i_{st}) and an earlier and faster activation of i_f current are responsible for a faster initial diastolic depolarisation. Later during diastole, depolarisation is further accelerated by the enhanced T-type and L-type Ca^{2+} currents.

i_{Kr} and i_{Ks} are enhanced by β-receptor stimulation; i_{Ks} via PKA-dependent phosphorylation [631] and i_{Kr} secondary to the rise in [Ca^{2+}]$_i$ and activation of PKC [434].

A shift of the activation curve of the i_f current in the positive direction [255,883] is caused by cAMP directly interfering with the channel in the SAN and by PKA-dependent phosphorylation in the Purkinje system.

Phosphorylation of the L-type Ca^{2+} channel [see 726] is responsible for the increase of the open probability during a depolarisation as well as of the number of functional channels. A direct effect of β -receptor stimulation on the T-type Ca^{2+} current has not been demonstrated but a facilitatory effect is possible secondary to the increase in $[Ca^{2+}]_i$ [1156].

2.1.1.1.2.2 Improved conduction through the atrioventricular node

Faster conduction of the impulse is primarily due to the enhancement of the L-type Ca^{2+} current, and secondarily to a better coupling between cells, following phosphorylation of the gap junction channel protein by PKA [954].

2.1.1.1.2.3 Change in action potential duration in atria and ventricles

The increase in i_{CaL} would normally prolong the action potential duration in atrial and ventricular cells, and this occurs at low concentrations (Fig. V.10). More i_{CaL} means also more elevated plateau. This larger depolarisation allows for greater activation of the two delayed K^+ currents, i_{Kr} and i_{Ks}, which are already increased in their conductance by β -receptor stimulation [555]. Stimulation of the Na^+ pump will further enhance the rate of repolarisation. The final effect is a higher plateau and shorter APD. During ischaemia, β -receptor stimulation causes activation of the $i_{K.ATP}$ and extra shortening of the action potential. Indeed, β -receptor activation stimulates extra consumption of subsarcolemmal ATP via stimulation of the Na^+/K^+ pump and cAMP synthesis and causes consequent ATP depletion.

2.1.1.1.2.4 Increased automatism in atrial and ventricular cells and generation of Ca^{2+}-mediated action potentials

Two different mechanisms can operate in atrial and ventricular cells to generate spontaneous activity in the presence of β -receptor stimulation: activation of i_f current and facilitation of triggered activity. The i_f current is present in Purkinje cells [132] but also in plain atrial [883] and ventricular cells [157,471]. In ventricular cells the threshold for activation is normally too negative. Remodeling however may cause a shift in the positive direction. Since β -receptor stimulation causes a further shift, threshold may be reached at the resting potential.

The second mechanism is triggered activity and is favoured by the Ca^{2+} overload which accompanies excessive β -receptor stimulation: Ca^{2+} influx is increased via the L-type Ca^{2+} channel and the amount of Ca^{2+} stored in the SR is enhanced by stimulation of the Ca^{2+} ATPase, secondary to phospholamban phosphorylation [see 547]. It is known that high SR Ca^{2+} content may result in spontaneous release of Ca^{2+} and genesis of DADs or EADs. Spontaneous release of Ca^{2+} is furthermore facilitated by hyperphosphorylation of the RyR, which causes leaky release channels as shown in heart failure [707].

The probability of arrhythmias can furthermore be enhanced by generation of slowly conducting action potentials. In depolarised cells, e.g. during ischaemia in the presence of increased $[K^+]_e$, enhancement of the Ca^{2+} current by catecholamines may generate Ca^{2+}-dependent action potentials [149]. Propagation of these action potentials is slow and creates conditions favourable for reentry.

2.1.1.2 α-receptor stimulation
2.1.1.2.1 α-receptors and transduction to effectors

Most of the α-receptors are of α1-type. Activation results in stimulation of different phospholipases [323]: PLC, PLD and PLA2. PLC activation which is the most important mechanism, increases turnover of inositol phospholipids and leads to formation of IP3 and DAG. DAG, also formed via PLD, in turn activates PKC. A different pathway is followed in PLA2 stimulation; it causes an increase in lysophospholipids and arachidonic acid (AA) with subsequent formation of leukotrienes; leukotrienes in turn may again activate PKC (Fig. V.11).

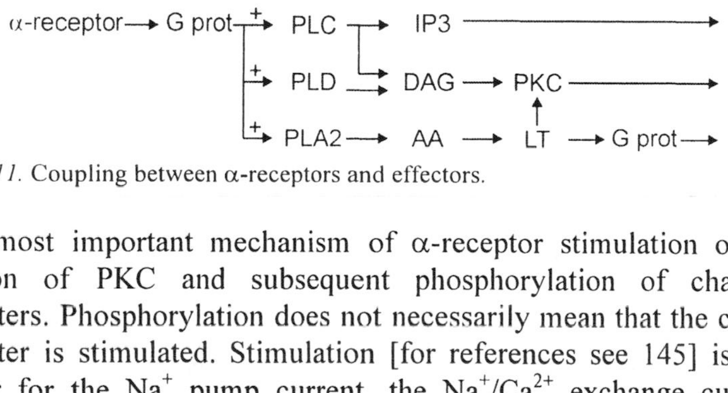

Figure V.11. Coupling between α-receptors and effectors.

The most important mechanism of α-receptor stimulation occurs via activation of PKC and subsequent phosphorylation of channels or transporters. Phosphorylation does not necessarily mean that the channel or transporter is stimulated. Stimulation [for references see 145] is the case however for the Na^+ pump current, the Na^+/Ca^{2+} exchange current and Na^+/H^+ transporter and has also been described for i_{CaT} and $i_{K.ATP}$. Inhibition occurs for i_{Na}, i_{K1}, i_{to}, i_{Kur} and gap junction channels. The effect on i_{CaL} and i_{Ks} is variable and species-dependent. Apart from PKC effects, the generated IP3 may cause a release Ca^{2+} from IP3-sensitive stores, while AA and leukotrienes can directly activate channels carrying outward current (e.g. $i_{K.AA}$ and $i_{K.ACh}$).

α2-receptors are negatively coupled to adenylate cyclase or positively coupled to a calmodulin-activated phosphodiesterase. In both instances activation leads to a decrease of cAMP. α2-receptor stimulation has thus opposite effects to that of β1-receptor stimulation.

> α-receptor activation results in
>   stimulation of transporters: Na⁺/K⁺ ATPase
>   Na⁺/Ca²⁺ exchanger
>   Na⁺/H⁺ exchanger
>   of currents: $i_{K.ATP}$, i_{CaT}
>   inhibition of i_{Na}, i_{to}, i_{Kur}, i_{K1}, i_{gap}

2.1.1.2.2   Electrophysiological aspects of α-receptor stimulation

2.1.1.2.2.1 Resting membrane potential and automaticity

α-receptor stimulation may cause depolarisation as well as hyperpolarisation of the resting potential. The reason is that two outward currents, which are important for determining the resting potential, are affected in opposite ways: pump current is increased but i_{K1} is inhibited.

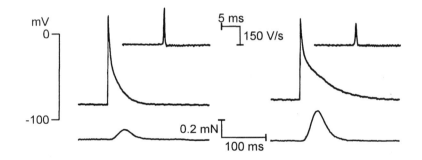

Figure V.12. Influence of phenylephrine (100 μM) (right) on action potential and upstroke velocity (upper traces), and force of contraction (lower trace), in the presence of β -receptor blockade. Note increase in force, prolongation of the action potential and decrease in maximum diastolic potential. Rat atrial preparation [510].

Depending on the relative contribution of these two currents the maximum resting potential may thus be increased (e.g. rat ventricle) or decreased (rat atrium) [311]. In Purkinje fibres a similar situation occurs with respect to promotion or inhibition of spontaneous activity; in younger animals the inhibition of i_{K1} seems to prevail and an increase of automaticity is the rule [933].

2.1.1.2.2.2 Action potential duration and triggered activity

In general the action potential is prolonged by α-receptor stimulation (Fig. V.12) [see323]. The underlying mechanisms are block of i_{to}, i_{Kur} and i_{K1}. The effect however, may show regional differences: in canine M cells the action potential is shortened, in contrast to the lengthening in epicardial, endocardial and Purkinje cells [125]. Slowing of repolarisation is often accompanied by the appearance of EADs. The effect on DADs is variable but in most cases they are potentiated. The mechanism is not clear but is probably related to the action potential prolongation which promotes Ca^{2+} load [330]. If Ca^{2+} overload is caused by Na^+ pump inhibition, DADs are reduced by the stimulatory influence on the pump.

The arrhythmogenic activity of α-receptor stimulation is especially pronounced in ischaemia and upon reperfusion. The density of α-receptors relative to β-receptors is increased in ischaemia-reperfusion and in heart failure. Following a first phase in which both receptors show an increased density (see Chapter VII), α-receptors become dominant. This is the result of a netto reduction in the number of β-receptors and a decrease in sensitivity towards transmitters following phosphorylation by receptor-kinase.

2.1.2 Parasympathetic stimulation

2.1.2.1 Acetylcholine and transduction to receptors
The effect of acetylcholine occurs mainly via stimulation of M2-receptors. They are linked to the effector in more than one way (Fig. V.13) [for references see 145]. The simplest way is a direct connection between a G protein and the channel protein as is the case for $i_{K.ACh}$ [503]. $i_{K.ACh}$ is well expressed in the SAN, AVN, atria but is also present in Purkinje and ventricular cells of certain species, including human.

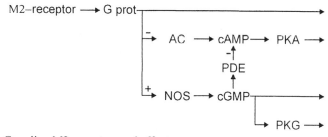

Figure V.13. Coupling M2-receptors and effectors.

Indirect inhibitory effects are caused by suppression of adenylate cyclase or by activation of nitric oxide synthetase (NOS). Activation of NOS results in a fall of cAMP and reduced phosphorylation by PKA or a rise in cGMP and increased phosphorylation by PKG. The final result is inhibition of i_{CaL}, i_f, i_{Cl} and the gap-junction channel conductance. Withdrawal of acetylcholine in the presence of β-receptor stimulation causes transient increases in i_{CaL} (accentuated antagonism).

M1-receptors are present in some species and are coupled to phospholipase and secondarily to PKC. They play a role in mediating the effect of ACh on the K.ATP channel activation and are responsible for some stimulatory effects at high concentrations [1006]; they seem to be absent however in the human [439].

2.1.2.2   Electrophysiological aspects of muscarinic receptor stimulation

In general, the effects of muscarinic receptor stimulation are opposite to those of β-receptor stimulation, but exceptions to this rule exist. M2-receptor stimulation by ACh results in slowing of the rate of diastolic depolarisation in pacemaker cells and reduction of frequency (Fig. V.9), slowing of AVN conduction, hyperpolarisation or stabilisation of the resting membrane potential, shortening of the action potential, inhibition of EADs and DADs [71,1065].

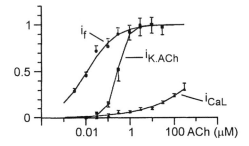

Figure V.14. Dose-response curves for i_f (shift of the activation curve), $i_{K.ACh}$ (steady-state current) and i_{CaL} (peak current) against ACh concentration, normalised to the maximum. Modified from [256].

In the SAN the rate is slowed and pacemaker shifts may occur. In AVN cells the upstroke of the action potential is inhibited resulting in conduction slowing or block. In clinical context, this blocking effect can be used to suppress paroxysmal supraventricular tachycardia [264]. The electrophysiological changes are the result of inhibition of i_{CaL} and i_f current, and activation of $i_{K.ACh}$ current.

L-type Ca^{2+} current is reduced by a decrease in the number of functional channels and a fall in open probability [898]. The i_f activation curve is shifted in the negative direction. This latter effect occurs at concentrations much smaller (K_d 20 nM) than required to open the K.ACh channel (0.5 μM) [257] or to inhibit i_{CaL} [1342] (Fig. V.14).

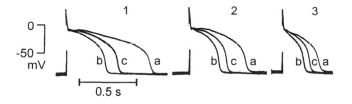

Figure V.15. Effect of ACh 10^{-6} M on the action potential of rabbit Purkinje fibres at three different rates of stimulation (0.2, 1 and 2 Hz, from left to right). a: control, b and c in the presence of ACh for 45 s and for 5 min (or steady-state); note desensitisation from b to c. Modified from [765].

In cells that express K.ACh channels, ACh induces hyperpolarisation and shortens the action potential duration (Fig. V.15). Both phenomena show desensitisation. As an antiadrenergic agent, acetylcholine suppresses catecholamine-induced early (EAD) and delayed afterdepolarisations (DAD) [1065] and thus acts as an antiarrhythmic. Antagonism for EADs is based on the inhibition of i_{CaL} and stimulation of outward K^+ current, thus preventing reactivation of i_{CaL} during the plateau. The same changes in currents are responsible for a decrease in Ca^{2+} load, for hyperpolarisation or stabilisation of the resting membrane potential and for inhibition of DADs.

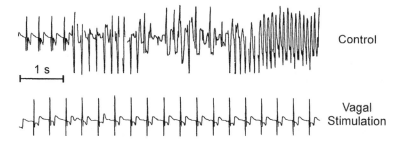

Figure V.16. ECG recordings in a conscious dog subjected to an exercise test and coronary occlusion for 70 s. Upper trace: ventricular tachycardia and fibrillation occurred in the control test. Lower trace: no arrhythmia occurred when vagal stimulation was applied during the occlusion. Modified from [1191].

Stimulation of M2-receptors reduces the occurrence of ventricular fibrillation in acute ischaemia and exerts a protective effect on reperfusion arrhythmias [1358] (Fig. V.16). The cardioprotective and stabilising activity of ACh is also evident from the fact that withdrawal of acetylcholine in the presence of increased adrenergic activity causes excessive lengthening of the action potential duration and induces delayed afterdepolarisations and spontaneous activity [1247]. In atrial cells, where the density of M2-

receptors is high, excessive shortening of the ERP may however favour reentry and lead to AF.

In contrast to the stabilising effects described above, excessively high concentrations of ACh induce a TTX-insensitive Na^+ current [718], with consequent rise in $[Na^+]_i$ and $[Ca^{2+}]_i$, and enhancement of Ca^{2+} transients and contraction [891].

2.2   Modulation by humoral factors

2.2.1   Purinergic receptor stimulation

Two types of purinergic receptors are present in the heart, P1 and P2, activated respectively by extracellular adenosine and ATP {Vassort, 2001 #4913}.

2.2.1.1   Adenosine
2.2.1.1.1   Release of adenosine, receptors and transduction to effectors

Adenosine is generated either intracellularly or extracellularly. Extracellularly it is formed from ATP under the influence of ecto-nucleotidases. In the cell it is normally formed from AMP under the action of 5'nucleotidase; this reaction is rapidly reversed under the influence of adenosine kinase. The breakdown and immediate reversal of the reaction seems to constitute a futile cycle but has the advantage to act as a fast signaling metabolic pathway in case of hypoxia. When oxygen tension is reduced below a critical threshold adenosine kinase becomes inhibited, adenosine genesis is amplified and adenosine is released from the cell. The high concentration reached, permits rapid vasodilation which counteracts the hypoxic stimulus {Decking, 1997 #3021}.

In the heart adenosine stimulates the A1-receptor, which is one of the four subtypes of P1-receptors. A1-receptors are linked to the effector in ways that to a certain extent are similar to the M2-receptors (Fig. V.17). A first possibility is a direct connection between a G protein and the channel protein. Similarly to ACh, adenylate cyclase is inhibited and NOS activated (see Fig. V.13). A supplementary indirect pathway connects the adenosine receptor to the activation of phospholipases and subsequently of PKC. This pathway is responsible for the activation of $i_{K.ATP}$ during preconditioning {Liu, 1996 #1630}.

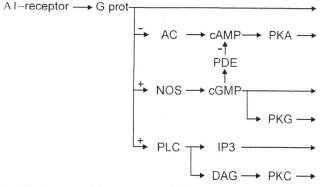

Figure V.17. Coupling between A1-receptors and effectors.

2.2.1.1.2 Electrophysiological effects of adenosine

To a certain extent the effects of adenosine and acetylcholine are comparable: hyperpolarisation of the diastolic membrane potential and shortening of the action potential, slowing of the rate of diastolic depolarisation in pacemaker cells, inhibition of EADs and DADs [71,1065]. The effect on ventricular action potential is species-dependent (Fig. V.18).

The electrophysiological changes are the result of K^+ current activation ($i_{K.ACh}$ and/or $i_{K.ATP}$) and inhibition of i_{CaL}, i_f and i_{Cl} current (see ACh). Of special importance is the effect of adenosine on the AVN. In AVN cells the action potential is inhibited resulting in conduction slowing or block. In clinical context, this blocking effect is used to suppress paroxysmal supraventricular tachycardia [264].

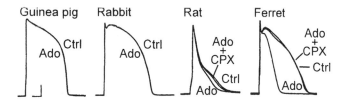

Figure V.18. Effect of adenosine (Ado 100 μM) on ventricular action potentials of different species. Ctrl: control records; CPX: selective A1 antagonist (8-cyclopentyl-1,3-dipropylxanthine). Calibration bar represents 20 ms and 20 mV for rat, and 50 ms and 20 mV for other species. Modified from [1064].

Adenosine should be considered a cardioprotective and stabilising agent. Mice overexpressing A1-receptors show an increased resistance against ischaemia evidenced by a longer delay to develop contractures and improved functional recovery upon reperfusion [713].

As an antiadrenergic agent adenosine suppresses catecholamine-induced early and late afterdepolarisations [1065]. This effect may play an antiarrhythmic role during ischaemia and reperfusion.

2.2.1.2   Extracellular [ATP]
2.2.1.2.1   Release of ATP, receptors and transduction to effectors

Extracellular ATP is generated from two sources: i) sympathetic nerve endings secrete ATP upon electrical stimulation together with noradrenaline; ii) as a metabolite ATP is released from cardiac cells exposed to hypoxia [240], from activated platelets, endothelial cells, smooth muscle cells and inflammatory cells [1195]. In the extracellular space the concentration of ATP may transiently reach the micromolar range and induce multiple functional changes in cardiac cells [see review 1195]. The time of action is limited because it is rapidly degraded to ADP, AMP and adenosine by ecto-nucleotidases.

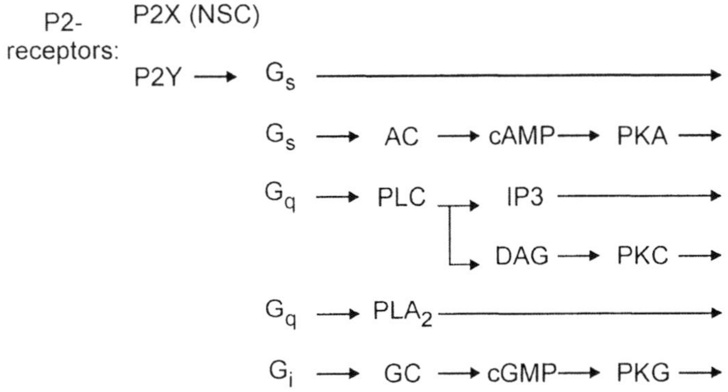

P2-   P2X (NSC)
receptors:
$\qquad$ P2Y $\longrightarrow$ G_s $\longrightarrow$

$\qquad\qquad\qquad$ G_s $\longrightarrow$ AC $\longrightarrow$ cAMP $\longrightarrow$ PKA $\longrightarrow$

$\qquad\qquad\qquad$ G_q $\longrightarrow$ PLC $\longrightarrow$ IP3 $\longrightarrow$
$\qquad\qquad\qquad\qquad\qquad\qquad\quad$ DAG $\longrightarrow$ PKC $\longrightarrow$

$\qquad\qquad\qquad$ G_q $\longrightarrow$ PLA$_2$ $\longrightarrow$

$\qquad\qquad\qquad$ G_i $\longrightarrow$ GC $\longrightarrow$ cGMP $\longrightarrow$ PKG $\longrightarrow$

Figure V.19. Coupling of P2-receptors with effectors.

ATP binds to specific P2-receptors (Fig. V.19). Distinction is made between ionotropic P2X-receptors, which are actually ligand-gated non-selective ion channels and metabotropic P2Y-receptors or G protein-coupled receptors. P2Y-receptors have been shown to be linked via a stimulatory G_s protein directly to the i_{CaL}, $i_{K.ACh}$ and i_{Ks} channels or activate indirectly i_{CaL} and i_{Cl} via activation of adenylate cyclase or PLC. The final result is a substantial increase in $[Ca^{2+}]_i$ and a positive inotropic effect. This rise in $[Ca^{2+}]_i$ may stimulate Ca^{2+}_i-dependent processes (e.g. increase of i_{CaT} [484] or i_{Ks} [1149]). In the ferret ATP inhibits i_{CaL}, [897] an effect that has been proposed to occur via the cGMP and PKG pathway [1195]. Whereas most of the activated currents are inward, stimulation of AC during ischaemia when the cell is already depleted of high-energy compounds may cause a further fall of ATP, activate $i_{K.ATP}$ and generate outward current [41].

2.2.1.2.2 Electrophysiological effects of extracellular ATP

Changes in electrophysiologic properties caused by extracellular ATP are different in normal and under ischaemic conditions. In normal conditions the overall initial effect of extracellular ATP in most preparations is depolarisation of the resting potential and prolongation of the action potential (Fig. V.20), except in the ferret ventricle where opposite changes are observed. The underlying mechanisms are activation of inward currents, more specifically i_{NSC}, i_{Cl} (fall in resting potential), and stimulation of i_{CaT} and i_{CaL} (prolongation of action potential). The depolarisation may be conducive to the generation of spontaneous activity and arrhythmias [1195,1197].

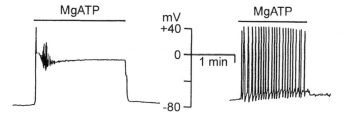

Figure V.20. Application of 10 µM MgATP to rat ventricular myocytes induces either sustained depolarisation or spiking. Modified from [1198].

In ischaemic conditions, with cells partly depleted of [ATP], stimulation of adenylate cyclase may further deplete local subsarcolemmal [ATP] and activate $I_{K.ATP}$ [41]. This will lead to hyperpolarisation and shortening of the action potential. Extracellular ATP may thus cause changes that are opposite in healthy tissue and in ischaemic cells. In vivo the effect is of short duration, because ATP is rapidly broken down to adenosine.

2.2.2 Histamine, serotonin and vasoactive intestinal peptide

Histamine, serotonin (5-hydroxytryptamine, 5-HT) and vasoactive intestinal peptide (VIP) have a common mode of action; they stimulate adenylate cyclase (AC) and secondarily activate PKA.

2.2.2.1 Histamine

Histamine acts as a neurotransmitter in histaminergic nerves of the hypothalamus and is produced in specific endocrine cells in the gastric tubular glands. In the heart it is present in mast cells and is released in immunological reactions [423,885].

2.2.2.1.1   Receptors and transduction to effectors

Histamine interacts with two types of receptors, H1 and H2. Both are present in heart cells but H2 is the most important. The distribution as well as the effects of both are somewhat comparable to that of α- and β- receptors of the sympathetic system [1144]. H3-receptors are present in sympathetic nerve endings and their activation leads to inhibition of noradrenaline release [697].

Activation of H2-receptors causes an increase of cAMP, activation of PKA [730]and stimulation of i_{CaL}, i_{Ks}, i_{Cl} and Na^+/K^+ pump current [637,1316]. The coupling of H1-receptors is less analysed; some evidence points to an intermediary activation of PKC. Such a mechanism may be responsible for the inhibition i_{to} and i_{K1} and stimulation of i_{Ks} in atrial cells.

2.2.2.1.2   Electrophysiological effects

Stimulation of H2-receptors results in positive chronotropic, dromotropic and inotropic effects. Increase in heart rate is due to stimulation of i_f, i_{CaL} and i_{Ks} currents. The action potential plateau is elevated and shortened consequent to the simultaneous stimulation of inward i_{CaL} current and outward currents through i_{Ks}, $i_{Na/K}$ and i_{Cl}. Conduction through the AVN is accelerated, and seen as a shortening of PR interval in the ECG [636].

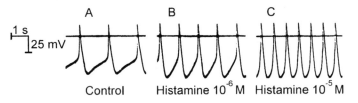

Figure V.21. Effects of histamine at 10^{-6} and 10^{-5} M on spontaneous action potentials in human right atrial fibre. Modified from [636].

Histamine has pronounced arrhythmogenic effects. Automaticity is induced or enhanced (Fig. V.21) in atria [636] or Purkinje fibres [156]. DADs are generated [1144] or enhanced [156]. In K^+-depolarised atria and ventricles Ca^{2+}-mediated action potentials are induced [730].

Dangerous side-effects at the electrophysiological level have been described for drugs interacting with histamine-receptors or their metabolism. H1-antagonists are widely used for allergic conditions, but a number of them also strongly block i_{Kr} in heart [see 143], which may lead to dangerous torsade de pointes arrhythmias.

2.2.2.2   Serotonin
2.2.2.2.1   Receptors and transduction to effectors
Most of the serotonin or 5-HT is found in the gastrointestinal tract and more specifically the enterochromaffin cells, in platelets and the CNS. The serotonin content in platelets is of special importance for the heart since it is released and can act on myocardial cells when platelets are activated.

The 5-HT4-receptor, which is the most important hydroxytryptamine receptor in heart, is not widely distributed but is present in the human atrium [735]. The receptors are positively coupled to AC and enhance i_{CaL} [511] and i_f [867].

2.2.2.2.2   Electrophysiological effects
Stimulation of 5-HT4-receptors result in positive chronotropic, dromotropic and inotropic effects, similar to those of histamine.

Dangerous side-effects at the electrophysiologic level have been described for drugs interacting with 5-HT-receptors or their metabolism. 5-HT-antagonists like ketanserin and cisapride prolong the APD, slow heart rate and may lead to TdP arrhythmias. These effects are not related to receptor activation.

Drugs that block the reuptake of serotonin are frequently used as antidepressant agents. These agents (e.g. fluoxetine) have important blocking effects on i_{CaL}, i_{Na} and i_{to} [836] and may cause serious rhythm disturbances.

2.2.2.3   Vaso-intestinal peptide
VIP, first discovered as a gastrointestinal hormone, is coreleased with ACh from vagal nerves, especially after excessive stimulation of the vagal system. It exerts important vasodilator effects.

2.2.2.3.1   Receptors and transduction to effectors
Activation of VIP1-receptors results in activation of AC resulting in stimulation of cAMP synthesis and positive effects on i_{CaL} [413,1146] and i_f in the SAN [3] and in the Purkinje system [164]. The corelease with ACh can be considered as a negative feedback and as safety factor in cases of excessive vagal activity [447,1037].

2.2.2.3.2   Electrophysiological effects
Stimulation of VIP1-receptors results in positive chronotropic, dromotropic and inotropic effects, similar to those of histamine. It is co-released with ACh during vagal stimulation and most probably responsible for the postvagal tachycardia [447]. Similar arrhythmogenic effects as for histamine may be expected to occur but information is not available.

2.3   Modulation by autocrine and paracrine factors: angiotensin, endothelin, atrial natriuretic peptide, bradykinin and thrombin

Endothelin, angiotensin, natriuretic peptide and bradykinin are produced mainly in the endothelium but also in cardiac myocytes. They have in common that synthesis and release are promoted in certain pathophysiological stress situations, such as pressure or volume overload, myocardial ischaemia [119], high frequency pacing, atrial fibrillation [1280], sympathetic stimulation [55], and Ca^{2+} overload [130]. Thrombin is a serine protease that normally is not present in the blood but formed in the final step during blood clotting.

2.3.1   Angiotensin

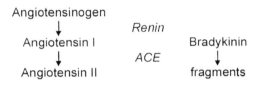

Figure V.22. Metabolism of angiotensin and bradykinin. Enzymes involved in italics.

Angiotensin II (Ang II) is formed from angiotensin I under the action of angiotensin converting enzyme (ACE). It is the last link in the renin-angiotensin system. ACE responsible for the formation of Ang II also causes breakdown of bradykinin (Fig. V.22).

2.3.1.1   Receptor transduction to channels and transporters

Fig. V.23 illustrates the receptors and effectors involved in the effects of Ang II on cardiomyocytes. Among AT1- and AT2-receptors for Ang II the most important are AT1 [180]. AT2-receptors are present in the fetal stage, but less in the adult; in pathologic situations they are upregulated [234]. AT1-receptors on the other hand, are downregulated in hypertrophy and heart failure [905].

Ang II stimulates phospholipid metabolism via the PLC pathway and activates PKC. The effects on channels (e.g. inhibition of i_{to}) and transporters (e.g. increase of Na^+/H^+ exchange) are comparable to stimulation of α-receptors. The AT1-receptors are also negatively coupled by a G_i protein to AC. Inhibition of AC occurs in parallel with PLC activation and opposes the influence of excessive β-receptor activation (accentuated antagonism), as shown in the case of i_{CL}.

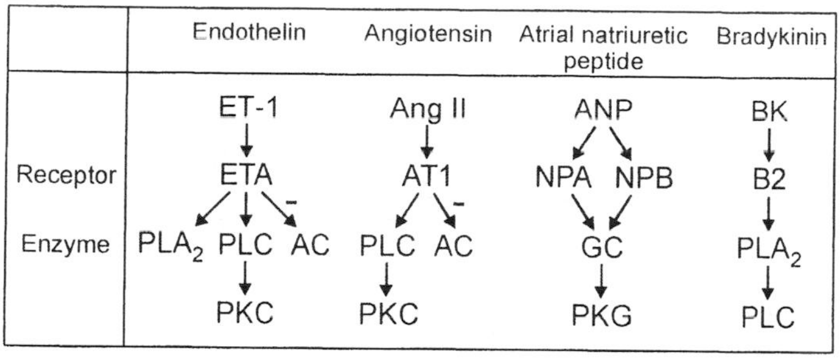

	Endothelin	Angiotensin	Atrial natriuretic peptide	Bradykinin
	ET-1 ↓	Ang II ↓	ANP ↗ ↘	BK ↓
Receptor	ETA ↗ ↓ ↘ —	AT1 ↗ ↘ —	NPA NPB ↘ ↙	B2 ↓
Enzyme	PLA$_2$ PLC AC ↓	PLC AC ↓	GC ↓	PLA$_2$ ↓
	PKC	PKC	PKG	PLC

Figure V.23. Coupling between receptors and effector-enzymes for endothelin, angiotensin, atrial natriuretic peptide and bradykinin in cardiac cells.

Ang II binds also to neuronal AT1-receptors and causes an intense release of NA from the endings of the sympathetic system and a concomitant inhibition of ACh secretion from the parasympathetic system. Since AC activity in the cardiomyocytes is simultaneously inhibited, the α-adrenergic effects of the sympathetic system will dominate.

2.3.1.2 Electrophysiological effects of angiotensin

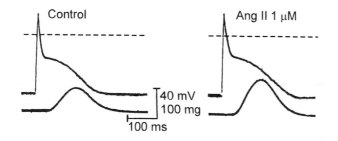

Figure V.24. Prolongation of the action potential and increase of twitch tension in rat ventricular myocytes following 10 min treatment with Ang II (1 µM). Modified from [1309].

The effect of angiotensin on the ventricular action potential is biphasic with an initial shortening, followed later by a lengthening [1309] (Fig. V.24). Ca^{2+}_i transients are increased [1256]. The action potential lengthening which is caused by block of i_{to} and i_{Ks} and activation of i_{Cl} [758], can be very pronounced and be accompanied by EADs. Similarly to adrenaline, Ang II can generate Ca^{2+}-mediated action potentials [349].

In animal models Ang II aggravates reperfusion arrhythmias, whereas ACE inhibitors protect against digoxin-induced and reperfusion-induced arrhythmias [349,655]. The effect of ACE inhibitors is due to a reduction of Ang II generation and a decrease of bradykinin degradation [655]. Consistent with the observations of improved Ca^{2+} influx, Ang II promotes

Cs-induced ventricular tachycardia and fibrillation [383]. On isolated cells exposed to ischaemic conditions, on the other hand, Ang II had no effect on the transient inward current (i_{ti}), which normally is responsible for DAD generation, but losartan, an ACE inhibitor reduced its incidence [679].

> Angiotensin: increased release of NA from nerve endings,
> decreased release of ACh from nerve endings
> Atrial natriuretic peptide: opposite effects of angiotensin

To understand the influence of Ang II on *in vivo* arrhythmias the increased release of adrenaline from the sympathetic system and the decreased secretion of ACh from the parasympathetic nerves [281] should be taken into account. The release of catecholamines from nerves and inhibition of ACh secretion has been shown to be due to angiotensin acting on neuronal AT1-receptors [281]. In animal models of ischaemia AT1-antagonists reduce NA overflow and the occurrence of ventricular fibrillation [709]. This indirect modulation is of special importance in myocardial infarction or heart failure [see 329] and explains the beneficial use of ACE inhibitors in those circumstances. In patients, ACE inhibitors reduce the concentration of plasma noradrenaline and increase sinus rate variability [431], indicative of a shift in favour of ACh over NA.

Ang II has pronounced effects on remodeling (see Chapter IX). It affects protein expression in myocardial cells and fibroblasts and causes adaptational changes during development, hypertension, atrial fibrillation and myocardial infarction. In cardiomyocytes important changes occur at the level of ionic channels. By reducing i_{to}, angiotensin treatment causes the typical notch of the subepicardial action potential to disappear, whereas treatment with a AT-1 antagonist generates a notch in the action potential of the subendocardial cell (Fig. V.25). These effects require hours to develop and are due to posttranslational changes of the channel protein, which affect primarily the recovery kinetics of the i_{to} current [1330]. During development of hypertension, angiotensin plays an important role in the long-term decrease of i_{to} and other K^+ currents, and the raised expression and kinetic changes of i_f. Use of AT1-receptor antagonists suppress this remodeling process [159]. In atrial fibrillation AT1-receptor activation is functionally important in the downregulation of i_{CaL} which is responsible for the shortening of ERP and its loss of rate adaptation. These changes are prevented by ACE inhibitors or AT1-antagonists [783].

In atrial fibrillation and also during the healing process of myocardial infarction, AT2-receptors are upregulated [375]. Activation of AT2-receptors plays a role in development and differentiation, induces apoptosis and inhibits growth [234]. Overactivity of AT2-receptors may thus be expected during the use of AT1-receptor antagonists but not during treatment with ACE inhibitors. From a therapeutic point of view different results in remodeling could be predicted for the use of the two drug types. In a comparative study (ELITE II) [875] of treatment with losartan, an AT1-antagonist, and captopril, an ACE-inhibitor (which prevents activation of both receptors), no definitive advantage for one of these treatments has been found however.

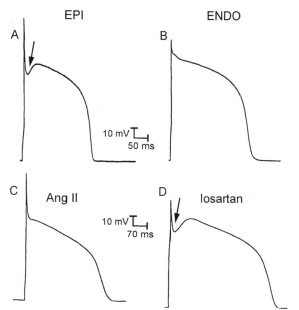

Figure V.25. Action potential from dog subepicardial (left) and subendocardial (right) ventricular cells under control conditions (A and B) or after pretreatment with angiotensin II (C) or losartan (D), an AT1-receptor antagonist. Arrow points at the notch in the repolarisation phase. Incubation with angiotensin II altered i_{to} in epicardial cells in such a way that their action potential resembles the endocardial type. Incubation of endocardial cells with losartan induced a phase 1 notch in the action potential. Modified from [1330].

Ang II not only affects the function of cardiomyocytes but has multiple effects on cardiac fibroblasts: it induces fibroblast proliferation, synthesis and secretion of adhesion molecules and extracellular matrix proteins, and expression of integrin adhesion receptors [985]. These processes are responsible for the fibrotic changes in the interstitial milieu associated with left ventricular hypertrophy, postmyocardial infarction remodeling and congestive heart failure.

2.3.2   Endothelin

2.3.2.1.1   Receptor transduction to channels and transporters

Among the three isoforms of endothelin, ET-1 is the most important for its effects on cardiac myocytes [1119]. The compound interacts with ETA-receptors [712] (Fig. V.23). ET-1 stimulates phospholipid metabolism via activation of PLA2 and PLC. The effects on channels (e.g. inhibition of i_{Kr} [690]) and transporters (e.g. increase of Na^+/H^+ exchange [550]) are comparable to stimulation of α-adrenergic receptors. ETA-receptors are also negatively coupled to AC by a G_i protein. Inhibition of AC occurs in parallel with PLC activation and opposes the influence of excessive β -adrenergic receptor activation (accentuated antagonism). The latter effect has been experimentally shown in the case of i_{CaL} [690] and i_{Ks} [1255].

Apart from its enzyme-mediated effects, endothelin binding to ETA-receptors activates $i_{K.ACh}$ directly via a stimulatory G protein (pertussis-toxin sensitive) [568]. However, when the channel is preactivated by a high concentration of ACh, ET-1 exerts inhibition via a pertussis-toxin insensitive pathway [1306] (Fig. V.26).

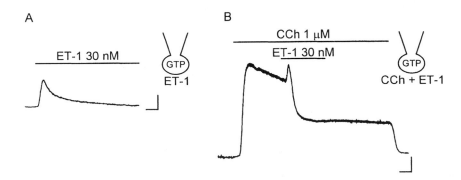

Figure V.26. Opposite effects of endothelin-1 (ET-1, 30 nM) on membrane currents of guinea pig atrial cells in the absence (A) and presence (B) of 1 μM of carbachol. Holding potential: -40 mV. Scale bars: 1 min and 100 pA. Modified from [1306].

2.3.2.1.2   Electrophysiological effects of endothelin

Negative as well as positive chronotropic effects have been described. Slowing of pacemaker activity is due to activation of $i_{K.ACh}$ [1306] and inhibition of i_f [1130]. This effect is accompanied by hyperpolarisation, shortening of the atrial action potential [1326] and slowing of AVN conduction [825]. The mechanism of positive chronotropy has not been analysed.

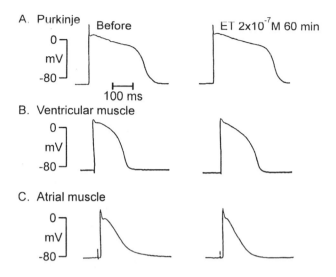

Figure V.27. Effects of endothelin-1 (ET) on action potentials recorded from Purkinje fibre, ventricular muscle and atrial muscle isolated from dog hearts. Pacing frequency: 1 Hz. Note prolongation of action potential in the Purkinje fibre and ventricular muscle, but shortening in the atrial preparation. Modified from [1326].

In contrast to the shortening of the atrial APD, the ventricular APD is lengthened [1326] (Fig. V.27), a result due to inhibition of i_{to} and the delayed i_K. QT prolongation in vivo can be accompanied by EADs and lead to arrhythmias [367,550]. Other factors involved in the arrhythmogenesis are: generation of IP3 and release of Ca^{2+} from intracellular stores, and induction of Na^+ and Ca^{2+} overload via stimulation of the Na^+/H^+ exchanger [see 295].

Endothelin is a very potent inotropic agent, an effect that has been correlated to the lengthening of the APD, enhanced Ca^{2+} influx and facilitated Ca^{2+} release. Ca^{2+} transients are increased. Direct measurements of i_{CaL} have yielded variable results depending on experimental conditions. An enhancing effect, following a short decrease, has been correlated to a PKC-mediated stimulation of Na^+/H^+ exchange and consequent intracellular alkalosis [1293] (Fig. V.28). i_{CaL} is indeed very sensitive to intracellular pH; alkalinisation furthermore increases the myofilament sensitivity to Ca^{2+} ions. Inhibition of i_{CaL} occurs when i_{CaL} is first augmented by β-receptor stimulation [1142]. The effect is due to suppression of AC activity via a G_i protein.

Interpretation of effects *in vivo* should take into consideration that ET-1 has pronounced vasoconstrictive effects on the coronary system, cause transient ischaemia and in that way, depress contraction and provoke arrhythmias.

Endothelin also plays a role in remodeling especially during cardiac hypertrophy and in heart failure [562]. The concentration of endothelin is increased in heart failure and blockage of the ETA-receptor exerts beneficial therapeutic effects [1284].

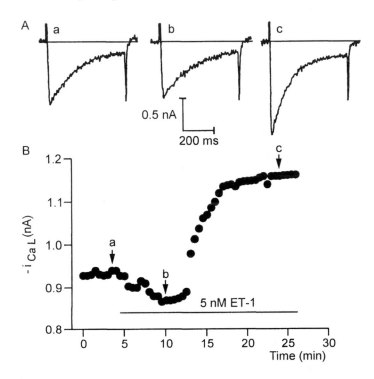

Figure V.28. Effects of endothelin-1 (ET-1) on i_{CaL} in a guinea pig ventricular myocyte. A: examples of i_{CaL} at times indicated in the lower graph. B: Time course of change in i_{CaL}: after a small decrease the current substantially increased. Horizontal bar: addition of endothelin. Modified from [1293].

2.3.3 Bradykinin

2.3.3.1 Receptors and transduction to effectors
Bradykinin (BK) is a nonapeptide released from kininogens; it is broken down by ACE (Fig. V.22). Its concentration is increased during ischaemia. Bradykinin-receptors in the heart are of the B2-type. Activation of myocyte receptors results in stimulation of PLA2 and secondarily of PLC, PKC and/or tyrosine kinase [962] (Fig. V.23). Receptors are also present on sensory [1002] and postganglionic [610,709,1003] sympathetic nerves and their activation leads to NA release.

2.3.3.2 Electrophysiological effects

Bradykinin applied to single atrial cells of the guinea pig causes an increase of i_{CaL} and a decrease of $i_{K.ACh}$. The effects are secondary to activation of PKC and/or tyrosinekinase [962] and lead to prolongation of the action potential. Lengthening of the action potential has also been seen in the rat [385].

In many studies BK has been shown to exert a positive chronotropic effect [651,678,962,1003]. The effect may be secondary to NA release by stimulation of BK2-receptors on sensory and postganglionic nerves [1002]. A direct effect however exists since an increase in rate is seen upon application of bradykinin to single atrial cells [962] and after application of β-receptor blockade [1138]. In a few studies a negative chronotropic effect [551,913] has been described and shown to be caused by stimulation of local cholinergic neurons [505].

It is not clear whether bradykinin's action should be considered arrhythmogenic or antiarrhythmic. As an adrenergic stimulans it could facilitate the genesis of arrhythmias. However, blockage of the breakdown of bradykinin by ACE inhibitors has been shown to be protective against ischaemia- and reperfusion-induced arrhythmias [444]. In this respect bradykinin's vasodilatatory action on the coronary system may be of primary importance. Less formation of Ang II also plays a role in this protection.

It is generally accepted that ACE inhibitors have beneficial effects in remodeling processes that occur in hypertension, myocardial ischaemia and heart failure. It is further evident that ACE inhibitors not only reduce the interference of Ang II but at the same time increase the concentration and the impact of bradykinin [466,849]. An enhancement of bradykinin formation by kallikrein gene delivery attenuates myocardial infarction and apoptosis upon reperfusion [1327]. Bradykinin prevents myocardial hypertrophy and ventricular dilatation in B2-receptor knockout mice [307]. Bradykinin also is one of the signaling pathways in the initiation of preconditioning [194,842].

2.3.4 Atrial natriuretic peptide

Among the natriuretic peptides three types are distinguished: brain natriuretic peptide (BNP), C-type or endothelium-derived natriuretic peptide (CNP) and atrial natriuretic peptide (ANP) [see 68]. Under normal conditions the ANP-type is synthesised and stored in the atria; under pathological conditions the concentration rises and the compound is released from the cells. In ischaemia [368] and heart failure [841] the peptide is also formed in the ventricle. Stretch and raised intracellular Ca^{2+} are initiators of the release phenomenon [130,635].

2.3.4.1   Receptor-effector transduction

ANP binds directly to NPA- and NPB-receptors on the cardiac myocyte. These receptors function as a membrane-bound guanylate cyclase, produce cGMP, activate PKG [189] (Fig. V.23) and inhibit i_{CaL} [622]. The receptor is also coupled to the i_{to} channel via an inhibitory G_i protein (human atrium [622]). A major effect occurs via inhibition of the sympathetic system and excitation of the parasympathetic system [189,1141].

2.3.4.2   Electrophysiological effects

ANP causes slowing of the pacemaker, hyperpolarisation of the resting membrane potential, shortening of the atrial action potential and slowing of AVN conduction. Catecholamine-induced action potentials are antagonized [189]. Consistent with this observation, ANP was found to inhibit Cs-induced arrhythmias [827]. The effect on ischaemia-induced arrhythmias is less clear and no change [1122] as well as inhibition of extrasystoles and ventricular tachycardia [1123] have been described.

Although ANP concentration is increased in atrial fibrillation, heart hypertrophy and infarction, its role in remodeling processes is less evident [776,960]. In neonatal rat heart cells ANP induces apoptosis [1296].

2.3.5   Thrombin

2.3.5.1   Receptors and transduction to effectors

Thrombin is a serine protease that catalyses the formation of fibrine from fibrinogen. Normally it is not present in the blood but formed in the final step during blood clotting. It has a role in hemostasis, inflammation and proliferative processes.

Thrombin hydrolyses PAR-1 (protease-activated receptor) by cleavage of its N-terminal exodomain, exposing a new amino-terminal sequence (SFLLRN) which acts as a ligand and binds intramolecularly to the body of the receptor [215]. The resulting G-protein activation stimulates phospholipid metabolism by activation of PLC and PLA2 [727]. The result is formation of IP3 and DAG and subsequent stimulation of PKC or generation of lysophospholipids and arachidonic acid.

Augmented Ca^{2+} influx in the cell occurs through L-type Ca^{2+} channels [12] and another not specified plasma membrane pathway [528]. Enhanced Na^+ influx induced by thrombin can occur via stimulation of Na^+/H^+ exchanger [1321] or be secondary to modification of fast Na^+ channels by release of lysophospholipids. Lysophosphatidylcholine induces repetitive spontaneous openings of the Na^+ channel at the resting potential and also activates a non-selective cation current. The final result is augmented Ca^{2+} load and Ca^{2+}_i transients [953].

2.3.5.2   Electrophysiology

Information on the electrophysiological aspects is sparse. Thrombin causes prolongation of APD, promotes the appearance of EADs and DADs and elicits spontaneous activity in depolarised cells [1097]. Arrhythmias especially upon reperfusion are frequently induced [509]. The importance of thrombin-receptor activation is further illustrated by the observation that acute regional ischaemia induced by thrombotic occlusion results in a greater incidence of malignant arrhythmias than mechanical obstruction by a balloon. Pretreatment with Na^+/Ca^{2+} exchanger blockers or α-adrenergic receptor blockers prevent or reduce the severity of these arrhythmias [1313].

Besides these electrophysiological effects thrombin also promotes the production of growth factors and activates MAP kinases, inducing cardiac hypertrophy [953].

2.4   Modulation by hormones

2.4.1   Insulin

Diabetes mellitus is a very common disease with major cardiac complications: cardiomyopathy, autonomic neuropathy accompanied by decreased perception of myocardial pain and prevalence of the sympathetic tone, coronary atherosclerosis and life-threatening arrhythmias. One distinguishes two forms, which have the common characteristic of an inadequate regulation of glucose homeostasis. Type I is insulin dependent and is caused by a deficient production of insulin in the pancreas β-cell. Experimentally it can be induced by streptozotocin which causes a selective destruction of the pancreatic β-cells. Type II is insuline-resistant with defects downstream to the binding of insulin to its plasma membrane receptor. Experimentally it is mimicked by chronic treatment with fructose-sucrose diet, leading to insulin overproduction and insulin resistance.

Diabetes
Type I: deficient production of insulin in the pancreas
Type II: deficient sensitivity of the membrane receptor to insulin

2.4.1.1   Receptor transduction to effector

Insulin binds tightly to a membrane receptor, a tyrosine kinase and its activation results in phosphorylation of target proteins. Insulin has two major effects: it modulates the activity of enzymes (including ion channels) and it regulates gene expression of enzymes and of ion channels. Anabolic processes and growth are promoted. The MAP kinase pathway is activated. At the ionic channel level insulin deficiency is accompanied by inhibition of

i_{to}, i_{Kur} and i_{CaL}, a significant depression in the activity of Na$^+$/K$^+$ ATPase, the Na$^+$/Ca^{2+} exchanger and the Na$^+$/H$^+$ exchanger [166] and a decrease in SR Ca^{2+}ATPase and RyR density [1139]. PKC expression and activity on the other hand are markedly enhanced [1025].

2.4.1.2   Electrophysiological effects

Information on electrophysiological changes is mainly derived from rat models and caution is required when extrapolating to the human condition.

In type I diabetes the prolongation of the action potential (Fig. V.29) is caused by a reduction of i_{to} and the steady-state current; i_{CaL} also is reduced but this change cannot be responsible for the prolongation of the action potential [166].

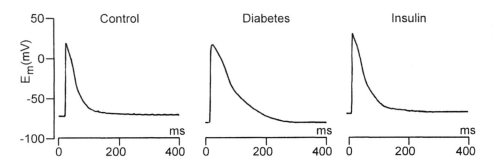

Figure V.29. Action potentials in rat left ventricular trabeculae, in a control animal, in the 4th week of experimental streptozotocin-induced diabetes and in the 2nd week of insulin treatment following 4 weeks of diabetic state. Stimulation at 0.5 Hz. Modified from [691].

Under normal conditions i_{to} current in the rat is more expressed in subepicardial than in subendocardial cells [1027] and causes a gradient in APD, with shorter APD in the subepicardial cells. This gradient is responsible for the positive T wave in the ECG. At elevated frequencies the gradient even increases due to a larger reduction of i_{to} in the subendocardial cells, because of the slower recovery from inactivation of the current. In type I diabetes i_{to} and its recovery from inactivation as well as the steady-state current are markedly attenuated [1020]; the changes in i_{to} are especially pronounced in subepicardial cells, narrowing in this way the dispersion in current amplitude and kinetics. The decrease in i_{to} and steady-state currents is responsible for the prolongation of the action potential, whereas the selective attenuation of i_{to} in the subepicardial cells explains the flattening of the T wave and the decrease in dispersion. Although the smaller dispersion is antiarrhythmic, a reversal of the repolarisation gradient diminishes the normal protection against reexcitation or retrograde conduction. In larger animals the importance of changes in i_{to} in determining QT or T wave is less pronounced.

The changes in i_{to} current are due to a deficient expression of the channel protein and/or increased phosphorylation by PKC. Insulin treatment can reverse the changes in i_{to} but requires the integrity of the subsarcolemmal cytoskeleton [1028], suggesting that new channels may be transported to the membrane via the actin or microtubule system. The reversal by insulin is blocked by inhibition of MAP kinase [1027]. An important modulator of i_{to} in diabetes is PKCε. PKC expression and activation normally results in inhibition of i_{to} and of steady-state current and the enzyme seems maximally expressed and stimulated in diabetes [1025].

Reduction of i_{CaL} current is accompanied by a fall in the Ca^{2+} content of the SR [166] and in smaller Ca^{2+}_i transients. The stimulatory effect of β - receptor activation on the Ca^{2+} content is less pronounced, explaining the diminished inotropic effect of sympathetic stimulation in diabetic hearts. i_{CaL} can be upregulated by insulin treatment [38]; the effect is dependent on PKA activation.

In heart vesicular preparations from diabetic animals, significant depressions in the activity of Na^+/K^+ ATPase, Na^+/Ca^{2+} exchanger and Na^+/H^+ exchanger have been described [166]. Normally the reduction of Na^+/Ca^{2+} exchanger is not accompanied by Ca^{2+} overload because of the concomitant fall in i_{CaL} [432].

In type II diabetes QT is not changed or slightly shortened. Steady-state current is increased while i_{to} is not affected. An exposure of cells to insulin for 5 hrs or longer causes similar changes [1027].

2.4.2   Estradiol

Based on clinical observations estradiol may have beneficial as well as detrimental effects on the cardiovascular system. Cardiac mortality is smaller in women and this difference may be due to a cardioprotective effect of estrogens. Some arrhythmias on the other hand, e.g. LQT-related arrhythmias are more frequent in women [172].

2.4.2.1   Receptors and effectors

Estrogen receptors are present in the female heart. In male rat ventricle the nuclear estrogen receptor is not expressed [77].

Some of the important effects of estrogens on the heart are indirect via modulation of the coronary vessel structure and function. Chronic treatment with estradiol stimulates angiogenesis [529], inhibits cardiac fibroblast proliferation and reduces collagen synthesis [286]. In the endothelium production of NO is increased, while synthesis of ET-1 is reduced.

Production of ACE and thus of Ang II is inhibited, whereas degradation of bradykinin is less: the balance of the renin-angiotensin system is thus shifted in favour of vasodilation [115].

The effects on heart cells are caused by activation of the nuclear estrogen receptor or directly via an action of the steroid molecule on channels or transporters. Direct effects on ionic channels have been observed in male animals in the absence of the female nuclear receptor, or are seen at high estrogen concentrations. The i_{CaL} is rapidly reduced within seconds; the effect is due to a shift of the inactivation curve in the negative direction and occurs even in the presence of isoproterenol or ET-1 [779,1129]. Outward currents are decreased in a direct way [1129] (Fig. V.30), and also indirectly following downregulation at the transcriptional level: this has been verified for i_{to} [77], i_{Ks} [779,1129] and i_{Kr} [779,1129].

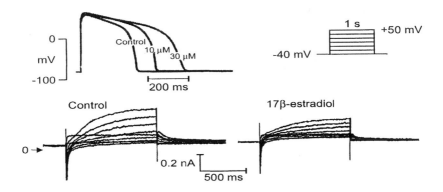

Figure V.30. Acute effects (5 min) of estradiol on action potential (upper traces; control, 10 and 30 μM superimposed) and voltage clamp currents (below; control and following exposure to 30 μM estradiol) in guinea pig ventricular myocytes. Modified from [1129].

2.4.2.2   Electrophysiological effects

Estradiol prolongs the ventricular [77,422](Fig. V.30), and shortens the atrial APD [779] (Fig. V.31). Prolongation in the ventricle is due to suppression of outward currents; it is most pronounced at low frequencies [77,1129] and may result in EADs [422]. The occurrence of EADs and arrhythmias is prominent in combination with class III drugs [172]. When the ventricular action potential is first lengthened under the effect of ET-1, prolongation is converted into shortening with concomitant block of EADs; the underlying mechanism is inhibition of i_{CaL}.

Block of i_{CaL} is responsible for the shortening of the action potential in the atrium and the inhibition of abnormal automaticity induced by isoproterenol [779].

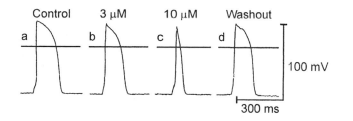

Figure V.31. Effects of 17β -estradiol at 3 and 10 μM concentration on action potential in guinea pig atrial myocyte stimulated at 0.2 Hz. Modified from [779].

2.4.3   Thyroid hormone

The primary action of thyroid hormone is on gene expression. Thyroxine and triiodothyronine enter the cell and bind to cytoplasmic protein receptors, which possess DNA binding parts. The binding transforms the receptors into transcriptional enhancers. Specific genes are then expressed, resulting in a direct modification of the number and function of channel and transporter proteins, their kinetics and signaling pathways modulating the effectors.

2.4.3.1   Receptor and tranduction to effectors
2.4.3.1.1   Transduction and the hyperthyroid state

One of the signaling pathways which is very sensitive to thyroid function is the β -receptor-PKA pathway. In the hyperthyroid state a category of specific genes is activated and results in what, from a clinical point of view, has been described as an hyperadrenergic state. Catecholamine levels are not increased, but the number of β -receptors is increased and the coupling with adenylate cyclase is facilitated. G protein levels are changed: G_{sa} levels are increased by reduced catabolism, whereas G_i levels are decreased by inhibition of transcription. The stimulatory pathway (isoproterenol) is thereby sensitised, while the inhibitory pathway (acetylcholine) is desensitised [43,114]. In contrast to β -receptors, α-receptors are decreased in number. The resulting hyperadrenergic state is different from what occurs with Ang II where the release of NA is increased and that of ACh decreased.

> Thyroid hormone and the sympathetic system
>
> Increase in numbers of β -adrenergic receptors
> Improved coupling to AC via enhanced level of G_{sa}

At the level of ionic currents the improved coupling of the stimulatory pathway is translated in changes of the amplitudes and kinetics of different currents: i_{CaL}, i_f, i_{st}, i_{Ks}, i_{Kur}, $i_{K.ATP}$ and i_{Cl}. Since basal i_{CaL} is already increased in the hyperthyroid state, the enhancing effect of administered isoproterenol may be minimal and only apparent as an increase in potency.

There is more however, than a shift towards an hyperadrenergic state: the expression and function of currents and transporters is directly modulated by the thyroid hormone. The i_{to}, i_{Kur}, and i_{K1} currents are for instance upregulated. In cultured neonatal cells treatment with triidothyronine induces a concentration-dependent increase in the density of i_{to} [589] and an acceleration of the recovery from inactivation, which is translated in a less suppressed current at elevated rates [1276]. The changes in current are conditioned by a shift in RNA and protein expression from $K_V.1.4$ to $K_V.4.2$ and $K_V.4.3$. Similar changes occur during postnatal development.

There is further an increased expression of SR Ca^{2+} ATPase, upregulation of α- and β-subunits of the Na^+/K^+ ATPase [1005,1275], enhanced expression of Na^+/Ca^{2+} exchanger [464,1292] and Na^+/H^+ exchanger proteins.

Increased i_{CaL} [603], elevated Ca^{2+} ATPase [904], greater number of ryanodine receptors [527] and upregulation of Na^+/Ca^{2+} exchanger [1292] can explain the enhanced Ca^{2+}_i transients. Excitation-contraction coupling is also promoted by a better structural conjunction of DHP-receptors with ryanodine receptors in the T-tubular system [1275].

HCN2 mRNA [837] and the i_f channel protein expression [911] are enhanced and result in a larger i_f current. In contrast to β-receptor stimulation, triidothyronine treatment does not induce a shift of the i_f activation curve, but such an effect can still be generated by stimulation of the sympathetic system.

2.4.3.1.2   Transduction and the hypothyroid state

In hypothyroidism the sensitivity of the β-receptor pathway is decreased. Deficiency of thyroid hormone results in a decrease of peak i_{to} and i_{Kur} in rats [1029,1114] and of i_{Ks} in guinea pig [107] (Fig. V.32, lower panel). The fall is greater in subepicardial than in subendocardial cells and recovery from inactivation is slowed in subepicardial cells. At elevated frequencies i_{to} thus will be especially lowered in subepicardial cells, making the repolarisation gradient much less expressed. The effect can be related to a greater expression and activity of PKCε (compare with insulin deficiency) [1025]. Among the transporters there is a marked reduction in Ca^{2+} ATPase and Na^+/K^+ ATPase activity [1275].

2.4.3.2   Electrophysiology
2.4.3.2.1   Electrophysiology and hyperthyroidism

Stimulation of the adrenergic system together with the direct effects of the hormone on channels and transporters result in a higher SAN rate, faster

AVN conduction, shorter APD, elevated Ca^{2+}_i transients and positive inotropic effects. There is a pronounced propensity to arrhythmias [415].

Sinus tachycardia is caused by the higher sympathetic tone and the enhanced expression of i_f. Larger outward currents, i_{to}, i_{Kur}, i_{Kr} and i_{Ks}, together with the higher sinus rate, are responsible for the shorter APD. Stimulation of i_{CaL} does result in a more positive plateau and greater activation of the delayed K^+ currents: the final result is a higher plateau but shorter APD. Clinically, paroxysmal AF is a frequent complication of hyperthyroidism. Short ERP, elevated i_{CaL} and high rate play an important role [603].

2.4.3.2.2 Electrophysiology and hypothyroidism

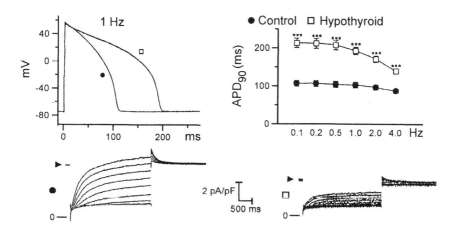

Figure V.32. Prolongation of action potential duration and decrease in delayed outward K^+ current in the hypothyroid state. Guinea pig ventricular myocytes. Top: Representative action potentials (left) and mean values of action potential duration (right) as a function of frequency in control (closed symbols) and in the hypothyroid state (open symbols). Bottom: Records of the delayed K^+ current under control (left) and in the hypothyroid state (right). Voltage clamp pulses from -50 mV to different depolarising levels up to +70 mV. Modified from [107].

At the electrophysiological level the effects are opposite to those of hyperthyroidism: SAN rate is down as well as AVN conduction, APD is prolonged [668] (Fig. V.32, upper panel). In the ECG this reflects in a longer QT interval. Due to different recovery processes of i_{to} in subepicardial and subendocardial cells the repolarisation gradient is reduced, the T wave becomes smaller and may even reverse direction. The hypothyroid state is antiarrhythmic and protects against electrically induced ventricular fibrillation [668] and arrhythmias secondary to myocardial infarction.

2.4.4   Adrenocortical hormones

2.4.4.1   Aldosterone

Aldosterone is the principal mineralocorticoid secreted by the adrenal glands and is responsible for the retention of Na^+ and excretion of K^+ from the body. Its secretion is activated by high plasma K^+ concentrations and by Ang II. In the cytoplasm it combines with a receptor molecule and diffuses into the nucleus where it affects the expression of the genome.

Aldosterone stimulates the Na^+/K^+ pump in the basolateral border of the kidney tubular cells. A different effect is seen in the heart. Voltage clamp measurement of Na^+ pump current in rabbit myocytes shows no change in maximal capacity but a fall in affinity for Na^+ [738]. Passive pathways for Na^+ entry in the cell, such as the Na^+/H^+ exchanger [595] and Na^+-K^+-Cl^- cotransport [737] are upregulated. The final result is an increase of $[Na^+]_i$ in heart cells.

In accord with the finding of Na^+ pump inhibition in heart, aldosterone was described to cause depolarisation and action potential prolongation in rabbit SAN and atrial preparations [237]. As a consequence spontaneous rate and excitability were decreased.

Hyperaldosteronism has deleterious effects on the cardiac function. These are caused by indirect effects such as hypertension and hypokalaemia, and direct enhanced fibrosis in the heart, and generate conditions which favour reentrant arrhythmias [900]. In a large clinical trial [876] the use of spironolactone, an aldosterone antagonist, has been shown to reduce death due to progressive heart failure and death due to ventricular arrhythmias.

2.4.4.2   Glucocorticoids

Among the glucocorticoids secreted by the adrenal glands, cortisol or hydrocortisone is the most important. It stimulates gluconeogenesis and mobilises lipids and proteins. Its secretion is enhanced in stress situations and inflammation, and depends on the release of ACTH from the anterior pituitary gland. Dexamethasone is a synthetic glucocorticoid, 30 times as potent as cortisol.

Experiments on cardiac preparations have been mostly performed with the synthetic and highly potent dexamethasone. Chronic treatment has been shown to modulate the expression and function (kinetics) of different channels. Among K^+ channels, $K_v1.5$ mRNA expression is upregulated in the rat ventricle, but not in the atrium [638,1125]. In the neonatal mouse dexamethasone has important effect on the developmental changes of ionic currents. In the neonatal period i_{Kr} normally decreases and disappears later (as can be measured by dofetilide binding [289]), whereas i_{to} becomes more expressed. These changes are inhibited by dexamethasone [1240]. At the same time the shortening of the action potential and the fall in dofetilide binding are prevented [289]. Dexamethasone also slightly increases i_{CaL} [1240] and changes the kinetics of i_{Na} [1127].

3.   MODULATION BY DRUGS

3.1   Drugs and antiarrhythmic activity

During the last 50 years many drugs that block Na^+, Ca^{2+} and K^+ currents have been used frequently as antiarrhythmic agents. The picture has changed completely since the Cardiac Arrhythmia Suppression Trial study (CAST) [493] demonstrated an increased mortality during chronic treatment with class Ic drugs or compounds that block the fast sodium channel with slow kinetics. Drugs blocking K^+ currents in a rate-independent way also have been found to provoke torsade de pointes arrhythmias and sudden death [922,1290]. Therapeutic interventions for antiarrhythmic activity have consequently shifted to implantation of cardioverter-defibrillator devices and ablation techniques, whereas the prescription and use of antiarrhythmic drugs has dramatically declined [1357].

With the exception of pure β-receptor blocking drugs, which do not act directly on ion channels, and Ca^{2+} channel antagonists in restricted indications, classical antiarrhythmics acting on Na^+ and K^+ channels are not used anymore in ventricular arrhythmias, especially when contraction function is impaired. The use of class I drugs is avoided in patients with heart failure, cardiac ischaemia or previous infarction. Amiodarone, which has inhibitory effects on many channels and is also antiadrenergic is preferred above lidocaine for the treatment of shock-refractory ventricular fibrillation [868]. It is used as an adjuvans after implantation of a defibrillator [907] but a demonstration of a significant reduction in mortality rate is absent.

The main indication of antiarrhythmic drug treatment remains atrial fibrillation [906], but even in this case the use of Na^+ channel blockers (flecainide, propafenone) and K^+ channel blockers (dofetilide, sotalol) has not been proven to reduce mortality. Drugs that prolong the action potential have been shown to be effective in acute chemical conversion, and to prevent paroxysmal AF or to maintain sinus rhythm after electrical conversion. Ca^{2+}-channel antagonists (verapamil) are indicated for the control of ventricular rate in AF and for the conversion or prevention of AVN reentrant tachycardia.

Basic concepts underlying the development of antiarrhythmic drugs are questioned. Can a drug acting directly on a channel exert antiarrhythmic activity without an obligatory concomitant arrhythmogenic effect? Can a drug that blocks only one current be of any beneficial use against arrhythmias of complex origin in patients with a different pathologic background? [1357]. Should one not rather promote the development of drugs acting on other channel and carrier targets, or acting upstream to the channel or drugs modifying the substrate on which arrhythmias are grafted?

Before discussing these future approaches, which are certainly valid on a theoretical level, it seems adequate to stress that there is still a need for compounds acting directly on channels. Whereas implantable cardioverter-defibrillators are life-saving, the defibrillator shocks are often reducing the quality of life [998] and antiarrhythmic drugs may be useful in reducing the number of required shocks. Drugs are still used in the chemical cardioversion of AF and its recurrence or as an adjuvans in electrical cardioversion [906]. It is amazing however that in this context drugs are used that are known to be strongly arrhythmogenic at the ventricular level. It is time to develop safe and efficient drugs. We presently have a good insight in the arrhythmogenic mechanisms: absence of selectivity for depolarised cells, absence of selectivity for cells stimulated at elevated rate, abnormally slow kinetics of binding and unbinding with consequent prolongation of the vulnerable period. A discussion of drugs acting directly on ion channels and the requirements to avoid arrhythmogenic effects is therefore useful and follows in the next section.

3.2   Presently available drugs

Drugs can interact directly with ionic channels and change their function. Function is increased (agonist action) or reduced (antagonist action) and this is the result of either a change in ion permeation or in gating [for a review see 148].

3.2.1   Agonist effects

For voltage-activated channels, an increase in function is normally the result of a change in gating: slowing of the inactivation time course increases the current, a shift of the voltage-dependence of inactivation processes in the depolarising direction makes more channels available. For ligand-activated channels modulation of the affinity of the ligand for the channel can cause gain of function: a decreased affinity for ATP will activate $i_{K,ATP}$.

Agonist-induced increase in Na^+ current (e.g. by ibutilide [628]) or in Ca^{2+} current (e.g. by Bay K-compounds [69]) cause prolongation of the action potential. Theoretically these agents should lengthen the wavelength in a reentry pathway, reduce the number of wavelets, and eventually block reentry. Ibutilide's action is not limited to elevated rates however, and excessive prolongation of the action potential at low rates may generate TdP arrhythmia [1179]. A further disadvantage of these agonists is possible Na^+ and Ca^{2+} overload and thus an increased propensity to develop EADs, DADs and to reduce gap junction conductance. A dissociation between the arrhythmogenic and antiarrhythmic effects of the Na^+ and Ca^{2+} channel agonists seems difficult to realise.

A typical example of agonist action on K^+ channels is activation of the K.ATP channel. The channel in the plasma membrane as well as the channel in the mitochondrial membrane are activated in ischaemic conditions [652]. The mitochondrial channel has been proposed to play an important role in preconditioning [670]. The development of drugs selectively activating the mitochondrial channel may be promising. Information on the final effectors in the process of preconditioning however, is still lacking, and extrapolation to the possible use of K^+ channel openers in preventing ischaemia must await further research.

3.2.2   Antagonist effects

Loss of channel function is caused by a change in gating or by an interaction with the permeation process. Binding to the pore causes a direct obstruction of the permeation pathway. The same effect can be obtained by binding outside the pore but causing a reduction in permeation via an allosteric effect. Most drugs that have been used as antiarrhythmics and did fall into discredit belong to the group of pore blockers. The reasons for their falling in discredit are manifold.

3.2.2.1 Na^+ channel blockers

The question of inherent arrhythmogenic activity is especially important with respect to Na^+ channel blockers (so-called class I drugs). By reducing conduction velocity, a unidirectional block may be converted into a bidirectional block with inhibition of the reentry circuit. However at the same time cells in which conduction is critically lowered may now become the site of a unidirectional block with re-induction of reentry. To be effective in inhibiting reentry arrhythmias, the drug should act in a very selective way on partially depolarised cells and should block only at high frequencies (prolongation of refractoriness) while not reducing the conduction velocity at moderate frequencies [467]. Prolongation of the ERP should also occur without prolonging the vulnerable window [1094]. This is the period following repolarisation during which an extra stimulus might result in unidirectional block, with conduction in the retrograde direction and block in the anterograde direction. As far as Na^+ channel blockers are concerned it may be difficult, perhaps impossible to design drugs that fulfil these requirements.

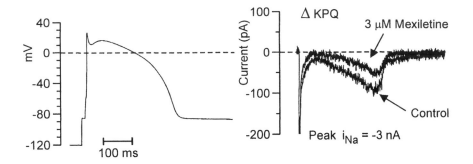

Figure V.33. Action potential clamp of a HEK cell expressing the ΔKPQ mutation of the *SCN5A* Na$^+$ channel before and during exposure of 3 μM mexiletine. Theoretical action potential waveform (left) used as voltage clamp waveform and superimposed Na$^+$ current traces (right) in the absence and presence of mexiletine. The late Na$^+$ current was suppressed by 50%; the peak Na$^+$ current (off scale) is much less inhibited. Modified from [1235].

Apart from the treatment of reentry arrhythmias, Na$^+$ channel blockers may also be used to shorten the action potential in cases where a slowly inactivating (persistent) Na$^+$ current causes prolongation of the action potential and leads to EADs (LQT3 syndrome, hypoxia [537], lysophosphatidylcholine exposure [126]). The aim is to reduce the persistent current without affecting the initial current responsible for the fast upstroke (Fig. V.33). Such an effect can be reached by blocking the open channel, with time constants in the order of tens of ms, combined with fast recovery from block during diastole [144,1235]. Upstroke velocity and conduction are not changed since the drug has no time to bind to the channel in the short and fast depolarisation phase of the action potential and no accumulation occurs with frequency. This antiarrhythmic activity may be important in cases where the persistent current is pronounced such as in reperfusion, and congenital or acquired long QT syndromes.

3.2.2.2   Ca^{2+} channel blockers

L-type Ca^{2+} channel blockers (class IV drugs) belong to three different groups: the dihydropyridines, the phenylalkylamines (e.g. verapamil) and the diltiazem group. Dihydropyridines preferentially block Ca^{2+} channels in the depolarised state, and are mainly used for their vascular effects. The phenylalkylamines and diltiazem show a pronounced use-dependency, which makes them efficient in cases of tachycardia with direct or indirect involvement of the Ca^{2+} channel, such as AVN reentry arrhythmias. In atrial fibrillation, Ca^{2+} channel blockers of this type are used to control ventricular rate by slowing conduction through the AVN. All Ca^{2+} channel inhibitors have the inherent disadvantage of negative inotropism.

3.2.2.3 K⁺ channel blockers

Inhibitors of i_{Kr} and i_{Ks} prolong the action potential (class III drugs) and may be expected to block reentry by increasing the wavelength of the impulse (short excitable gap). The vulnerable window is normally not prolonged, because conduction and recovery from excitability are not changed. And yet the same substances may cause dangerous ventricular arrhythmias, torsade de pointes and sudden cardiac death. The reason is excessive prolongation of the action potential at low frequencies, with accompanying appearance of EADs [469]. Prolongation of the action potential does not show rate-dependence or the wrong rate-dependence, with greater prolongation at low rates and marked dispersion of the APD ("reverse use-dependence"). The underlying mechanism is block of the channels in a state-independent way or block of the open channel with slow recovery during diastole. In some instances recovery does not occur at all and the drug is trapped in the channel during deactivation [141,142].

To avoid the complication of TdP, drugs should be developed that block the open channel with a time constant longer than the duration of the action potential and a recovery from block during diastole that allows for preferential summation at high frequencies [144]. If the time constant of the block is too short, block will be complete within a single action potential and prolongation of the action potential maximal at low frequencies. If the recovery is absent or very slow (trapping), block of the channel becomes frequency-independent, and prolongation of the action potential then shows the reverse rate-dependence.

The two other outward currents, i_{to} and i_{Kur}, are important in generating repolarisation in atrial cells, less or not in ventricular cells. Their role at elevated rates is less evident since both currents undergo slow inactivation. When blocked, one of the consequences is elevation of the plateau, with faster activation of i_{Kr} and i_{Ks} and sometimes unexpectedly a shorter APD.

3.2.2.4 Block of more than one current?

Certain drugs that block more than one current, e.g. amiodarone, are less arrhythmogenic than drugs blocking only one current and are presently preferred for therapeutic intervention. Should the development of this type of drug be promoted? In favour of this thesis is the complexity of different arrhythmic situations. On the other hand it is not enough realised that the apparent advantage of these drugs is mainly due to the compensation of negative side effects: complication of excessive prolongation of the action potential and appearance of EADs at low frequency by block of i_{Kr} is avoided by block of i_{CaL}. It seems more logical to develop drugs which, first of all, lack the negative side effects.

3.3   Future approaches

3.3.1   Other channel and carrier targets

Time is ripe to develop drugs acting on other currents than Na^+, K^+ or Ca^{2+} currents. Such other candidates are stretch-activated currents, the SR release channel, the Na^+/H^+ exchanger, Na^+/Ca^{2+} exchanger, the SR Ca^{2+} ATPase, the i_f current.

Stretch is an important causal factor in the genesis of arrhythmias by causing depolarisation [544,1346] and eventually Ca^{2+} overload. Stunned cells are passively elongated during the active contraction of viable cells in acute ischaemia. In the chronic stage or during development of cardiac failure stretching occurs in Purkinje cells overlying the infarct or in cells close to the borderline.

Ca^{2+} overload favours the occurrence of EADs and DADs and can be expected to occur during reperfusion. Important pathways for Ca^{2+} overload are: non-selective cation channels, Ca^{2+} leak channels, deficient Na^+/Ca^{2+} exchanger or reduced uptake by the SR Ca^{2+} ATPase. Block of the Na^+ leak through the non-selective cation or of the persistent Na^+ current during the plateau of the action potential has already been mentioned as an antiarrhythmic intervention. Because of the acidosis in ischaemia Na^+ influx through the Na^+/H^+ exchanger will contribute to Na^+ overload. Block of the exchanger may thus be a useful intervention to reduce Na^+ overload and has been shown to be antiarrhythmic [639].

3.3.2   The upstream approach

Drugs can indirectly affect the function of a channel, by acting on membrane receptors or their G protein coupling to intracellular signaling pathways. This type of signaling normally results in phosphorylation or dephosphorylation of the pore unit or subunits (see this Chapter, section 2). Examples in this category of substances that have proven their utility, are β - and α-receptor blockers. Their antiarrhythmic activity is based on the avoidance and prevention of the hyperadrenergic state and Ca^{2+} overload.

In recent years it has become evident that long-term changes in ion channel function develop in pathological situations. They are caused by modified expression of channel proteins or of subsidiary molecules involved in the modulation of channels, a process called remodeling (see Chapter IX). Instead of modifying the function of the channel and hoping to stop an arrhythmia it may become possible in the near future, to change the transcriptional signaling that generates the substrate of the arrhythmia and/or to import directly and locally transcription factors and stem cells [832]. β - blockers for instance, not only reduce the sympathetic drive and affect the modulation of channels, but seem to prevent hypertrophy and dilatation, the substrate for failure and life-threatening arrhythmias [1357]. Remodeling is probably also the mechanism underlying the promising results obtained by ACE inhibitors [328]. However, before any logic development of this type of drugs can be made, it is necessary to obtain more information on the advantages-disadvantages of particular aspects of remodeling and more important, on the mechanisms underlying the remodeling processes. In this way unnecessary arrhythmogenic complications can be prevented.

3.3.3   Pharmacogenomics

Pharmacogenomics is the study of the relationship between the genome of an individual and his pharmacological response to drugs. Polymorphisms and mutations in the human genome are not exceptional and are responsible for modulation of disease processes and for the variability in the response to drugs. This kind of variability is generated by changes in genes that control drug metabolism and clearance, or are responsible for the expression of ion channels, transporters and receptors, molecules that are targeted by drugs [923]. Variability is further generated at the protein level by alternative splicing of transcripts, or extensive posttranslational processing [35].

The genetic background implied in the genesis of heart failure for instance, is currently under study and a number of genes have been identified which play a role in dilated cardiomyopathy [165]. The hypothesis is under study that some mutations represent a "forme fruste" of the congenital LQT syndromes and are responsible for part of drug-induced arrhythmias of the torsade de pointes type [787]. Allelic variants of MiRP1, which functions as a subunit for the i_{Kr} channel, contribute to a significant fraction of cases of drug-induced LQTs. Detection of these variants by molecular screening may allow identification of individuals and their family members who are at an increased risk to develop life-threatening arrhythmias when taken a given drug for the first time [1001].

A better knowledge of pharmacogenomics will replace former empirical strategies which were used to avoid side-effects and complications of drug therapy. Information on the genetic determinants of the disease process or the response to drugs will lead to an appropriate, personal treatment scheme and prevent for instance dangerous arrhythmias and sudden death.

Chapter VI

Electrophysiological basis of the electrocardiogram

1.   BIO-ELECTRIC POTENTIALS AND DIPOLES

The electrocardiogram (ECG) is a very useful tool to investigate the electrical activity of the heart. Electrical activity of cells generates short-circuit currents in the extra- and intracellular environment. According to Ohm's law such short-circuit currents cause electrical potential differences also in the extracellular environment. Studying these potentials can give important information about the underlying processes.

The cardiac current sources can be approximated by a dipole as was introduced by Einthoven in 1913 [303], and current interpretation of the electrocardiogram is still based on this model.

In the resting state of a cardiac cell, the cell is polarised, but since the polarisation is uniform over the whole cell no potential differences are present between different points in the extracellular environment.

When part of the cell or tissue is depolarised while the other part is still at rest, differences in charge density exist not only in the intracellular medium but also in the extracellular environment. Extracellular potentials are directly related to the spatial distribution of the intracellular potential. Although the exact relationship is described by a rather complex function [1072], in case of one-dimensional conduction at constant velocity the time course of the extracellular potential near the preparation is approximately proportional to the second time derivative of the intracellular potential. The boundary between the part of the cell or tissue that is electrically active at a certain moment in time and the part which at that moment is still at rest can be seen as a wave front. The part that is activated contains an excess of negative charges in the extracellular space, while the part at rest contains an extracellular excess of positive charges. The charge separation at the boundary between the activated and the rested part of the tissue can thus be seen as an electric dipole (two charges of equal magnitude but opposite sign at a small distance of each other). During the activation a dipole vector is thus present pointing in the direction in which the activation proceeds (Fig. VI.1). When several cells are simultaneously being activated, the resulting potential is the superposition of contributions of the different cells, and the resulting dipole vector can be approximated as the vector sum of the individual dipole vectors, and the size of the dipole vector is thus proportional to the size of the wave front.

In nerve and skeletal muscle the depolarisation phase of the action potential is immediately followed by repolarisation. The repolarisation also introduces spatial inhomogeneity in the electric field. The direction in which the repolarisation wave proceeds in these cells is the same as the direction of the activation wave. Since the vector points in a direction from cells at the resting potential towards depolarised cells, the repolarisation vector in these cells is opposite to the activation vector (Fig. VI.1 left panels).

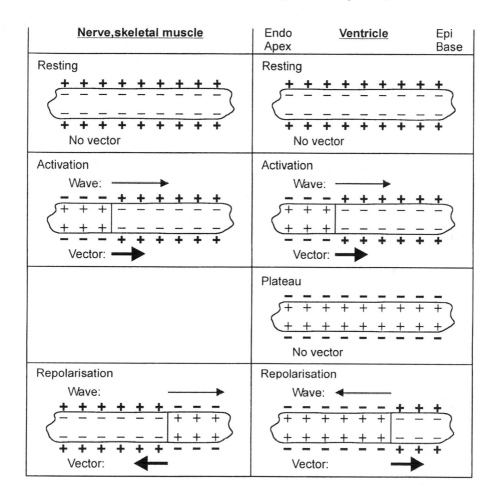

Figure VI.1. Propagation of electrical activity and dipole vector. Left panels: Propagation in nerve or skeletal muscle cells. Right panels: Propagation in ventricular myocardium. In ventricular myocardium the repolarisation wave proceeds in opposite direction as the activation wave. While activation starts from the apical endocardial surface and proceeds towards the epicardial surface at the base of the ventricle, repolarisation starts from the epicardial surface at the base of the ventricle. This causes the vector during ventricular repolarisation to point in the same direction as the activation vector.

In ventricular cells the long plateau phase of the action potential causes the repolarisation to be delayed, so that for some time all ventricular cells are depolarised. When the whole ventricle is depolarised, the extracellular electric field is uniform and no potential differences exist in the extracellular space. The plateau of the ventricular action potential is followed by the final repolarisation phase. In the cardiac ventricle however (unlike in nerve, skeletal muscle or atrial cells) the last cells to be activated are the first cells to repolarise, so that the general direction of the repolarisation wave is opposite to that of the activation wave (as will be discussed later in relation with the T wave of the ECG). This causes the vector during the ventricular repolarisation to point in the same direction as the vector during activation of the ventricle (Fig. VI.1 right panels).

2.   DIPOLE THEORY

Two charges (+Q and –Q) with the same magnitude but opposite sign and at a small distance (d) of each other form a dipole. Such a dipole can be characterised by a dipole vector. The magnitude of the dipole vector is equal to the product m = Q . d. The vector has its origin in the centre of the dipole and points in the direction of the dipole, from the negative to the positive charge (Fig. VI.2).

2.1   Dipole and dipole vector model

The presence of a dipole in a conducting field surrounding the dipole will cause current flow in the surrounding medium, which will cause differences in electric potential at different places. The potential (V_P) at a point in a homogeneous field surrounding a dipole can be expressed as a function of the size, orientation and distance of the dipole vector with respect to the recording electrodes: $V_P = m.\cos \alpha / 4\pi\varepsilon r^2$ where V_P is the potential at point P, m is the magnitude of the dipole vector, α is the angle between the dipole vector and the axis defined by the position of the recording electrodes, r the distance between recording electrodes and the dipole, and ε the dielectricity constant of the medium (the equation can be derived by subtracting the potentials of the two point charges and making a few approximations based on the very small distance between the two point charges with respect to the distance between recording electrodes and dipole (Fig. VI.2)). The equation predicts that *the potential is proportional to the projection of the dipole vector on the axis of registration, and inversely proportional to the square of the distance of the recording electrode to the dipole*. The measured potential therefore reflects the size of the dipole, and the proximity and orientation of the dipole with respect to point P.

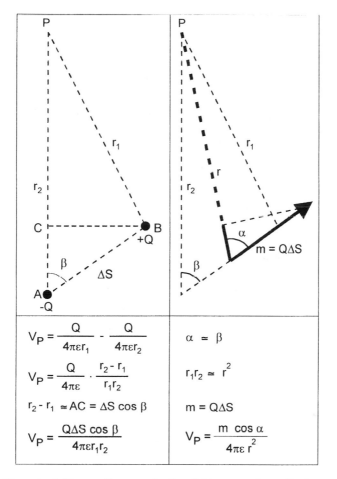

Figure VI.2. The potential in a uniform conductive field surrounding a dipole.

The dipole model (which is the most simple model of the cardiac current generator, and which proves to be a very useful model) presents a two-dimensional analysis of the potential in the field around a dipole. In applying the dipole model to electrocardiographic source, the wave front is approximated by a single dipole vector representing the dipoles in the extracellular medium. The magnitude of the dipole vector is proportional to the size of the wave front, and the direction corresponds to the average direction of the propagation of the wave front. The sense of the dipole vector (from negative to positive extracellular charges) is from the cells that are depolarised to the cells that are at the resting potential.

2.2   Solid angle model

An alternative approach (the solid angle model), treats the electrical sources in a three-dimensional space. Although the model is also based on dipoles, it does not need explicit reference to a dipole vector, but directly relates potential to wave front properties.

For a uniform conducting field surrounding an activation front which can be represented as a uniform electric double layer, it can be demonstrated that *the magnitude of the potential at any point P is proportional to the solid angle (Ω) under which the activation front is seen from this point* [see 946] (a solid angle is defined as the area of the intersection of a cone originating at P with a unit sphere centred at P). The solid angle at which an activation front is seen from a point P is proportional to the size of the activation front, and also reflects its proximity and orientation relative to the point P (Fig. VI.3). The solid angle theory can thus be viewed as a three-dimensional extension of the dipole vector representation, and gives essentially equivalent predictions, without the need to introduce a dipole vector (the size and direction of which can be only qualitatively related to the existing wave front).

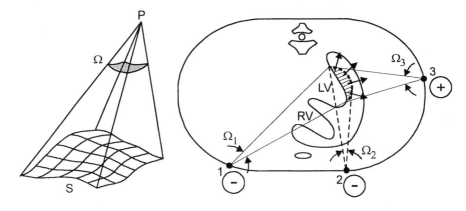

Figure VI.3. Activation front, solid angle and measured potentials. The potential measured at a point (P) in the field of a propagating front (S) of electrical activity is proportional to the solid angle (Ω) under which the front is seen from this point. The right panel shows the projection on the transverse plane of an activation front and the solid angles under which it is seen from three points. The activation wave front is proceeding in the general direction of point 3. The potential at point 3 is positive since point 3 is on the positive side of the dipoles (the average dipole vector pointing rather towards than away from point 3). The activation wave front is receding from points 1 and 2, resulting in negative potentials at these points.

2.3   Limitations of the models

The models have of course their limitations:
It is clear that the simple single dipole model, which treats the electrical sources as a single two-dimensional uniform double layer with its dipole perpendicular to the activation front, or the solid angle model, which also treats the sources as uniform double layers, are very crude approximations of the electrical activity of the heart (e.g. curvature of the wave front, multiple wave fronts, anisotropic propagation). Also considering the body as a uniform conductor, neglecting its three–dimensional structure and its non-uniform distribution of conductive properties (e.g. fat and air-filled body cavities acting as insulators), appears to be a grossly inaccurate representation of reality. Nevertheless theoretical analysis demonstrates that the body inhomogeneities do not add important complexities to the general pattern of the body surface potential distribution, but causes a smoothing of surface potential distribution and a reduction of spatial resolution [947] [for an overview see 946], and that capacitative effects can be neglected, which validates the quasi-static approximation. Also practical experience demonstrates that in most conditions the potentials recorded in ECG registrations can be very well approximated as representing the projections of a single dipole vector, or related to the solid angle.

–   While the models are extremely useful for relating cardiac activity to ECG, it should be noted that the applicability of the models is reduced when the activation front is due to a point source such as an ectopic focus: due to propagation in longitudinal as well as transverse direction, the effect of myocardial anisotropy becomes more important, so that approximating the wave front as a uniform double layer approaches its limitations. Other models have been proposed combining axial and transverse components, such as the oblique double layer model [877, see 946]. While these models are very important for gaining insight in the relation between electrical events in the heart and body surface potential, their importance for practical electrocardiography is limited.

–   The models are also limited in their ability to provide detailed information on local electrical activity in the heart, such as the exact origin of ectopic foci. Body surface ECG recordings from many points, analysed by computer can provide more detailed information, although the spatial resolution remains limited. Intracardiac recordings of the ECG, as used to localise reentry pathways prior to ablation, provide much more detailed information, about the localisation of electrical events. However models considering activation fronts as two-dimensional planes are not suitable for studying potentials in the vicinity of the wave front.

3.   ECG STANDARD LEAD SYSTEM

The ECG is the registration of the extracellular body surface potentials, which are due to the propagation of cardiac action potentials. For the registration standard electrode positions in the frontal and transversal planes are generally used.

3.1   Frontal plane

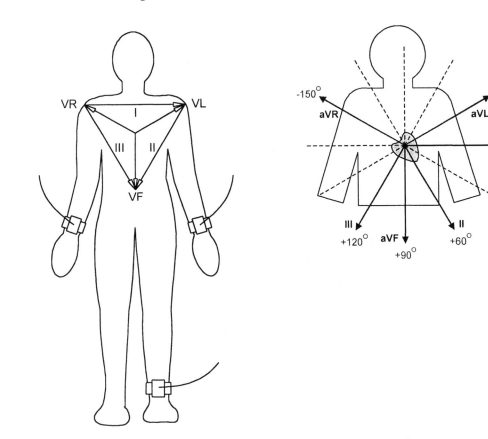

Figure VI.4. Frontal plane derivations. Left panel: Right arm (VR), left arm (VL) and left foot (VF) derivation, and the Einthoven triangle. Right panel: Frontal plane axes defined by the Einthoven triangle for the three augmented unipolar derivations (aVR, aVL and aVF), and for the three bipolar derivations (I, II, III).

Electrodes are connected to right arm (VR), left arm (VL) and left leg (VF). In addition a grounding electrode is connected to the right leg. Using these electrodes, six different registrations are made: three (augmented) unipolar registrations, which measure the potential at one point with respect to zero potential (see section 3.1.1), and three bipolar registrations, which measure the potential difference between two points (see section 3.1.2).

The positions of the three recording electrodes define an (approximately) equilateral triangle, the Einthoven triangle (Fig. VI.4). In an equilateral triangle the distance from each of the corners to the centre of the triangle is the same. Choosing an equilateral triangular reference system therefore has the advantage that differences in the size of the registered potentials in the frontal plane are not due to differences in distance between registration electrode and the dipole, and thus only depend on the projection of the dipole vector (see section 2.1).

3.1.1   Unipolar derivations

The unipolar leads VR, VL and VF are the potentials in each of the three leads with respect to the "Central Terminal of Wilson", with is obtained by summing the potentials of the three unipolar frontal leads. This average potential equals zero (since the sum of the amplitudes of projections of one vector on three axes (in the same plane) with angular separation of 120° is zero). The sum of the potentials of the three unipolar derivations can thus be used a reference point at zero potential.

In the standard ECG practice augmented unipolar leads are used, instead. In the augmented leads (indicated as aVR, aVL and aVF) the potential in one lead is taken with respect to the average potential of the two other frontal leads, instead of using the central terminal of Wilson as the reference. E.g. $aVR = VR - (VL + VF)/2$. This results in the augmented unipolar signal being equal to 1.5 times the corresponding non-augmented lead.

This can easily be seen since

$aVR = VR - (VL + VF) / 2 = VR - (VR + VL + VF) /2 + VR/2$

Since $VR + VL + VF = 0$ (central terminal of Wilson) $aVR = 3/2 \ VR$

3.1.2   Bipolar derivations

The bipolar derivations I, II and III (also called D1, D2 D3) use the difference between the potentials in two leads

$I = VL - VR$

$II = VF - VR$

$III = VF - VL$

The six leads together establish an axial reference system consisting of six axes. The sides of the equilateral triangle define the three bipolar axes, while the connection from the centre of the triangle to the corners define the three unipolar axes. The potentials registered in a lead correspond to the projection of the dipole vector on the axis corresponding to that lead. The vector can be constructed from two bipolar or from two unipolar projections.

From the definitions it is easily seen that II = I + III, which also can be obtained from the second law of Kirchoff, stating that the total potential difference in any closed circuit is zero.

3.2   Transverse plane

The potentials in the transversal plane are registered by means of six chest (precordial) electrodes positioned as shown in Fig. VI.5. The precordial registrations are unipolar with as reference the central terminal of Wilson. The six precordial leads define an axis system in the transversal plane.

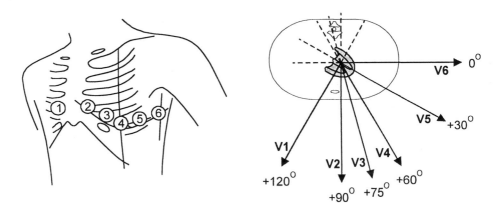

Figure VI.5. Transverse plane derivations and ECG axes in the transverse plane

Since the distance of the electrodes to the heart is small and not equal for the different electrodes, the size of the recorded signal is not comparable, so that the vector in the transversal plane cannot be constructed. The direction of the vector can however be found by determining the transition zone. This is the area between two recording electrodes where the recorded potential changes sign. The vector is perpendicular to the transition zone. The sense of the vector is then easily determined by verifying that it is consistent with the sign of its projection on anyone of the axes in the transverse plane.

4. GENESIS OF THE ECG WAVES

Table 1. Approximate normal values of action potential and conduction parameters in different parts of the heart. dV/dt_{max} = maximal upstroke velocity, APD = action potential duration (at 90% repolarisation), CV = conduction velocity, CT = conduction time. (* = strongly frequency-dependent).

	dV/dt_{max} (V/s)	APD (ms)	CV (m/s)	CT (ms)
SAN	1 - 10	100 – 200	< 0.05	45
Atria	100 - 200	100 – 200	0.3 – 0.5	40
AVN	5 - 15	100 – 200	0.05 – 0.1	100
His Purkinje system	600 - 800	200 – 500 *	2 – 5	30
Ventricle	100 - 200	200 - 400 *	0.3 – 0.5	50

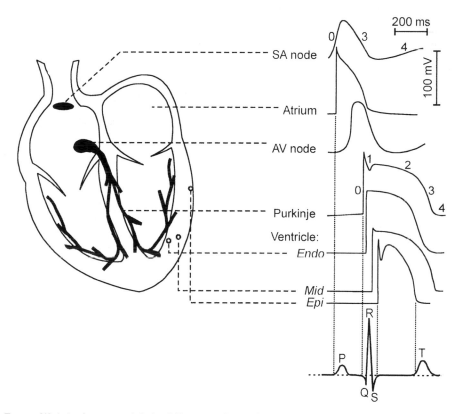

Figure VI.6. Action potentials in different regions of the heart and their relation to the ECG.

Normal electrical activity of the heart starts by spontaneous activity in the sinoatrial node (SAN) and propagates through the atria towards the atrioventricular node (AVN). From there it propagates via the ventricular conduction system (His bundle Purkinje system) to the ventricular myocardium. Action potentials in different parts of the heart sequentially activate and show typical measurable delays (Table 1).

Also the action potential configuration is not uniform over different areas of the heart. Fig. VI.6 illustrates the configuration and temporal relation of action potentials in different regions of the heart and their relation to the electrocardiogram. A brief historical overview of the naming of the ECG waves and a brief account of their genesis was given by Hurst [483].

4.1   The P wave

The normal depolarisation sequence starts with Ca^{2+} action potentials in the SAN, and spreads over both atria towards the AVN. Conduction in the atria is provided by Na^+ action potentials. The normal conduction velocity in the atria is about 0.8 to 1.0 m/s. Propagation of the atrial activation, which takes of the order of 100 ms to depolarise both atria, produces the P wave of the ECG. The first half of the P wave is largely due do the right atrium, while the second half largely corresponds to left atrial depolarisation. The average vector in the frontal plane is generally downward and to the left.

From the atria propagation proceeds towards the AVN. Propagation through the AVN occurs via Ca^{2+} action potentials and is very slow (conduction velocity of the order of 0.1 m/s) so that it takes about 70 ms to activate the His bundle. Because of its small size, electrical activity of the AVN fails to register on surface electrocardiograms, and the segment between the end of the P wave and the beginning of the QRS complex on the surface ECG largely corresponds to the AVN conduction time.

4.2   The QRS complex

The fast conduction of the His bundle Purkinje system (2 – 5 m/s), which is due to a high density of Na^+ channels, ensures rapid activation of the ventricles. The activation wave in the His bundle Purkinje system first reaches the left side of the interventricular septum. At the same time the His Purkinje system causes a fast propagation of the activation towards the apex from where the activation spreads over the endocardial side of the ventricular myocardium towards the epicardial side. From the endocardial surface the activation spreads through the myocardium to the epicardial side at a speed of about 0.3 m/s, by means of Na^+ action potentials. Because of the larger size of the left ventricle, the last part of the heart to be activated is the epicardial surface at the postero-basal side of the left ventricle [294].

Since activation is rapid due to the presence of the fast conduction system, the normal QRS complex is narrow (< 100 ms) and large (Fig. VI.6).

The complex activation sequence of the ventricle results in a vector that shows large changes in amplitude and direction. This causes the registered potentials during the ventricular activation to have the appearance of a complex (the QRS complex) with alterations between upward and downward deflections, typical of the QRS complex, and containing multiple peaks in most of the leads. Since initially the activation front propagates from left to right into the septum the initial vector of the ventricular activation points normally to the right. As the depolarisation spreads towards the apex, the vector has a downward direction. From the apex the activation spreads towards the base of the ventricles and from the endo- to the epicardial surface; the last part of the ventricle to be depolarised is the basal portion of epicardium of the left ventricle. The average vector of the QRS complex (the electrical axis) is normally directed in a downward and leftward direction, in general being slightly more leftward than the morphological axis defined by the interventricular septum. The deviation between the morphological and electrical axes is due to the larger mass of the left ventricle, which provides a larger contribution to the resultant vector.

The QRS segment in normal ventricle is followed by a rather long period where all ventricular cells are depolarised during the plateau of the action potential. At this moment no net electrical dipole is present. The QRS complex present in the normal ECG is therefore followed by an isoelectric interval, the ST segment, lasting a few hundreds of milliseconds, starting at the end of the QRS complex, marked by the so-called J point, and ending at the beginning of the T wave, which signals the ventricular repolarisation.

A number of pathological situations, such as acute ischaemia and Brugada syndrome give rise to non-isoelectric ST segments. Unlike direct current (DC) electrograms recorded by non-polarisable electrodes, normal ECG recordings make use of alternating current (AC)-coupled amplifiers. The baseline of the ECG therefore does not correspond to a true zero potential level. Therefore ST segment elevations on surface electro-cardiograms can be due to a real change of the level of the ST segment, but also to an opposite change in the level of the diastolic baseline (TQ segment depression), or a combination of both. While the ST elevation in the Brugada syndrome is caused by dispersion of the ventricular action potentials and therefore is a true ST denivellation (see section 5.1.5.1), the ST elevation seen during early ischaemia is due to a combination of a shift of the ST segment and an opposite shift of the TQ segment. The shift of the TQ segment during acute ischaemia is due to the presence of ischaemia-induced changes in resting potential, resulting in electrical gradients during the ventricular diastole. The ischaemia-induced shift of the ST segment is due to dispersion in plateau level and duration of the ventricular action potential [for review see 585]. The ST segment elevations during myocardial ischaemia have been related to opening of sarcolemmal ATP-sensitive K channels [652].

4.3   The T wave

The plateau of the ventricular action potential is followed by a phase of repolarisation propagating through the ventricle, which produces the so-called T wave in the ECG (Fig. VI.6). Since the duration of the plateau of the ventricular action potential strongly depends on action potential frequency (see Fig. VI.7), the duration of the QT interval (measured from the beginning of QRS to the end of the T wave) is also strongly frequency-dependent. In order to evaluate the duration it needs to be corrected for frequency. Such corrected QT interval is denoted as QTc. Different equations are used to correct QT for frequency but often the equation of Bazett is used: QTc = QT interval / $\sqrt{}$ RR interval [65].

In normal hearts the start of the T wave is caused by the decline of the plateau of the epicardial action potential, while the peak of the T wave correlates in time with the full repolarisation of the epicardium. The next region that repolarises is the endocardium, while the last region to repolarise is the midmyocardial region. The end of the T wave thus coincides with the repolarisation of the midmyocardial M cells (Fig. IV.6). Since the epicardial cells have the shortest action potential duration (APD) and the midmyocardial cells have the longest action potentials, the time interval between the peak and the end of the T wave represents the transmural dispersion of repolarisation [25].

The average direction of the T wave vector is similar to the average direction of QRS vector. This is due to the shorter epicardial action potential, which causes the repolarisation wave to start at the epicardial surface at the base of the ventricle. The general direction of propagation of the repolarisation wave in the normal heart is therefore roughly the opposite of the propagation of the activation wave. Since the dipole vector points from cells that are depolarised to cells at the resting potential, the general direction of the repolarisation vector is towards the epicardium. The repolarisation and activation vectors therefore point in similar directions, causing the polarity of the T wave in most ECG derivations to be similar to the average polarity of the QRS complex (Fig. VI.6). Changes in the direction of the T wave occur in a several pathological conditions, e.g. ischaemia, hypothermia, arrhyhmias, and remodeling (cardiac memory) (See Chapters VII, VIII, IX).

4.4 The U wave

A diastolic deflection, the so-called U wave, is often seen in normal conditions as a separate deflection following the end of the T wave. The normal U wave is usually monophasic and directed similarly to the T vector. Three theories have been proposed as explanation for the normal U wave [for review see 1115]:

– One theory [1258] explains the U wave as due to the repolarisation of the His Purkinje system. However the small mass of the His Purkinje system is not easily reconciled with the size of U waves reported in the literature, especially since in experiments in canine left ventricle the repolarisation of Purkinje fibres thus far failed to register on the ECG, so that no direct evidence for this hypothesis has been obtained from simultaneous measurements of action potential and ECG (see e.g. Fig. VI.9) [1311].

– Another hypothesis explains the U wave as due to late repolarisation of a region of ventricular myocardium. With the discovery of midmyocardial M cells, with action potential duration longer than subendocardial and subepicardial cells (see Chapter I, and section 5.1), it was proposed that the repolarisation of M cells is responsible for the U wave. Drouin found a concordance between changes in time of repolarisation of human M cells and changes in QTU interval, providing support for the hypothesis that the M cells contribute to the U wave on the ECG [280]. From experiments with potential recordings from arterially perfused canine left ventricular wedge preparations, however Antzelevitch [1311] provided evidence that the repolarisation of the M cells correlates with the end of the T wave (Fig. VI.9).

– According to the mechanoelectric feedback hypothesis, the U wave would be due to afterpotentials caused by ventricular stretch [see 1115]. While no proof for the hypothesis has been obtained thus far, the main support for the theory rests on the timing of the U wave, which is largely concomitant with the rapid ventricular filling phase, and on experiments with ventricular stretch applied at the end of the action potential.

Since thus far for none of the hypotheses conclusive evidence could be obtained, the nature of the normal U wave remains unresolved.

5. IMPORTANCE OF DISPERSION OF ACTION POTENTIAL CONFIGURATION

Dispersion of action potential duration and recovery of excitability is known to favour the development of ventricular fibrillation. Differences in action potential duration are present between different parts of the ventricle (spatial dispersion) [for review see 129], but beat-to-beat differences can occur at the same site (temporal dispersion), resulting in T wave alternans.

5.1   Spatial dispersion of the action potential shape

Action potential shape is different in different regions of the ventricle. Differences are found between left and right ventricle, and between base and apex of the ventricle. Also transmural differences are found in the ventricle and in the atria. In general action potentials are longer at early activation sites and shorter at late activation sites.

5.1.1   Differences between right versus left ventricle

Ventricular action potentials show differences in shape and duration between left and right ventricular myocardium. Action potential notch and i_{to} are much larger in right versus left ventricular epicardium from dog heart [248]. Also action potentials in midmyocardial cells from the right ventricle have shorter duration, deeper notches and less prolongation of the action potential at lower pacing rate, than in midmyocardial cells from the left ventricle. The effects can be related to the larger density of i_{to1} and i_{Ks} in the right ventricle as compared to the left ventricle [1222]. The authors conclude that arrhythmogenic electromotive gradients could also arise at the septal junction of the right and left ventricle, and suggest that the contribution of the right ventricle to the formation of J waves in the ECG may be larger than previously assumed.

5.1.2   Differences between apex and base of the ventricle

Cheng et al. [175] demonstrated that rabbit ventricle action potentials from cells at the base of the ventricle have shorter duration than action potentials at the apex, and that the difference is due to a different distribution of i_{Kr} and i_{Ks}. Both i_{Kr} and i_{Ks} densities are significantly smaller in apical than in basal myocytes, and while i_{Kr} is the largest component in apical cells, i_{Ks} is the dominant component at the base. The shorter duration op the action potential at the base causes the repolarisation of the ventricle to proceed from base towards apex. As already mentioned, this is the reason for the polarity of the T top in the ECG to be similar to the average polarity of the QRS complex. Since the dispersion of APD and refractoriness is a substrate for reentrant arrhythmias, the inhomogeneous distribution of i_{Kr} and i_{Ks} between apex and base could be important for the effects of class III antiarrhythmics blocking i_{Kr}, and β agonists and antagonist which mainly affect i_{Ks} [see 1181].

5.1.3   Transmural dispersion

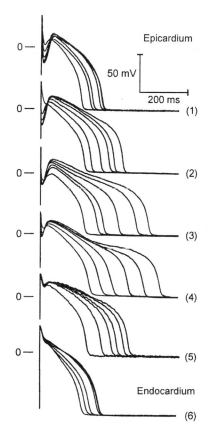

Figure VI.7. Spatial dispersion and frequency-dependence of the shape and duration of the ventricular action potential, showing that APD and its spatial dispersion is rate-dependent. Action potentials were recorded from myocytes from different transmural regions of the canine left ventricular myocardium: epicardium (1), endocardium (6), while M cells (3 and 4) and transitional cells (2 and 5) were obtained from the midmyocardial region. Basic cycle length was varied between 300 ms (shortest action potentials) and 8000 ms (longest action potentials. Modified from [665].

Studies in isolated tissues and myocytes demonstrated differences in action potential duration and configuration across the ventricular wall: the APD shows a so-called "transmural dispersion" (Fig. VI.7). It is shorter in subepicardial than in subendocardial cells, a finding which has been obtained in several animal species, including cells isolated from the human left ventricular wall [772]. The longest action potentials are found in the so-called "M cells" of the midmyocardial wall [1039], and the presence of M cells has also been demonstrated in human ventricle [280,647]. Transmural inhomogeneity is due to differences in expression of ion channels and transporters (see Chapter IV): transmural differences in i_{to1}, i_{Kr}, i_{Ks}, i_{Na}, and Na^+/Ca^{2+} exchanger have been described [for a review see 26] [1364].

It is still controversial whether transmural repolarisation gradients are present in vivo and are relevant to humans: due to cell coupling, local electrotonic currents would tend to mask differences in action potential duration between adjacent cell groups. A recent study failed to find transmural repolarisation differences within the human ventricle [1121].

Epicardium

Subepicardial cells have a short APD and a pronounced phase 1, resulting in a notch and a spike - dome appearance of the action potential. The short APD is due to a pronounced slow component of the delayed outward current i_{Ks}, while the notch is due to the presence of prominent transient outward current i_{to} [660,772,1270]. The i_{to} related spike - dome morphology of the subepicardial action potential is absent in neonates and develops with age [314], [for a review see 22].

Endocardium

Subendocardial cells lack the prominent notch and spike - dome appearance of the subepicardial cells. The absence of a prominent notch in subendocardial cells is a consequence of differences in i_{to} [185,324,354,660]. The transient outward current is about fourfold smaller in human subendocardial cells than in subepicardial cells [772,1270]. Also the kinetics of i_{to} is different: recovery from inactivation is much slower in subendocardial cells than in subepicardial and midmyocardial cells [647,772]. The difference was found to be due to differences in i_{to} isoforms expressed in subendocardial versus subepicardial cells, while also differences exist from apex to base [112].

Midmyocardium

The duration of the ventricular action potential is longest in the midmyocardial region, which contains the so-called M cells [27], which have been described in ventricles of many species including human ventricle [280,647] [for review see 26]. M cells have features intermediate between Purkinje and ventricular cells, but differ is several ways from Purkinje cells, e.g. by their lack of diastolic depolarisation. The M cells are characterised by long duration action potentials with a large maximal rate of depolarisation of phase 0, and a phase 1 with a notch, giving the action potential a spike-dome configuration. Their APD shows a steep frequency response. The M cells are found mostly but not exclusively in the midmyocardium of the left and right ventricle. They contribute to the ECG characteristics in different species including humans [29,45,121,280,647,1092].

The long APD of the M cells is due to a smaller i_{Ks} [26,29,664] [21], and a large Na^+/Ca^{2+} exchange current [1364]. Also the late Na^+ current appears to play a role for the dispersion of the APD across the ventricular wall [21], although different results have been described in M cells from different species. In dogs M cells have a larger persistent Na^+ current than subendo- or subepicardial cells [1039]. The finding that guinea pig M cells have a smaller persistent i_{Na} [963] is still controversial [21]. The spike - dome appearance of M cells, which contrasts with the absence of a notch in subendocardial cells, is due to a large i_{to} [671,1039].

5.1.4   Factors affecting transmural dispersion

As already pointed out the duration of the ventricular action potential is strongly frequency-dependent. However, the different types of ventricular cells have different frequency-dependence, resulting in rate-dependence of the transmural dispersion of ventricular APD (Fig. VI.7). The long APD of the M cells, which is related to a small net repolarising current, makes the potential duration of the M cell very sensitive to a small decrease of outward currents or an increase of inward currents. The prolongation of the APD in response to a slowing of rate is much more pronounced in the M cells than in subendocardial or subepicardial cells [24,26], and this effect is at the basis of development of QT dispersion, T wave alternans, long QT intervals, and cardiac arrhythmias, such as torsades de pointes. The magnitude of the transmural dispersion of the APD in the ventricle is rate-dependent (Fig. VI.7).

APD is also strongly dependent on external K^+ concentration: lowering $[K^+]_e$ prolongs the action potential and the effect is most marked in M cells, causing prolonged QT, flattened T waves with larger QT dispersion, and the eventual appearance of prominent U waves (see section 5.1.5.3) appearing after the end of the T wave in the ECG [1311].

Action potential simulations show that a decrease of i_{Kr} (such as occurs in the presence of sotalol, almokalant and other class III antiarrhythmic drugs or antihistamines such as terfenadine, or in LQT2) or an increase in late i_{Na} (as eg. in LQT3) causes a more pronounced prolongation of the action potential of the M cells than of subepi- or subendocardial cells [1219] which makes these cells much more vulnerable to development of EADs, DADs and triggered activity than subendocardial or subepicardial cells [1040]. The M cells therefore are thought to play an important role in arrhythmias associated with abnormal repolarisation, such as LQT and torsades de pointes [26,28,1023]. i_{Ks} block causes prolongation of the action potentials but decreases the spatial dispersion, since expression of i_{Ks} is less pronounced in M cells, which have the largest APD [1219], but dispersion rises with β-adrenergic stimulation [1024].

Not only the large APD of the M cells, but also the presence of a large i_{to} in subepicardial cells can cause transmural dispersion. Large subepicardial i_{to} has been shown to predispose to all-or-none repolarisation of the subepicardial action potential at the end of phase 1 of the subepicardial action potential and thereby can create important transmural potential gradients that result in ST segment elevation or idiopathic J waves in the electrocardiogram (Fig. VI.8). The transmural dispersion can lead to phase 2 reentry-based life-threatening arrhythmias. Experimental models show electrocardiographic characteristics similar to those of the Brugada syndrome [28,1310].

Changes in potential gradient between subendo- and subepicardium also occur during cardiac memory, which refers to the changes in T wave induced by and persisting after long time high frequency pacing. It has been demonstrated that i_{to} changes can provide at least a partial explanation for this phenomenon [1331].

5.1.5   ECG manifestations of spatial dispersion

The T wave in the ECG signals the ventricular repolarisation, and the duration of the ventricular action potential determines the QT interval. Transmural dispersion of repolarisation therefore contributes to amplitude, polarity and duration the T wave and to the duration of the QT interval and QT dispersion. It can result in ST segment elevation, QT dispersion and pathological U waves. Phase 1 of the action potential corresponds to the beginning of the ST segment, which is marked by the J point, defined as the point where the QRS complex joins the ST segment. Dispersion in the notch and spike - dome configuration of the ventricular action potentials can result in the presence of J waves and ST elevation.

5.1.5.1   ST elevation
Failure of the dome to develop can occur when the outward currents (principally i_{to}) overwhelm the inward currents (i_{Ca} and i_{Na}) during the plateau of the action potential. The loss of action potential dome in the right ventricular epicardium in the presence of a marked plateau of the subendocardial action potential creates a potential gradient during the plateau that is manifested as an ST segment elevation in the ECG as seen in the Brugada syndrome (Fig. VI.8) (see also J wave) [see 15,22]. While the ST elevation caused by dispersion of the ventricular action potential is a true ST denivellation, the ST elevation seen during early ischaemia is due to a combination of true ST elevation (due to changes in action potential

duration) and QT depression (due to changes in resting potential) (see section 4.2).

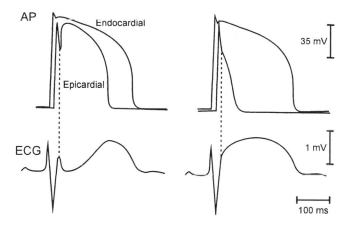

Figure VI.8. Loss of the action potential dome in the right ventricular epicardium but not the endocardium underlies ST segment elevation seen in the Brugada syndrome. Failure of subepicardial action potentials to develop spike - dome configuration gives rise to ST segment elevation as in the Brugada syndrome. Modified from [15].

5.1.5.2   QT dispersion

The QT interval, QT dispersion, the T wave peak-to-end interval, and the width and amplitude of the T wave, while often changing in parallel, contain different information. The measurement of QT dispersion, although it is dependent on the spatial dispersion of the duration of the action potential, does not represent an accurate quantitative measure of heterogeneity of refractoriness [61,347,601,629,696,786,961].

5.1.5.3   The abnormal T-U complex

Abnormal U waves occur in several pathological conditions, such as ischaemia, infarction and ventricular hypertrophy. In non-physiological types of QT prolongation such as LQT, notched T waves or prominent pathological U waves (so called T-U complexes) are often present. According to the M cell hypothesis, the U wave would be due to the late repolarisation of the M cells. From experiments with potential recordings from arterially perfused canine left ventricular wedge preparations, Antzelevitch [1311] provided evidence that the repolarisation of the M cells correlates with the end of the T wave (Fig. VI.9), and claims that the forces that give rise to pathological U waves, such as occur e.g. in LQT syndromes, are different from these responsible for the normal U wave. The pathological T-U complex is likely to be due to the presence of a second component in an interrupted T wave, resulting from potential gradients along the transmural axis on either side of the M region. The abnormal T-U complex therefore appears to be related to dispersion of action potential duration, while this does not appear to be the case for the normal U wave. In the presence of marked QT prolongation it is therefore necessary to make a distinction between a notched T wave (T-U complex) and a normal U wave.

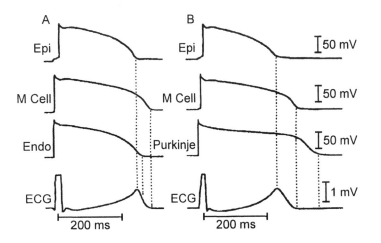

Figure VI.9. Cellular basis for the normal T wave. Simultaneous measurements from transmembrane potentials and transmural ECG in dogs show that the top and end of the T wave coincide with repolarisation of subepicardial respectively midmyocardial M cells. Modified from [1311].

5.1.5.4   The J wave

J waves (also called Osborne waves [see 483]), which are large deviations of the J point from the baseline, can be present in the ECG in certain conditions such as hypothermia, hypercalcemia or Brugada syndrome. A more prominent i_{to}-mediated spike - dome action potential morphology in the epicardium than in the endocardium has been proposed as the basis for J waves. Direct evidence for this hypothesis has been obtained from simultaneous registrations of transmembrane action potentials from several sites across the ventricular wall together with a transmural ECG [1310]. J waves are therefore thought to provide an index of the prominence of the spike - dome morphology of the epicardium. Volders et al. [1222] described that marked differences are present in i_{to}-mediated notches between M cells in right and left ventricle. These authors concluded that arrhythmogenic electromotive gradients could also arise at the septal junction of the right and left ventricle, and suggested that the contribution of the right ventricle to the formation of J waves in the ECG may be larger than previously assumed. (see Fig. VI.8 left panel).

5.2 Temporal dispersion and T wave alternans

Not only does the APD show spatial non-uniformity across the ventricular myocardium, it can also show marked beat-to-beat changes (temporal dispersion) alternating between short and long action potentials. These alternations coincide with beat-to-beat changes in amplitude of the T wave of the ECG (T wave alternans) and promote reentrant ventricular tachycardia [44,78,514,520,843,844,1022,1267]. The alternations in APD may be uniform across the myocardium (concordant alternans). However they may also be 180 degrees out of phase in different areas, the APD being short in some areas while being at the same time long in other areas. This causes beat-to-beat alternations in magnitude and direction of spatial gradients (discordant alternans). It results in enhanced dispersion of repolarisation and T wave, and can cause unidirectional block in the absence of a structural barrier, which can lead to polymorphic ventricular tachycardia. Structural barriers facilitate discordant alternans by electrically uncoupling neighbouring regions of myocardium, and can serve as an anchor for stable reentry resulting in alternans-based monomorphic ventricular tachycardia [44,78,844].

Spatial heterogeneity of repolarisation can form a substrate for unidirectional block and reentry provoked by a premature stimulus [44,620]. In the presence of spatial dispersion of APD and refractoriness, a premature beat can generate temporal dispersion of repolarisation. The spatio-temporal dispersion can result in a zone of functional conduction block causing a premature beat to propagate unidirectionally and can thereby initiate reentry. Spatio-temporal dispersion of refractoriness provides a unifying mechanism that can explain a broad range of cardiac arrhythmias.

Chapter VII

Acute ischaemia

1.   CHANGES DURING ISCHAEMIA

1.1   Biochemical changes

1.1.1   Shift from oxidative metabolism to anaerobic glycolysis

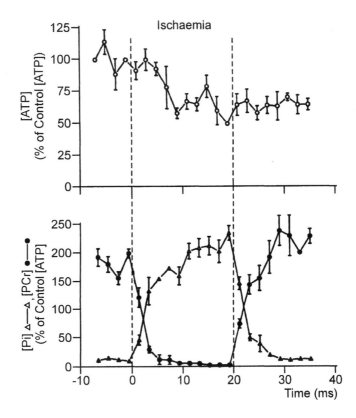

Figure VII.1. Metabolic consequences of ischaemia on intramitochondrial levels of ATP, inorganic phosphate (Pi) and phosphocreatine (PCr). Values are expressed as percent of control [ATP] obtained from 31P-NMR spectra in perfused ferret hearts. Modified from [702].

Acute interruption of blood flow causes a substantial fall in oxygen tension in the cytoplasm. In normal cells the turnover rate of high energy phosphates is so elevated that the time limit for exhaustion of the store is less than a minute [390]. When oxygen falls below a critical level the process of H$^+$ ejection in the mitochondrion stops and the energy stored in the proton electrochemical gradient becomes insufficient to synthesize ATP in sufficient amount. As a consequence the [ATP] may be expected to fall (Fig.

VII.1) and that of [ADP] and [Pi] to increase. The cell however has efficient means to maintain the [ATP] level: i) energy demand falls very rapidly during the first 30 s of ischaemia as a consequence of contraction failure, ii) phosphocreatine (PCr) is continuously used to restore ATP from ADP with concomitant increase in inorganic phosphate, iii) anaerobic glycolysis starts and intensifies.

Although the concentration of [ATP] stays remarkably constant, the free energy change upon hydrolysis of ATP immediately falls because of the rise in concentration of ADP and of Pi [337]. This has important consequences for a number of ATP-driven transporters such the Na^+/K^+ ATPase and the Ca^{2+} ATPase. The anaerobic glycolytic process is also self-inhibiting because of excessive generation of acidosis. Under those conditions the ATP synthase may act as a ATP hydrolase when the energy stored in the proton electrochemical gradient becomes too small [249]) (Fig. VII.2). The energy of this ATP hydrolysis is used to keep the mitochondrion polarised. If this process becomes deficient the mitochondrial membrane becomes depolarised and the mega channel or transition pore in the inner membrane is activated [874]. This leads to irreversible changes.

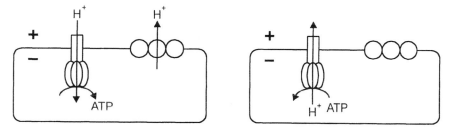

Figure VII.2. When the electron transport is deficient (right panel), the ATP synthase starts acting as an ATPase to keep the mitochondrial membrane polarised by extruding H^+ from the mitochondrial matrix.

In the next section a discussion is made of deleterious consequences of the block in oxidative metabolism, more specifically the disturbances in lipid metabolism, generation of free radicals, release of catecholamines and of purinergic substances.

1.1.2 Disturbances of lipid metabolism, generation of radicals, release of catecholamines, ATP and adenosine

1.1.2.1 Lipid metabolism

The arrest of β-oxidation caused by the anaerobic conditions, results in accumulation in the cytoplasm of fatty acids carnitines or long chain acyl carnitines (LCAC) (Fig. VII.3) and with some delay in a 4-7 times increase of fatty acids (FA). The metabolism of phospholipids is drastically disturbed by activation of a number of lipases [see 1177]. Arachidonic acid (AA) is released. Concomitantly, inositoltrisphosphate (IP3), diacylglycerol (DAG), lysophosphoglycerides (LPG) and specifically lysophosphatidylcholine (LPC) concentrations increase [728].

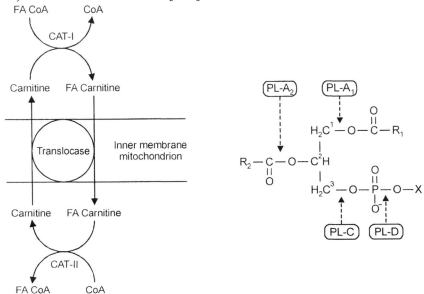

Figure VII.3. Left: Under aerobic conditions FA CoA is transformed to FA carnitine at the outer mitochondrial membrane and the reverse reaction occurs inside under the influence of carnitine acyltransferase (CAT). These reactions stop when oxygen is absent. Right: Phospholipases attack phospholipids at different sites.

All these substances accumulate in the plasma membrane, the gap junction membrane and intracellular membranes of the sarcoplasmic reticulum (SR) and the mitochondrion. LCAC and LPG are amphiphiles and act as zwitterions or cations at physiological pH; fatty acids (including AA) are negatively charged. The different physicochemical properties explain why they exert quite different effects on the function of channels and carriers. Changes occur at three different levels [398]: i) the channel or transporter protein, ii) the phospholipids surrounding the channel and iii) the whole lipid composition of the membrane. They consist in modifications of the electrical charge with accompanying modulation of channel gating and of the local concentration of permeating ions. The interaction with the whole lipid bilayer may be of a more general, non-specific detergent nature and result in an increase of membrane fluidity.

1.1.2.2 Radicals

Oxidative stress results from the excessive generation of radicals, peroxides and singlet oxygen on one hand, and from the deficiency of protective mechanisms (enzymes and scavengers) which normally eliminate these radicals on the other hand.

Free radicals are a normal product of the metabolic chain and, in some instances, functionally very useful (e.g. NO). In aerobic metabolism, between 1 and 5 % of total oxygen is reduced to superoxide during the oxidation of NADPH to $NADP^+$ [70]. In the presence of sufficient superoxide dismutase (SOD), the superoxide anion is directly transformed with H^+ to the less toxic hydrogen peroxide (Fig. VII.4). During aberrant metabolism (ischaemia or reperfusion) however, when high energy electrons leak out of the metabolic chain, radicals are formed to a higher degree [606]. The danger arises when superoxide radical, the NO radical and H_2O_2 are produced in excessive amounts and lead to the formation of the very reactive hydroxyl radical and secondary to lipid peroxylradicals (Fig. VII.4).

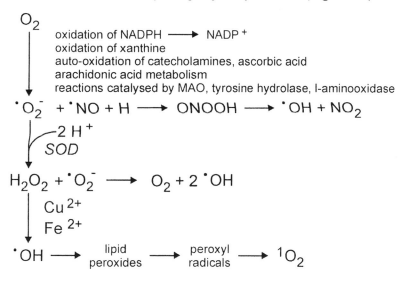

Figure VII.4. Schematic representation of possible reactions for radical production during ischaemia.

A second important factor in the genesis of oxidative stress is deficiency in the protection. The cell is protected against abnormal generation or too long persistence of radicals by a number of reactions catalysed by superoxide dismutase, catalase, glutathion oxidase and peroxidase. Radicals are further neutralized by anti-oxidants or scavengers: examples are vitamine E or α-tocopherol, vitamine C, glutathion, histidine and other aminoacids, carotenoids, flavinoids. In ischaemia and reperfusion these enzymes and scavengers are less available.

Radicals attack proteins and lipids [90]. Sulhydryl groups of proteins are oxidized and disulfide groups are formed, resulting in disturbances of the ion permeation or gating of ion channels, decrease of transport capacity of carrier molecules, and activation of enzymes. Membrane lipids, cholesterol and polyunsaturated FAs undergo peroxidation and change indirectly the behaviour of channels.

1.1.2.3   Release of catecholamines, ATP and adenosine

Ischaemia causes the appearance of high concentrations of catecholamines in the circulation and in the space surrounding the cardiac cells. An immediate release in the systemic circulation occurs following stimulation of pain receptors and afferent nerve fibres in the ischaemic zone (depolarisation due to increased $[K^+]_e$ and shortage of O_2) and is of short duration. At that time the local release in the ischaemic zone is negligible [797]. Around 10-15 min a second local and "metabolic" release phase starts which is quantitatively much more important (100 to 1000 times larger). The underlying mechanism (Fig. VII.5) of this phase is different from the first "exocytotic" phase and is accompanied by a reversal of the Na^+-dependent carrier which normally is responsible for the transmitter reuptake in the nerve endings [986]. Due to shortage of metabolic energy the Na^+/K^+ ATPase is blocked, $[Na^+]_i$ rises and causes the Na^+-dependent uptake transport to reverse. The increase in $[Na^+]_i$ is amplified by an acidosis-enhanced Na^+/H^+ exchange. At the same time the storage of the neurotransmitter in the vesicles falls to low levels because of inhibition of the H^+ ATPase.

The effect of this excessive release of catecholamines is amplified by increases in α- and β-receptor densities during acute ischaemia. The underlying mechanism for β-receptor upregulation is a translocation from an intracellular pool to the plasma membrane [692]. For α- receptors it is not a translocation but an uncovering process by the increased level of LCACs and consequent increase of membrane fluidity [214].

Although β-receptor density is upregulated early during ischaemia, synthesis of cAMP is finally reduced by stimulation of β-receptor kinase, which inactivates or desensitises the receptor [1169]. Initially during ischaemia AC activation may be increased, but later and certainly in the chronic stage density of the receptors is decreased and desensitisation takes over.

The concentration of extracellular ATP is increased by release from nerve endings and directly from the cardiac cells. Although micromolar concentrations can be reached, ATP is rapidly degraded to ADP, AMP and adenosine by ecto-nucleotidases. Adenosine is also released from the cardiac cell. It can reach high concentrations, permitting rapid signaling (see Chapter V).

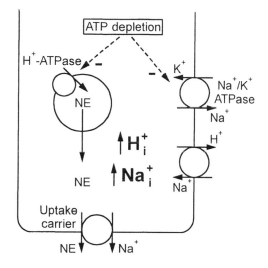

Figure VII.5. The massive release of catecholamines after 10 - 15 min of cardiac ischaemia is due to the reversal of the Na^+-dependent carrier which is normally responsible for the reuptake in nerve endings. Modified from [986].

1.2 Electrical changes

1.2.1 Description of electrophysiological changes

The most important electrical changes that occur upon acute and complete block of the circulation are summarised below [for review see 520,1288]:

- Fall in diastolic potential: depolarisation
- Initial lengthening, followed by shortening of the action potential, fall in amplitude and maximal rate of depolarisation
- Effective refractory period is prolonged relative to action potential duration: postrepolarisation refractoriness
- Fall in conduction velocity
- Excitability: initial increase followed by decrease to inexcitability
- Arrhythmias: phase Ia (2 - 10 min); phase Ib (20 - 30 min).

Arrest of blood flow results within 2-3 min in depolarisation of the normal resting potential from -85 to -60 mV. The initial fall in diastolic potential is accompanied by a slight increase in excitability. With further depolarisation, the amplitude and maximum rate of depolarisation during the upstroke of the action potential become reduced and excitability decreases. The upstroke, which normally shows a smooth time course may now be subdivided into more than one component and conduction gradually becomes depressed [519] (Fig. VII.6). Activation of the ventricles which is normally complete in 80 - 100 ms now requires 200 - 300 ms. Delayed activation is especially prominent in the subepicardium, whereas activation of the subendocardial layers is relatively unaffected.

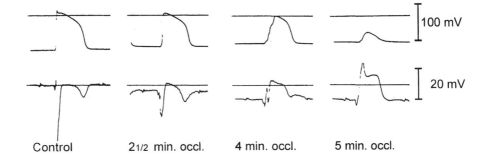

Control   2½ min. occl.   4 min. occl.   5 min. occl.

Figure VII.6. Transmembrane potentials (top traces) and local extracellular electrograms (lower traces; direct current records) from an isolated perfused pig heart before, at 2.5, 4 and 5 min after occlusion of the left anterior descending coronary artery. In the electrogram the fall in resting potential is seen as a depression of the TQ segment; the decrease in action potential amplitude and in upstroke velocity causes delayed intrinsic deflection; the fall in plateau height results in ST segment elevation. Modified from [519].

Initially the duration of the action potential (APD) is slightly prolonged [1212] but changes rapidly to a shortening. Typical for the ischaemic condition is the long effective refractory period (ERP) which follows the shortened action potential. APD and ERP thus change in opposite direction. This phenomenon causes the so-called postrepolarisation refractoriness (Fig. VII.7).

Between 7 to 10 min the APD may show beat-to-beat alternations with quasi-normal APD following very short durations (Fig. VII.8). Complete unresponsiveness follows very soon.

After 15 to 20 min however, cells in the middle of the infarction may temporarily regain their excitability although the upstroke and amplitude remain depressed. This is the time that catecholamines are massively released and the collateral circulation becomes operative [986]. After about

30 min however, the cells further depolarise and conduction is completely blocked. When ischaemia persists, irreversible phenomena occur [210].

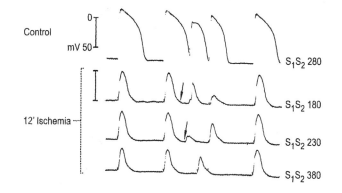

Figure VII.7. Postrepolarisation refractoriness. Stimuli were delivered 1 mm from the recording site. S1S2: coupling interval between control pulse and extra stimulus in ms. In control situation, recovery of excitability closely follows repolarisation. After 12 min of ischaemia, the heart responded to a test stimulus applied 100 ms earlier than in the control situation. However, the latency between stimulus and response is more than 100 ms. For a stimulus interval of 230 ms there is a minimal latency but a very small response. Reasonable action potentials without latency occurred only when the coupling interval was increased to 380 ms, well after completion of repolarisation. Modified from [273].

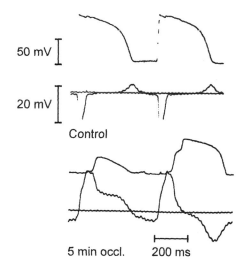

Figure VII.8. Alternation in action potential configuration 5 min after coronary occlusion in the pig heart. Top traces: transmembrane potentials; lower traces: DC electrograms. Note separation of the upstroke into two components in lower right potential. Modified from [586].

All these changes do not occur uniformly over the infarcted myocardium, and heterogeneity is especially pronounced at the border zone. The border zone is the zone which limits the infarct in the plane of the ventricular wall but also in the transmural direction. The existence of marked differences is not unexpected: dispersion of the action potential duration exists already under normal conditions and gradients for action potential duration occur from subepi- to subendocardium [27], between apex, free wall and septum [381], and between right and left ventricle [1222]. In contrast to the existence of postrepolarisation refractoriness in the middle of the infarct zone, the dissociation between APD and ERP is less present or absent in the border zone of the infarct; in this region both APD and ERP shorten to the same extent.

Also excitability is differently affected in the border zone compared to the central zone. On both sides of the border [306], excitability can be increased: at the ischaemic side because of a small rise in $[K^+]_e$, and at the non-ischaemic side because of the existence of an injury current, both resulting in moderate depolarisation (Fig. VII.9). A reduction of 20% in threshold has been measured in a 1-2 mm width adjacent to the ischaemic border. At the endocardial border zone injury current may affect the Purkinje system in such a way that diastolic depolarisation which did not reach threshold now results in spontaneous activity. Injury current is generated by the difference in membrane potential between two zones: a maximum is obtained when activation of the ischaemic zone occurs at the moment the normal zone already repolarises.

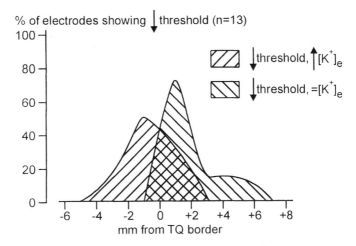

Figure VII.9. Spatial distribution of electrical threshold and $[K^+]_e$ over the border zone of an ischaemic zone. Threshold is decreased in a substantial number of sites (electrodes). This increase in excitability may occur with or without concomitant change in $[K^+]_e$. Modified from [213].

For an electrode facing the ischaemic zone, the fall in resting potential during the first minutes of ischaemia is reflected in an initial depression of the TQ segment in the electrocardiogram recorded with a DC amplifier [532] (Fig. VII.6). In the classic ECG this is seen as a ST segment elevation. The intrinsic deflection is delayed and the QRS broadened. After about 5 min the ST segment becomes further elevated because of the shorter action potential in the ischaemic part of the heart [519]. Later, when activation in the ischaemic region is seriously delayed, the ST segment becomes markedly elevated and is followed by a pronounced inverted T wave. After 8-15 min local activation transiently recovers and is often accompanied by T wave alternans [387]. When cells in the central zone of an infarct become inexcitable the electrocardiogram shows monophasic derivations.

Arrhythmias are a serious complication of acute ischaemia [1288]. In most animals a first burst of tachycardia is seen between 2 and 10 min (called phase Ia, see Fig. VII.10) [1057]; evolution into ventricular fibrillation during this phase is rare. This is followed by a 10 min period of relative quiescence. A second phase (phase Ib) of arrhythmias appears between 20 and 30 min. The percentage of animals showing these arrhythmias is less than in phase Ia, but the evolution towards ventricular fibrillation and death is more frequent. For a more complete analysis see Chapter VIII.

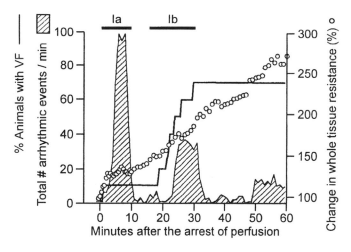

Figure VII.10. Two phases of arrhythmias (Ia and Ib, solid horizontal bars) can be distinguished during acute cardiac ischaemia. Plot shows percentage of pigs with ventricular fibrillation (VF; solid line, left axis) during a 60 min ischaemic period; on the same axis is shown total number of arrhythmogenic events per 1 min period. Open circles (right axis) indicate mean percentage change in tissue resistance. Major increase occurs during Ib period and is accompanied by increased probability of VF. Modified from [1057].

1.2.2   Mechanisms underlying the electrophysiological changes

1.2.2.1   Mechanisms responsible for the changes in resting potential
1.2.2.1.1   Rise of extracellular K⁺

The major cause of the large depolarisation during ischaemia is an increase in $[K^+]_e$ (Fig. VII.11). As explained in Chapter II, the membrane potential in the absence of an action potential is mainly determined by the equilibrium potential for K^+ ions, E_K, and will thus fall as $[K^+]_e$ rises.

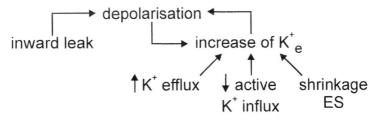

Figure VII.11. The fall in resting potential or depolarisation is caused by accumulation of extracellular $[K^+]_e$ and the existence of net inward current. (ES: extracellular space).

K^+ loss during acute ischaemia occurs in three phases [1282] (Fig. VII.12). A first phase starts during the initial 20 s after the occlusion of a coronary artery when the external $[K^+]_e$ rapidly rises and reaches values to between 8 and 20 mM after 3 to 10 min. The concentration then stabilises at a plateau for 5-10 min, during which the $[K^+]_e$ is constant or slowly changing in the positive or negative direction. Later, after 15-20 min a secondary and irreversible rise occurs.

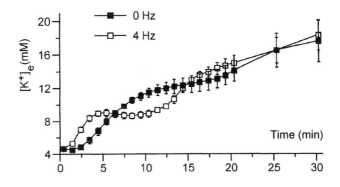

Figure VII.12. Increase in $[K^+]_e$ during ischaemia in Langendorff-perfused quiescent and stimulated (4 Hz) rat hearts, measured with K^+-sensitive electrodes inserted in mid-left myocardium. Note faster rise but lower plateau during stimulation; the effect on the plateau has been interpreted as being due to activation of the Na^+/K^+ pump. Modified from [1282].

The time to reach the plateau and the actual levels of $[K^+]_e$ differ widely among species, and depend on the rate of beating (Fig. VII.12) and on the degree of activation of the sympathetic nervous system. The changes in $[K^+]_e$ are far from homogeneous, with higher concentrations in the centre of the infarct, and in the subepicardium as compared to subendocardium [981].

The mechanisms responsible for the rise in $[K^+]_e$ are increased K^+ efflux, decreased K^+ influx and shrinkage of the extracellular space (Fig. VII.11). Shrinkage is essentially due to the intracellular breakdown of complex molecules into smaller units, followed by water absorption in the cell. The resulting shrinkage of the extracellular space is only responsible for a few % of the observed rise in $[K^+]_e$ [1312]. Of major importance is the increased efflux of K^+ ions through specific K^+ channels which become activated during ischaemia, such as $i_{K.ATP}$ [for review see 1137], and possibly $i_{K.Na}$ and $i_{K.AA}$. Activation of these channels raise the K^+ conductance of the membrane. By itself this change in K^+ conductance would hyperpolarise the membrane, bring the membrane potential close to E_K and thus limit further K^+ efflux. However, as long as the preparation remains excitable and action potentials are generated, the mean membrane potential remains markedly positive to E_K and causes net K^+ efflux from the cells. When the cell becomes inexcitable the rate of K^+ loss slows down and remains only dependent on the existence of an inward leak current. The importance of K.ATP activation in causing depolarisation has recently been convincingly demonstrated by the use of transgenic mice with a knockout of the K.ATP channel [652]. While induction of ischaemia in wild type mice did result in a typical ST denivellation (the ECG sign of depolarisation), this was not the case in the mutant animals (Fig. VII.13).

The second main reason for K^+ loss is a fall in active K^+ influx, caused by inhibition of the Na^+/K^+ pump. From the maximum capacity of the Na^+ pump [782] and the size of the extracellular space it can be estimated that complete inhibition of the pump can result in a rise of 18 mmol $K^+.l^{-1}.min^{-1}$. A partial inhibition of active K^+ influx is thus more than sufficient to account for the accumulation of $[K^+]_e$. Such moderate inhibition of the pump during ischaemia is plausible: LCAC [1013] and oxygen free radicals [1007] have been found to reduce pump activity. Availability of metabolic energy needed to fuel the pump furthermore, becomes deficient. This is not due to the absolute fall in [ATP] alone but much more to the increase in [ADP] and [Pi] which cause a substantial fall in the energy delivered from ATP hydrolysis, called the phosphate potential. According to estimations [373] the phosphate potential may drop to such low values that the pump stops functioning at the resting potential. In accord with the assumption of a partial block of the pump activity recent measurements reveal substantial increases in $[Na^+]_i$ (see section 1.2.2.2).

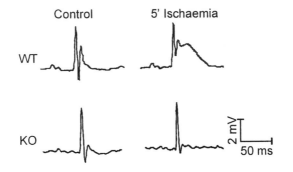

Figure VII.13. Electrographic phenotypes of wild type and homozygous Kir6.2 knockout mice (Kir6.2 codes for the pore forming unit of the K.ATP channel). Typical electrocardiograms from wild type (top) and knockout (bottom) mice in control and during ischaemia: ST denivellation is present in wild type, but not in knockout animals. Modified from [652].

1.2.2.1.2   Inward leak current

Apart from the rise in $[K^+]_e$ and the accompanying fall in E_K, inward background current is an additional source for depolarisation (Fig. VII.11). The importance of this leak current for K^+ loss has already been emphasized. The inward background current is mainly carried by Na^+ and Ca^{2+} ions. Na^+ channels are modified by LPC in such a way that they open and show continuous activity at the resting potential level [1168]. Inward current via non-selective cation channels can be induced by a multitude of factors: stretch [220], extracellular [ATP] [350], free radicals [506], long chain fatty acids [477], and a rise in $[Ca^{2+}]_i$ [204]. Chloride channels could eventually also contribute to inward current since E_{Cl} is positive to the resting potential. Cl⁻ channels are activated during ischaemia via β -receptor stimulation, a rise in $[Ca^{2+}]_i$, hypotonic volume distention, and $[ATP]_e$. However their role in generating an inward current is poorly investigated [478].

1.2.2.2   Mechanisms of changes in upstroke velocity and action potential amplitude

The decrease in upstroke velocity and amplitude of the action potential is caused by a fall in Na^+ current through the fast Na^+ channel and for a minor extent to the simultaneous increase in outward current causing a short-circuiting effect. This outward current is mainly carried by $i_{K.ATP}$.

> **Fall in Na$^+$ current: i$_{Na}$= N.p$_o$.g.(E$_m$ - E$_{Na}$)**
> i)   inactivation: less Na$^+$ channels available (N.p$_o$)
> ii) fall in conductance: less permeation (g)
> iii) reduction of electrochemical gradient: (E$_m$ -E$_{Na}$)

Three factors play a role in reducing the fast Na$^+$ current. i) the fall in resting potential, due to the rise in [K$^+$]$_e$, is the most important and is responsible for a substantial inactivation of the Na$^+$ channels; ii) a direct decrease in conductance of the channel is caused by interaction with amphiphiles, FAs, oxidative stress and acidosis [1261] causing a reduction of peak Na$^+$ current. Interestingly as mentioned already, some of these agents modify a small proportion of the Na$^+$ channels in such a way that they open repetitively and generate a persistent current which carries inward current at the resting potential and during the plateau of the action potential; iii) a third factor causing a decrease in Na$^+$ current is the fall in the electrochemical gradient due to the depolarisation and simultaneous increase in [Na$^+$]$_i$.

When inward current of Na$^+$ ions is critically lowered, current carried by Ca^{2+} ions may take over and be responsible for a slow Ca^{2+}-mediated upstroke (see below Fig. VII.15). Release of catecholamines favours the genesis of Ca^{2+}-mediated action potentials [150].

Intracellular sodium and ischaemia.
Cytoplasmic free [Na$^+$] concentration varies between 5 and 10 mM for different animal species [1206]. Higher values have been noted in the rat and mouse ventricle (15-16 mM). In general [Na$^+$]$_i$ is greater in subepicardial than subendocardial cells [206]. In each cell restricted diffusion seems to exist in the narrow subsarcolemmal space, called fuzzy space [140,627,1110]. In this fuzzy space the concentration can be higher or lower than in the bulk solution. During ischaemia or metabolic inhibition [Na$^+$]$_i$ increases two to fivefold, with actual values of 20 to 25 mM after 15 to 20 min ischaemia [272,865].

The rise in [Na$^+$]$_i$ is caused by an increased passive influx at the resting potential and a decreased active efflux. A complete block of the pump is estimated to result in an increase of 13.5 mmol.l^{-1}.min^{-1}; a partial block during early ischaemia, which is highly likely, is more than sufficient to explain the rise in [Na$^+$]$_i$ (see 1.2.2.1.1).

In mitochondria the concentration of [Na$^+$] is estimated to be only half the cytoplasmic value, although the matrix of mitochondria is negative [272,1269]; this is due to an efficient Na$^+$/H$^+$ exchange. During ischaemia [Na$^+$] is assumed to increase to the same extent as in the cytoplasm.

1.2.2.3   Mechanisms of changes in action potential duration

Changes in APD consist of an initial lengthening followed by a marked shortening. The transient prolongation of the action potential during the first initial seconds of ischaemia has been related to a drop in local temperature

(> 1°C) [920]. Other mechanisms involved may include an acute inhibition of i_{to} [1212], a fall in i_{K1} as a consequence of intracellular acidosis and a reduction in electrogenic pump current.

The prominent shortening of the action potential which follows very rapidly is caused by an increase in outward current, carried mainly by K^+ ions (partly by Cl^- ions), with only a minor role for the changes in inward Na^+ and Ca^{2+} currents.

Under ischaemic conditions a number of K^+ currents, such as $i_{K.ATP}$ (review [1137]), $i_{K.Na}$ [541,685] and $i_{K.AA}$ [1230] become activated. They carry large time-independent currents and do not show inward rectification. Therefore, outward current increases during depolarisation and the effect is most marked on the plateau of the action potential. The K^+ currents, that are normally active under physiological conditions, such as i_{to} [1212], i_{K1} [504] and i_{Kr}, are inhibited by ischaemic conditions, especially acidosis, but the effect is counteracted by the elevated $[K^+]_e$.

Cl^- currents are activated during ischaemia by osmotic swelling, mechanical stretch, external [ATP], $[Ca^{2+}]_i$ and by β-receptor stimulation, secondary to catecholamine release. Because E_{Cl} is around -30 mV, activation of Cl^- channels will carry outward current at potential positive to -30 mV and promote repolarisation from the peak of the action potential to the plateau. At the resting potential however, they will carry inward leak, and contribute to depolarisation.

A shortening of the action potential also occurs in the non-ischaemic border zone. It is mainly due to "injury current" or short-circuit current generated by the difference in membrane potential between ischaemic and normoxic myocardium and much less to changes in ionic current [557]. This injury current causes a small depolarisation during diastole, but reverses direction during electrical activity and causes enhanced rate of repolarisation.

1.2.2.4   Mechanisms of changes in excitability and effective refractory period

Excitability. In the centre of the infarct excitability is increased during the first minutes of ischaemia: threshold potential remains unchanged, but less current is needed to reach the critical level because of the existing depolarisation [271]. Later, excitability gradually decreases mainly because of inactivation of the Na^+ channel by the depolarisation, which shifts the threshold to more positive values. This reduction in excitability is faster and more pronounced in the subepicardial than in the subendocardial fibres [370].

After 15 min of ischaemia some cells regain excitability; this recovery has been related to some hyperpolarisation, as the result of washout of extracellular K⁺ consequent to the opening of collateral circulation and/or redistribution of K⁺ secondary to stimulation of the Na⁺/K⁺ pump, which may occur following the massive release of catecholamines [987] and the rise in $[Ca^{2+}]_i$ [360]. Catecholamines also facilitate the occurrence of Ca^{2+}-mediated action potentials in depolarised cells by increasing the Ca^{2+} conductance [149]. The recovery of excitability has also been related to an increase in intercellular resistance and gain of safety factor. Experimental results [930] as well as theoretical calculations [1011] have shown that the safety factor for generating a conducted action potential can paradoxically increase when gap junction coupling is reduced, because of reduced load (see Chapter III). Under normal conditions activation of Ca^{2+} channels cannot cause propagation because the current is too small and the threshold for activation too positive. However when gap junction conductance is decreased and the resting potential depolarised, Ca^{2+}-mediated action potentials may take over and be responsible for propagation of the impulse.

A second phase of inexcitability starts after about 30 min and is due to a secondary increase in K⁺ loss from the cells (Fig. VII.12), concomitant with a fall of [ATP] to very low levels. Na⁺ as well as Ca^{2+} channels are further inactivated and cells become uncoupled.

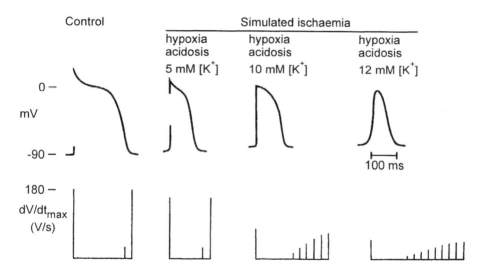

Figure VII.14. Schematic representation of changes in transmembrane action potentials (upper panel) and upstroke velocity (dV/dt $_{max}$) (lower panel), following an action potential in control conditions and in three conditions simulating ischaemia. Modified from [1288].

Refractoriness. In the ischaemic zone, the effective refractory period (ERP) is prolonged (Fig. VII.7) in contrast to the shorter APD. The prolongation of ERP is due to slowing of recovery from inactivation of Na⁺

channels secondary to the depolarisation caused by the high $[K^+]_e$, to block of Na^+ channels by acidosis [1261], LCAC, LPC [1168], and oxygen radicals [91], and to the short-circuiting effect of the opening of K^+ and Cl^- channels. The role of high $[K^+]_e$, acidosis and hypoxia as important contributors to the fall in Na^+ conductance and slow recovery from inactivation has been convincingly demonstrated on *in vitro* preparations (Fig. VII.14) [see 1288].

In the non-ischaemic border zone both the ERP and APD are shortened. The effect is due to the existence of injury current which is depolarising during diastole but hyperpolarising during the plateau of the action potential. Although the Na^+ channels might be slightly inhibited by the small depolarisation during diastole, the increase in resting conductance is absent and limits the fall in excitability. The total duration of the ERP is short and recovery of excitability following the repolarisation is fast [213]. A marked dispersion in ERP thus exists over the border zone, a condition which favours the occurrence of reentry arrhythmias. Sympathetic stimulation increases this type of dispersion [830].

1.2.2.5   Mechanisms of conduction changes

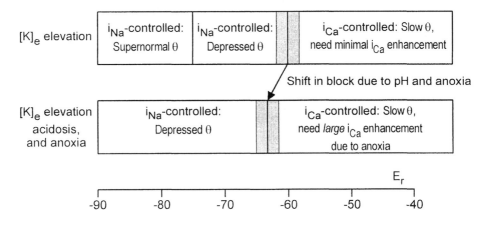

Figure VII.15. Characteristics of propagating action potentials and ionic currents under elevated $[K^+]_e$ only (top) and combined ischaemic conditions (bottom) over a range of $[K^+]_e$ - induced changes in resting potential (E_r). Results are based on calculations using the Luo-Rudy model of action potential. Shaded zone corresponds to region in which biphasic upstrokes are apparent. The bold line in each shaded zone indicates the least depolarised E_r at which conduction fails when i_{CaL} is not enhanced. Modified from [1010].

Under normal conditions, conduction velocity is determined by active properties of the cell (amplitude and upstroke velocity of the action potential) and passive cable properties of the muscle bundle (see Chapter III). During early ischaemia these parameters change and affect conduction velocity in a negative way. At the start, the decrease in amplitude and in rate of rise of the action potential are most important, together with the increased resting conductance of the membrane and the rise of extracellular resistance secondary to blood vessel collapse and cell swelling [583]. The increase in $[K^+]_e$ reduces Na^+ current in a potential-dependent way and slows its recovery. At moderate increases of $[K^+]_e$, conduction is mediated by Na^+ current but at more depolarised levels it becomes dependent on Ca^{2+} current. The simultaneous acidosis shifts the dependence on Ca^{2+} current activation in the negative direction and raises the requirement for elevation of the Ca^{2+} conductance to maintain conduction (Fig. VII.15). Enhancement of Ca^{2+} conductance is made possible by the massive release of catecholamines.

At a later stage (>15 min) cell resistance increases dramatically and results in a marked fall of conduction. This change is due to the closing of gap junctions, following the joint rise in $[H^+]_i$ and $[Ca^{2+}]_i$ [127,811,1272], the effect of LCAC [1297,1305] and a further fall in [ATP]. The existence of transjunctional potentials may cause additional inactivation of the gap junction conductance [1236]. Modifications in gap junctions are not uniform over the whole infarct zone and this heterogeneity represents an important factor in the genesis of arrhythmias.

Changes in $[H^+]$ and $[Ca^{2+}]_i$

Important parameters in the closing of gap junctions are the changes in $[H^+]$ and $[Ca^{2+}]_i$. Under normal perfusion and oxygenation intracellular pH is slightly more acidic than extracellular pH. During ischaemia, carbonic acid retention and net production of protons shift the intracellular as well as the extracellular pH in the acidic direction [187] (Fig. VII.16). External pH has been described to change rapidly and monotonically from 7.4 to values as low as 6.0. Results on intracellular pH differ, but in general the fall in pH_i is reported to be less pronounced, an effect which has been correlated to the higher buffering capacity of the intracellular medium.

Free cytoplasmic $[Ca^{2+}]$ during diastole and at low stimulation frequencies is of the order of 100 nM (from 50 to 200 nM) [133]. During systole this value may increase to between 500 and 1000 nM or even higher values depending on the Ca^{2+} load in the SR [81]. The resting free Ca^{2+} concentration represents only 0.03% of the total calcium, inclusive stores. During activity the free $[Ca^{2+}]_i$ ion fraction rises to 0.1%.

During metabolic inhibition, the change in systolic $[Ca^{2+}]_i$ is biphasic: an increase during the initial 3-5 min is followed by a secondary fall after a delay of 5-10 min (Fig. VII.17) when diastolic free $[Ca^{2+}]_i$ rises [566,702]. The rise in diastolic $[Ca^{2+}]_i$ precedes the development of contracture and the uncoupling of gap junctions. It is caused by four different mechanisms: 1) Ca^{2+} is displaced from binding sites by the increased H^+ concentration [358], 2) Ca^{2+} uptake in the SR is reduced, secondary to inhibition of the Ca^{2+} ATPase [547], 3) Ca^{2+} is less efficiently removed from the cell via the Na^+/Ca^{2+} exchanger, because of the rise in Na^+ concentration [410] and functional modification by radicals [192] and acidosis [269,861] and

4) an increased inward leak of Ca^{2+}, via background channels activated by radicals [506] and via non-selective cation channels activated by $[ATP]_e$, mechanical stretch and by a rise in $[Ca^{2+}]_i$ itself.

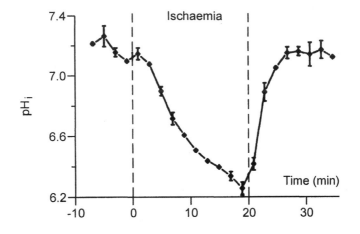

Figure VII.16. Gradual fall of intracellular pH (pH_i) during ischaemia and fast recovery upon reperfusion. Measurements by 31P-NMR in ferret hearts. Modified from [702].

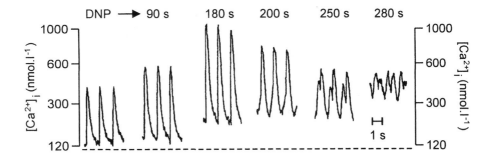

Figure VII.17. Changes in free $[Ca^{2+}]_i$ measured by indo-1 fluorescence in guinea pig myocytes upon metabolic inhibition by exposure to 0.1 mM dinitrophenol (DNP). Cells were voltage clamped with pulses to 0 mV. Systolic $[Ca^{2+}]_i$ increased transiently, before declining and becoming oscillatory. Diastolic $[Ca^{2+}]_i$ gradually increased. Temporary increase in $[Ca^{2+}]_i$ transient has been explained by a block of Ca^{2+} absorption in the mitochondria which normally takes place during systole. Modified from [498].

2. CHANGES DURING REPERFUSION

2.1 Reversible phase

2.1.1 Biochemical changes

If reperfusion occurs following an ischaemic period which does not exceed 30 min, oxygen consumption rapidly recovers with concomitant decrease of the $[NADH]/[NAD^+]$ ratio. After brief (5 to 10 min) ischaemic bouts, PCr concentration quickly returns to normal; recovery of [ATP] however is slow (Fig. VII.1). Following longer periods of ischaemia (not exceeding 30 min), [PCr] still recovers within 5 min but [ATP], which may have dropped to 50%, stays at this low level for 30 min or more [703].

When oxygen tension is restored, the pre-ischaemic pattern of substrate utilisation is normalised, meaning that oxidation of fatty acids is the main contributor to ATP synthesis; the level of glycolysis however, remains elevated in the early period of reperfusion and is important for ATP generation and the normalisation of $[Na^+]_i$ and $[Ca^{2+}]_i$ [663]. FAs are present in high concentration; when their concentration is too high, a stop of glycolysis at the pyruvate level may occur with continuous production of lactate and overproduction of protons. This is a disadvantageous situation which can result in aggravation of Ca^{2+} overload and release of intracellular enzymes [675].

In some instances oxygen consumption rate can be abnormally high early after reperfusion. Futile cycles related to Na^+ and Ca^{2+} transport in the mitochondria may be responsible [225]. As already explained, the energy generated by the electron transport and stored in the proton gradient is used for ATP synthesis but also for maintaining normal $[Na^+]$, $[Ca^{2+}]$ and $[K^+]$ levels in the mitochondria. In the case of Na^+ and Ca^{2+} overload, more energy will be deviated in keeping mitochondrial $[Na^+]$ and $[Ca^{2+}]$ at a low level. When mitochondrial $[Ca^{2+}]$ is critically augmented the mega channel may intermittently open [103]. The leak thus created causes breakdown of the mitochondrial electrical gradient and release of Ca^{2+}. Activation of the mega channel may propagate from mitochondrion to mitochondrion, creating a Ca^{2+} wave in the cytosol [487]).

2.1.2 Electrical changes and recovery of ion concentrations

Upon reperfusion the concentration of $[K^+]_e$ falls very rapidly and may even decrease transiently below the control level [11]. Washout of the extracellular space together with stimulation of the active Na^+/K^+ pump are the main mechanisms. Concomitant to the normalisation of $[K^+]_e$, $[Na^+]_i$

decreases monotonically and normalises within 5 min. A transient slight increase at the very start of the reperfusion is possible (Fig. VII.18). The fast recovery of [Na$^+$]$_i$ upon reperfusion is somewhat unexpected since washout of protons from the extracellular space should stimulate Na$^+$/H$^+$ exchange and lead to a net Na$^+$ influx. This occurs when H$^+$ ions continue to be produced in excess, as is the case when glycogen is still available. In those instances inhibition of the exchanger improves recovery of contractile activity [490] and prevents arrhythmias [866]. Activation of the Na$^+$/K$^+$ pump however seems mostly to prevail over Na$^+$/H$^+$ exchange in determining [Na$^+$]$_i$.

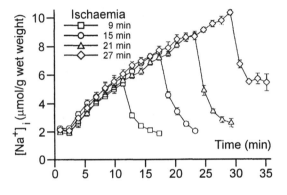

Figure VII.18. Evolution of intracellular [Na$^+$]$_i$ during ischaemia and upon reperfusion in isolated rat heart. ^{23}Na NMR measurements. Recovery of intracellular [Na$^+$]$_i$ became incomplete after ischaemia periods longer than 21 min and was correlated with deficient recovery of contractile activity. Modified from [490].

Washout of external K$^+$ quickly restores the resting potential to normal values (Fig. VII.19). There may even be a transient pronounced hyperpolarisation accompanied by the reduction of [K$^+$]$_e$ below the control value. The mechanism is an early and extra stimulation of the Na$^+$/K$^+$ pump [1178], secondary to the [Na$^+$]$_i$ load. It illustrates nicely that [Na$^+$]$_i$ is more important than [K$^+$]$_e$ in determining pump activity. The action potential however stays very short. This leads to a paradoxical situation where a short action potential is combined with a low [K$^+$]$_e$ [212]. The short action potential is due to the outward current generated by the pump; the low [K$^+$]$_e$ would normally oppose this effect through a reduction of the i$_{K1}$ channel conductance, but pump current seems to be more pronounced. Hyperpolarisation and shortening of the action potential is further caused by open K.ATP channels that may remain activated as long as the ATP concentration is not normalised. Since reopening of the vasculature and recovery of pump activity and ATP synthesis is not homogeneous, marked heterogeneity may exist in APD and ERP.

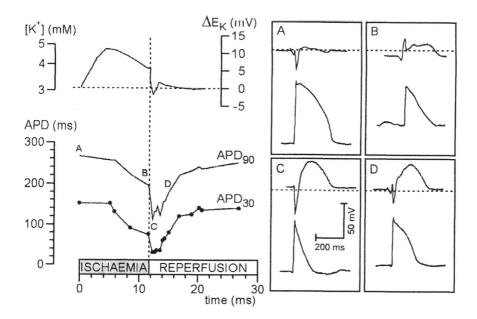

Figure VII.19. Left panels: Evolution of extracellular $[K^+]_e$ and action potential duration (APD) during ischaemia and during reperfusion in an isolated pig heart. Right panels: examples of electrograms and intracellular action potentials at times indicated by letters in the lower left graph. Note the undershoot in $[K^+]_e$ and APD and the peaked T waves in the early phase of reperfusion. Modified from [212].

Excitability is depressed due to incomplete recovery of $[Na^+]_i$ and $[H^+]_i$ concentrations. Spontaneous activity may occur, probably as a consequence of DADs and EADs, which are related to the persistence of Ca^{2+}_i overload. In the reversible phase the change in diastolic $[Ca^{2+}]_i$ can follow two different time courses, depending on the level that had been reached during ischaemia and the extent of recovery of the SR Ca^{2+} ATPase [547,764] and the Na^+/Ca^{2+} transporter activity: i) a rapid decline to the normal value [703]; ii) a initial fall to an intermediate value followed by oscillations, which can end with a return to normal or be followed by a secondary increase [952,1041] (Fig. VII.20). In this last case membrane potential oscillations may be present and trigger arrhythmias [769].

Arrhythmias can occur immediately upon opening of the vasculature or after a delay of 2 to 7 min. The immediate arrhythmias degenerate frequently in ventricular fibrillation. Dispersion of APD and excitability are important parameters in the genesis of reentry [212]. Delayed arrhythmias are of the tachycardia type and are less dangerous. They originate probably in the Purkinje system overlying the infarct zone and are initiated as DADs and EADs [9].

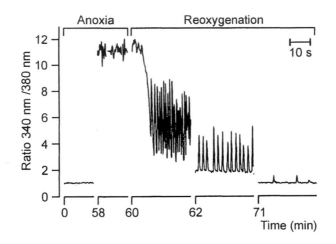

Figure VII.20. Intracellular [Ca²⁺] in relative units at the start, at 60 min of anoxia and during the first ten min of reoxygenation. Intracellular [Ca²⁺], which was importantly increased, recovered rapidly during the first minutes, but showed transient decelerating oscillations before returning to normal levels. Isolated adult rat myocytes. Modified from [1041].

2.2   Irreversible phase

In some cases, even if reperfusion occurs before 30 min of ischaemia, removal of the coronary obstruction does not result in an efficient perfusion. The cause is oxidative stress leading to secondary vasoconstriction and the so-called no-reflow phenomenon. Recovery then becomes substantially retarded or is absent. Reperfusion after more than 30 min may still lead to an important recovery of oxygen consumption but the recovery is only transient, while contractile function remains severely and persistently depressed.

Irreversibility is consequent to a rise of cytoplasmic $[Ca^{2+}]_i$ above 1 µM during ischaemia, which does not recover upon reperfusion [1041,1132]. Reactivation of the Na^+/K^+ pump fails, due to shortage of ATP. Not only cytoplasmic $[Ca^{2+}]_i$ increases to abnormally high levels causing contracture, but also the $[Ca^{2+}]$ concentration in the mitochondria climbs to excessive levels and leads to opening of the mega channel or transition pore [749].

In the mitochondrion free Ca^{2+} concentration at rest or during diastole is somewhat below the cytoplasmic Ca^{2+} concentration or close to it. Although a much higher matrix Ca^{2+} concentration is expected from the negative potential (estimations vary between −150 and −180 mV), mitochondrial [Ca^{2+}] is kept at a low level via the Na^+/Ca^{2+} and Na^+/H^+ exchangers (Fig. VII.21).

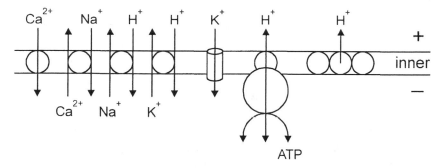

Figure VII.21. The electron transport in the mitochondria generates a proton gradient and an electrical gradient. From the negative matrix potential a high intramitochondrial [Ca^{2+}] concentration is expected. This does not occur because of Na^+/Ca^{2+} and Na^+/H^+ exchangers, which utilise the proton gradient to keep the [Ca^{2+}] concentration in the matrix at a low level. In ischaemia, because of the decreased proton gradient, mitochondrial [Ca^{2+}] will rise.

During ischaemia the Ca^{2+} concentration in mitochondria follows the change in cytosolic Ca^{2+} and net absorption occurs in the mitochondria when the cytoplasm becomes overloaded with Ca^{2+}. This takes place even when the electron transport is inhibited, because the cell will keep the mitochondrial matrix at a negative potential and maintain a proton gradient by reversing the activity of the ATP synthase so that it acts as an ATPase.

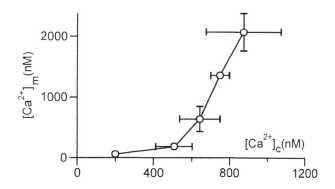

Figure VII.22. Relationship between mitochondrial (ordinate) and cytoplasmic (abscissa) Ca^{2+} concentration. In normal conditions the ratio of the two concentrations is smaller than 1.0. During ischaemia this ratio increases and may become larger than 1.0. Modified from [750].

It has been shown experimentally that the gradient of mitochondrial over cytoplasmic [Ca^{2+}] is less than unity when the cytoplasmic [Ca^{2+}] is below

500 nM; at higher cytoplasmic $[Ca^{2+}]$ levels the mitochondrial $[Ca^{2+}]$ increases in an exponential way and the ratio reverses, with more Ca^{2+} in the mitochondrion than in the cytoplasm [750] (Fig. VII.22). Net absorption of Ca^{2+} in the mitochondria is furthermore favoured by the increased cytoplasmic $[Na^+]_i$ which impedes the Na^+/H^+ exchanger and secondarily the Na^+/Ca^{2+} exchanger.

The presence of such an abnormally high $[Ca^{2+}]$ together with low [ATP], high phosphate, LCAC, acidosis and oxidative stress may cause the massive and steady opening of the mitochondrial mega channels [225,288]. Following such activation all mitochondrial gradients disappear and the final result is hypercontracture and cell death [288,393]. On the microscopic level, cells appear necrotic and later important fibrosis develops.

Chapter VIII

Arrhythmias

1.   BASIC MECHANISMS OF ARRHYTHMIAS

Automatism, triggered activity and reentry are the main mechanisms for generating arrhythmias. Automatism or triggered activity frequently initiate the arrhythmia and reentry most often is responsible for its perpetuation.

1.1   Automatism

In the early embryonic stage all cells are spontaneously active. With development the expression of channel proteins responsible for automatism becomes restricted. In the adult heart automatism is present in the SAN, which is the normal pacemaker centre, but can also be seen in other parts of the heart [495,806]. Diastolic depolarisation is normally present in AVN cells and Purkinje fibres but does not reach threshold. Diastolic depolarisation is also seen in myocardial cells deep in the pulmonary veins [176] and around the orifice of the sinus coronarius [1286]. In pathological conditions a return to the embryologic scheme of protein expression is often seen and spontaneous depolarisation during diastole then occurs in atrial and ventricular myocardial cells.

Three events are responsible for the diastolic depolarisation in SAN cells: deactivation of delayed K^+ current (i_{Kr} or i_{Ks}) [823], activation of the "pacemaker" current i_f and activation of the transient Ca^{2+} current, i_{CaT}. All three effects cause time-dependent depolarisation: i_f and i_{CaT} directly because they carry inward current, i_{Kr} or i_{Ks} deactivation indirectly allowing background currents to depolarise the membrane. Background currents which carry inward current are i_{st}, a sustained inward current (only present in SAN) [403], Na^+/Ca^{2+} exchange current, i_{Cl}, non-selective cation current, and stretch-activated currents.

In AVN and Purkinje cells i_f is present but its activation occurs at negative potentials; diastolic depolarisation is too slow to reach the threshold for the Na^+ channel before an impulse arrives from the sinus. In case of AV block or when the rate of diastolic depolarisation is enhanced by low $[K^+]_e$ or β-receptor stimulation, threshold is attained and automatism starts from the Purkinje system. A special type of automatism occurs in Purkinje cells when they are depolarised to the plateau level (-40 mV) as e.g. in a post-infarct period or upon perfusion with low external $[K^+]_e$. Stimulation of the Ca^{2+} conductance by adrenaline may then generate automatic activity which is dependent on deactivation of delayed K^+ current(s) and reactivation of i_{CaL} (Fig. VIII.1). In plain atrial and ventricular cells spontaneous activity is inhibited mainly because of the presence of a high K^+ conductance, i_{K1}, which keeps the membrane at a hyperpolarized level. i_f current is absent or its activation voltage range is too negative. In pathologic situations however, e.g. ventricular hypertrophy, i_f may become expressed again or its activation curve shifted in the positive direction.

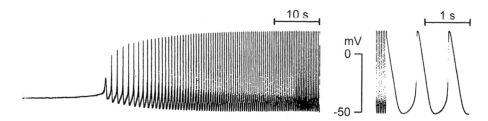

Figure VIII.1. Adrenaline-induced oscillations in a sheep cardiac Purkinje fibre depolarised in a solution with 1.35 mM $[K^+]_e$. Modified from [840].

1.2 Triggered activity

In contrast to automatism, triggered activity is characterised by the obligatory presence of an action potential. Two types of triggered activity can be distinguished: early afterdepolarisations (EAD) [221] and delayed afterdepolarisations (DAD) [222,332].

1.2.1 Early afterdepolarisations (EAD)

Early afterdepolarisations are secondary depolarisations that originate during the plateau or final repolarisation of the action potential (Fig. VIII.2). The main mechanism of EAD is a regenerative increase in Ca^{2+} conductance during the slow phase of the plateau [452,521]. When repolarisation is slow, Ca^{2+} channels can already recover from voltage-dependent and/or Ca^{2+}-dependent inactivation during the plateau phase of the action potential [1047]. In the narrow voltage range where the activation and inactivation processes overlap, Ca^{2+} channels can reactivate and lead to a new depolarisation. Activation of the Na^+/Ca^{2+} exchange current following a secondary release of Ca^{2+} from the SR and the accompanying depolarisation, acts in many cases as a conditioning process for this reactivation process of the Ca^{2+} current [1345]. EADs are thus frequently seen at low rates, following a sinusal pause and in the presence of drugs that block outward K^+ current(s). Under those conditions the action potential is prolonged, with a very slow rate of repolarisation during the plateau, allowing Ca^{2+} channels to recover and to be reactivated [1345].

EADs however can also be induced by acceleration of the stimulation rate [124], especially when the cell is Ca^{2+} overloaded (see Fig. V.7). The underlying mechanism seems to be a secondary release of Ca^{2+}

and extra stimulation of the Na^+/Ca^{2+} exchange current. Usually Ca^{2+} release is restricted to the initial period of the systole. In Ca^{2+} overload, the system's gain or the probability of Ca^{2+} release is enhanced and a second spontaneous release may occur late in the repolarisation process (late plateau and final repolarisation) [58]. This extra release stimulates the Na^+/Ca^{2+} exchanger, causing an extra inward current so that reactivation of i_{CaL} is possible.

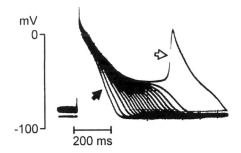

Figure VIII.2. Quinidine-induced early afterdepolarisation in a canine Purkinje fibre. A number of superimposed traces are shown. Black arrow: control; white arrow: triggered action potential. Modified from [926].

1.2.2   Delayed afterdepolarisation (DAD)

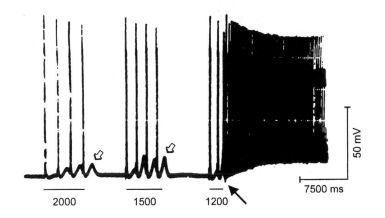

Figure VIII.3. Delayed afterdepolarisations (white arrows) elicited at different rates of stimulation in an atrial fibre of a canine coronary sinus preparation. The preparation was superfused with a Tyrode solution containing noradrenaline. The cycle length and the periods of stimulation are indicated by the horizontal bars. At a cycle length of 1200 ms triggered activity occurred at a high frequency (arrow). Modified from [1286].

Delayed afterdepolarisations follow full repolarisation and are due to the generation of a composite inward current, called transient inward current [332,554]. Depending on the preparation, species or experimental condition, three currents participate to a different extent: the Na^+/Ca^{2+} exchange current, the non-specific cation current, and the Ca^{2+}-induced Cl^- current [204,554,1365]. All three currents are activated by intracellular $[Ca^{2+}]_i$ and carry inward charge at hyperpolarised levels. The Na^+/Ca^{2+} exchanger is certainly the most important component [984].

When the resulting depolarisation is large enough to reach threshold for i_{Na} a propagated extrasystolic action potential is evoked. The situation may become self-replicating and cause runs of extrasystoles or paroxysmal tachycardia (Fig. VIII.3).

The trigger for DADs is spontaneous release of Ca^{2+} from the SR in situations of Ca^{2+} overload. Ca^{2+} overload can be the consequence of block of the active Na^+/K^+ pump by digitalis or hypokalaemia, or be the result of an increase in Na^+ or Ca^{2+} influx caused by high concentrations of catecholamines (Fig. VIII.3), elevated frequency of stimulation, stretch, or administration of Ca^{2+} channel agonists. Increase of passive Na^+ influx or block of active Na^+ efflux will elevate $[Na^+]_i$ and cause the cytosolic $[Ca^{2+}]$ level to rise via the modulated Na^+/Ca^{2+} exchange process.

1.3   Reentry

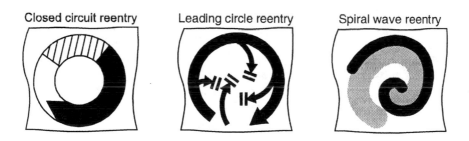

Closed circuit reentry   Leading circle reentry   Spiral wave reentry

Figure VIII.4. Schematic representation of three types of reentry, based on models proposed by Mines [740], Allessie [16] and Pertsov [855].

In reentry an impulse is travelling along a more or less circular pathway and instead of dying out, it reexcites the previously active cells [see 520,1287]. The pathway can be constant (ordered reentry; closed circuit reentry) or variable in size and location (random reentry), of small microscopic or large macroscopic dimensions. The pathway can be determined by an anatomical substrate (Fig. VIII.4) (abnormal junction between auricular and ventricular tissue, orifice of vessels, bifurcations of the Purkinje system, junctions between Purkinje fibres and the ventricular wall) or is entirely determined by functional characteristics (leading circle reentry, anisotropic reentry, spiral wave reentry [1071,1174]) (Fig. VIII.4).

1.3.1   Start of the reentry

Reentry can be started when together with an extra stimulus one of the following conditions is fulfilled: a unidirectional block exists or conduction is slowed to such extent that reflection becomes possible.

Unidirectional block: important parameters
    source-sink mismatch
    vulnerable period
    dispersion: slope of restitution; phase 2 reentry
Bidirectional conduction but critically low: **reflection**

1.3.1.1   Unidirectional block
Different ways of generation of unidirectional block have been discussed in the literature (see Chapter III: 4.2.3).

Source-sink impedance mismatch. When an action potential is generated the action potential not only depolarises the site where it is initiated but also acts as a source of current to depolarise neighbouring cells, which thus act as current sink. In order to obtain normal propagation the total number of positive charges entering the cell at the source should be larger than the positve charges leaving the cells at the sink. Source-sink impedance mismatch can be caused by geometrical factors and can occur when the wave propagates through junctional sites with an important increase in number of cells to be depolarised, e.g. at the interface between Purkinje fibres and ventricular myocardium. More recently it was realised that also the curvature of the wave front is an important source of impedance mismatch. When the wave front is convexly curved, the area of the wave front becomes progressively larger and causes a gradual increase in sink (for a discussion of different factors affecting the curvature see Chapter III, section 4.2.3).

A second important mechanism to generate unidirectional block is related to the existence of a **vulnerable period**. Each action potential is followed by a critical time- (and voltage-) window, during which an extra stimulus can induce unidirectional conduction. Stimulation during this period results in block of conduction in the anterograde direction, because the cells are still refractory, whereas recovery of the Na^+ conductance has proceeded far enough to allow conduction in the retrograde direction [1009].

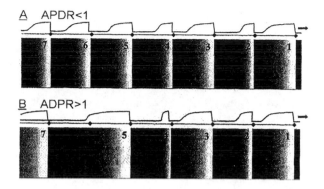

Figure VIII.5. Modelled electrical restitution and wavelength oscillations in a two-dimensional tissue paced at a fixed cycle length (diamonds). Wave front (AP upstroke) is white, wave back (repolarisation) is dark grey. The AP is travelling over the two-dimensional tissue from left to right. With APD restitution slope <1 (A), APD alternans progressively attenuates, but when APD restitution is > 1 (B), amplification occurs until the diastolic interval is too short for the next (sixth) wave to propagate. All these changes occur uniformly over the tissue (concordant alternans). Modified from [1265].

Dispersion in the action potential duration (APD) increases the likelihood to generate unidirectional conduction. Dispersion is normally present in the transmural direction [27], but also exists between apex, septum and the free wall [381] and between right and left ventricle [1222]. Dispersion can become pronounced for extrasystolic stimulation especially when restitution of the APD is fast [915]. When the slope of the relationship between APD and cycle interval is smaller than one, eventual differences in APD for successive stimuli are progressively smoothed out. However when the slope is greater than one, a small change in cycle length becomes amplified into a larger change in APD, generating temporal dispersion [1265] (Fig. VIII.5). The beat-to-beat alternation of APD is accompanied in the ECG as a beat-to-beat alternation in the amplitude of the T wave (T wave alternans). From clinical observations it is well known that ST-T alternans is associated with a higher tendency to ventricular fibrillation [387]. The alternations in APD may be uniform across the myocardium (concordant alternans) because conduction also is uniform. However they may also be 180 degrees out of phase in different areas, the APD being short in some areas while being at the same time long in other areas. This causes beat-to-beat alternations in magnitude and direction of spatial gradients (discordant alternans). The underlying mechanism is disuniform conduction, which can occur e.g. when a stimulus arrives before full recovery of the Na^+ conductance. Conduction velocity then is not constant but changes as the action potential propagates because of the change in diastolic period. Disuniform conduction also occurs when in certain areas cells are partially depolarised cells by elevated external K$^+$ or ischaemia. In those cases the APD does not only show temporal but also an important spatial dispersion. It is thus understandable that under those conditions the likelihood for unidirectional block and for reentry arrhythmia is drastically increased.

An example of extreme dispersion is "phase 2 reentry" [686]. Due to an abnormal increase in i_{to} and/or decrease in i_{CaL}, phase 2 or plateau of the subepicardial action potential may be absent, resulting in an early full repolarisation and marked difference of APD in subepicardial and subendocardial layers. The short-circuit current generated between depolarised and fully repolarised cells has been directly implied in the generation of an extra excitation. The phenomenon is most often pronounced in the right ventricle, because i_{to} is especially outspoken in subepicardial cells of the right ventricle. This type of reentry may be operative in the Brugada syndrome [117] (see later).

1.3.1.2   Reflection

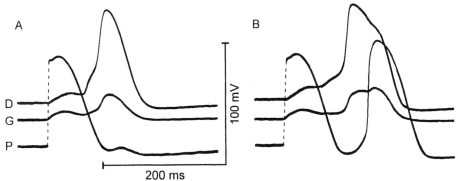

Figure VIII.6. Transmembrane potentials recorded from a feline epicardial ventricular muscle strip placed in a three-compartment bath. Proximal (P) and distal (D) segments were superfused with normal Tyrode, the middle segment gap (G) with a solution containing 35 mM [K$^+$]$_e$ that made the segment inexcitable. The proximal segment was stimulated at a cycle length of 1 s. In B the delay between activation of the proximal and distal element made it possible to reexcite the proximal element (reflection across the inexcitable gap); in A the delay was insufficient. Modified from [942].

A special case of an initiating process is reflection (Fig. VIII.6). In reflection, conduction in a linear pathway is slowed to such extent that a delay is generated which is of the order of the duration of an action potential. This means that at the time a propagated action potential is generated downstream, the membrane upstream has become excitable again, so that the short-circuit currents generated by the action potential in the distal segment trigger an action potential in the proximal segment. In such a way the excitation is "reflected". Reflection requires conduction to be bidirectional but depressed to a critically low level [23]. Experimentally such situation has been created by superfusing a multicellular preparation in a three-compartment system with the middle segment made inexcitable by elevated external $[K^+]_e$.

1.3.2 Stabilisation of reentry

1.3.2.1 Anatomical substrate

To enable an impulse to circle in an anatomically defined closed pathway, conduction must be slow enough and refractory period short enough to avoid the impulse reaching tissue that is still refractory. The wavelength, determined by the product of conduction velocity and refractory period, should be shorter than the length of the pathway [740]. The excitatory wave is followed by a relative refractory period and eventually an excitable gap. The centre of the circuit is inexcitable. The circuit time (inverse of frequency) equals the path length divided by conduction velocity. Reentry is stopped when conduction velocity is increased or refractoriness prolonged to such extent that their product (the wavelength) becomes longer than the length of the pathway.

The inexcitable centre of the circuit can be of relatively large dimensions creating a macroscopic reentry pathway such as may occur at the junction of Purkinje fibres with plain ventricular tissue or when a substantial scar formation has occurred following an infarct. However conduction barriers may also exist in a bundle of apparently normal tissue, generating a microscopic reentry pathway (Fig. VIII.7).

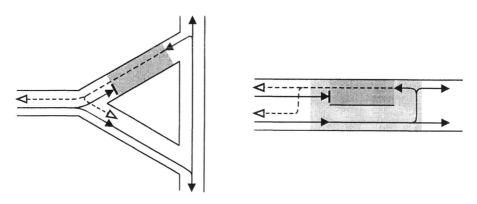

Figure VIII.7. Schematic illustration of macro-reentry and micro-reentry. Conduction is critically lowered in the shaded area. The impulse is blocked in the orthograde direction (full lines). Retrograde conduction is still possible (dashed lines).

1.3.2.2   Functional reentry
1.3.2.2.1   Leading circle reentry

Reentry arrhythmias are possible without a fixed anatomical pathway. Allessie and collaborators [16] were the first to describe and analyse in detail a functional type of reentry arrhythmia in an animal model of atrial fibrillation. According to this analysis the excitation wave is travelling along a functional circle determined by the wavelength (Fig. VIII.8). The centre of the circle is continuously depolarised by impulses originating from the circle. Rate is determined by the refractory period and there is no fully recovered excitable gap. Increase in conduction velocity causes the wave to move outwards, increasing the length of the path, and the converse happens with fall in conduction velocity. In either case, as long as refractoriness is not changed, the rate remains constant.

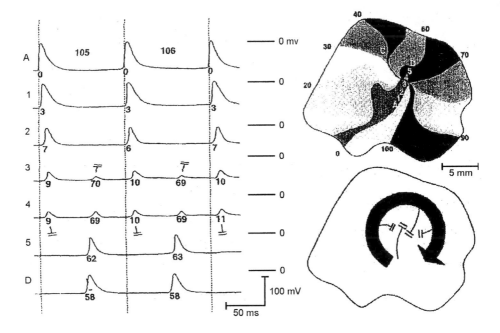

Figure VIII.8. Leading circle reentry. Action potentials (left) and activation map with times of activation in ms (upper right), obtained during steady-state tachycardia in an isolated rabbit atrial preparation. Cells in the central area of the reentrant circuit show double potentials of low amplitude (tracings 3 and 4). A schematic activation pattern is shown on the lower right. Double bars indicate block; black part is absolutely refractory, white cells between head and tail are relatively refractory. Typical for the leading circle reentry is the central core that is permanently kept in depolarised state by centripetal wavelets. Modified from [16].

1.3.2.2.2 Anisotropic reentry

Conduction is far from uniform even under normal conditions, it is faster in the longitudinal than in the transverse direction: the tissue is anisotropic [see 1079]. The orientation of the cells and the distribution of gap junctions influence the conduction of the electrical impulse through the myocardium and is responsible for its anisotropic properties. As long as anisotropy is uniform, conduction will proceed in an orderly fashion; the advancing wave front is smooth in all directions.

Remodeling of gap junctions (see healing and healed infarct) may generate non-uniform anisotropy. The excitation wave under those conditions can circulate around a functionally determined line of block, with very slow conduction at the edges of the line of block. Block in the transverse direction occurs when the coupling resistance becomes too elevated (see example Fig. VIII.12). Conduction block can also occur in the longitudinal direction [1011]. When the current produced by the depolarisation is critically lowered due to insufficient Na^+ current, longitudinal conduction is blocked (sink-source mismatch). The line of block then is perpendicular to the axis of the fibres. In pathological situations both longitudinal and transverse conduction may be lowered.

1.3.2.2.3 Spiral wave reentry and restitution

Experiments on atrial fibrillation have shown that the rate appears to be determined by the refractory period rather than by the wavelength, which is consistent with the leading circle concept [789]. Contrary to the predictions of this model however, high-resolution mapping of electrical activity using voltage-sensitive dyes revealed the existence of vortex-like activity with a central core which remains excitable [489]. Such behaviour supports spiral wave theory.

Spiral wave activity can be demonstrated in different non-linear systems such as chemical reactions (catalytic oxidation of malonic acid by bromate), changes in Ca^{2+} distribution in oocytes, electrical activity in brain or heart. A transient perturbation of the excitation wave results in vortex-like activity, during which the excitation wave acquires the shape of an archimedean spiral (Fig. VIII.9). The wave front has a variable curvature and thus also variable conduction (see Chapter III). At a certain point, called wave break, the depolarising front fuses with the repolarising tail. Its trajectory follows a circle and circumscribes the core which remains excitable. [233].

Evolution from a regular ventricular tachycardia (VT) to irregular ventricular fibrillation (VF) is important, because VF rapidly results in complete stop of the circulation. The change from a spiral wave (regular VT) into multiple wavelets (self-perpetuating VF) is promoted by the existence of a steep restitution curve (slope >1) leading to a large dispersion and alternans of APD [1265] (Fig. VIII.9). The reason is that a small change in CL is magnified in a larger change of APD. This results in an alternation of short and long APD (see also Fig. VIII.5). T wave alternans is well known to be related to the evolution from VT to VF. At a critical time the difference between long and short APD becomes so large that the wave cannot propagate any more and wave break is the result, with splitting up in different wavelets and evolution to VF [1265].

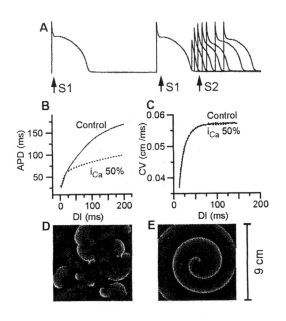

Figure VIII.9. Electrical restitution and spiral wave stability. Simulations on the basis of the Luo-Rudy model [688]. A: Method of double pacing (S1S2) for measuring restitution of action potential duration (APD) by introducing a progressively more premature stimulus (S2) in the normal pacing interval. B: APD restitution: APD as a function of diastolic interval (DI). Dashed line: a 50% block of i_{CaL} markedly reduces the slope of the relationship. C: Conduction velocity (CV) restitution; the recovery is determined by i_{Na} recovery; a fall in i_{CaL} has no effect. D: Spiral wave break-up (fibrillation) several seconds after initiation of a spiral wave in an homogeneous 2-dimensional cardiac tissue. White are depolarised, black repolarised cells. Conditions for restitution as in B control. E: Stable spiral wave (tachycardia) when slope of APD restitution curve is reduced by blocking 50% of i_{CaL}. Modified from [1265].

Reducing the slope of the APD restitution curve may thus be a possible therapeutical approach to prevent the evolution from VT to VF. Interventions affecting i_{Na} or i_{Ca} may change this slope and inhibit multiple wavelet fibrillation. Verapamil for instance has been shown to act in this way. Procainamide on the other hand, does not change the slope and has no regularising effect on VF or does not prevent it [915].

At the present time it is not always clear which of the three functional models is the most appropriate to explain the different forms of arrhythmic activity that have been described in the heart.

2.   MECHANISMS OF SPECIFIC ARRHYTHMIAS

2.1   Arrhythmias and cardiac ischaemia

2.1.1   Acute reversible ischaemia

2.1.1.1   Phase I arrhythmias

In most animals two successive phases (phase Ia and Ib) can be distinguished for arrhythmias generated during the acute phase of ischaemia (see Fig. VII.10); in some cases, phase Ia is absent [548,1057].

Phase Ia arrhythmias (2-10 min) are mostly of the tachycardia-type and rarely evolve into ventricular fibrillation. Tachycardia is often preceded by T wave alternans and deeply negative T waves, which are generated by the marked differences in activation and repolarisation. Mapping studies at the organ or multicellular level have demonstrated the reentry nature of these arrhythmias [880], with the abnormal impulse following a fairly long circuit within the ischaemic zone, or two wave fronts traveling around an area of conduction block in the form of a figure eight. In the period preceding the arrhythmia, activation is slowed, especially in the subepicardial region, much less in the subendocardium: diastolic bridging, i.e. continuous, fractionated electrical activity between two successive QRS complexes is frequent [548]. Conduction delay is markedly increased (Fig. VIII.10). Delayed activation is more pronounced when the ischaemia is caused by thrombus obstruction of the coronary circulation (in contrast to vasoconstriction alone). The difference is due to the release of thrombin in case of thrombus obstruction and consequent α-receptor stimulation [211,379].

At the cellular level slow conduction is related to the rise in $[K^+]_e$ which causes depolarisation with inactivation of Na^+ channels resulting in a decrease of ionic current during the upstroke of the action potential. The rise in $[K^+]_e$ also increases K^+ conductance, which negatively affects the safety factor for conduction. In the peri-infarct zone however, excitability may be increased: at the boundary of the infarct, $[K^+]_e$ accumulation and thus depolarisation is less than in the centre; outside the border of the infarct a small depolarisation is caused by the existence of an injury current between normal and ischaemic tissue [213,1128].

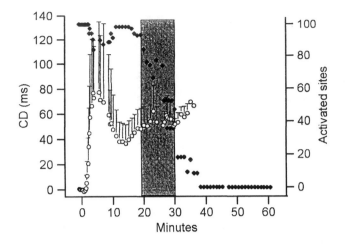

Figure VIII.10. Conduction delay and presence of local activation in the centre of an infarct in the in situ pig heart. Multiple electrodes were placed in the centre of the infarct. Conduction delay (CD, open circles) and % sites that show activation (diamonds) are shown at different times following infarction. Conduction delay increased early during ischaemia (phase Ia) with only 10-15% of electrodes showing block of activity. Later conduction improved. A secondary increase of conduction delay occurs at 20 to 30 min (phase Ib) coincident with high frequency of fibrillation (shaded area) and increase of the number of electrodes showing complete block. Modified from [1057].

A second factor important for the genesis of reentry is dispersion of refractoriness [829]. Although repolarisation is markedly accelerated in the centre of the infarct, the effective refractory period (ERP) is not shortened but rather prolonged because of the existence of postrepolarisation refractoriness [591] (see Fig. VII. 7 and Chapter VII, section 1.2.2.4). Postrepolarisation refractoriness is due to elevated $[K^+]_e$, acidosis, LCAC, LPC and oxygen radicals, all factors that cause normally a fall in recovery of Na^+ channels from inactivation. In the border zone a different situation exists [213]: injury current causes shortening of the action potential and of the effective refractory period. The shortening occurs in cells on the outer side of the border and thus in the absence of elevated $[K^+]_e$, acidosis, LCAC, LPC and oxygen radicals. ERP remains short. Dispersion in ERP creates favourable conditions for unidirectional conduction and reentry. This type of inhomogeneity is further amplified by β-receptor stimulation causing opposite effects on the action potential and refractoriness in normal versus ischaemic tissue: shortening the ERP in normal but prolonging ERP in the diseased cells [829].

Phase Ia is followed by a quiescent period. Between 20 to 30 min after coronary occlusion, a second phase of arrhythmias (phase Ib) occurs. During this phase, evolution to VF is more frequent (shaded area in Fig. VIII.10).

The mechanism of Ib-type arrhythmias is less well known, but is associated with an increase in gap junction resistance (closure of gap junctions) [67,1057], a second phase of $[K^+]_e$ rise and accompanying depolarisation [582], worsening of Ca^{2+} overload and secretion of catecholamines [988]. The site of arrhythmia genesis is probably the border zone; cells in the centre become inexcitable, as shown by the decrease in the percentage of activated sites in Fig.VIII.10, and go into irreversible contracture.

2.1.1.2 Reperfusion arrhythmias

The incidence of arrhythmias during reperfusion depends on the duration of the preceding phase of ischaemia and can be described by a bell-shaped curve. The frequency of arrhythmias increases for ischaemic insults lasting up to 30 min. Longer duration of ischaemia causes the frequency of arrhythmias to decrease again [46,548]. The decrease in incidence with prolonged ischaemia may explain why arrhythmia-related complications are rare following thrombolysis in hospital conditions: thrombolysis normally occurs after more than one hour of ischaemia.

Two periods of reperfusion arrhythmias are seen: an immediate phase developing frequently in VF and, in the absence of VF during this phase, a delayed (after 2-7 min) arrhythmia of the tachycardia-type, with multiple premature beats [46].

The starting stimulus of immediate or early reperfusion arrhythmia occurring within a few seconds after reperfusion, is located within the reperfused zone. The arrhythmia often evolves rapidly into multiple wavelet reentry. Despite circumstantial evidence in favour of EADs and DADs, the nature of the starting stimulus remains a matter of debate [212,1205]. In sites with an efficient reperfusion the action potentials are very short and start from a hyperpolarised membrane potential. In other sites, the membrane stays depolarised and conduction remains slow. Dispersion of APD and ERP thus remains pronounced.

Delayed reperfusion arrhythmias originate probably in the Purkinje system overlying the infarct zone [879,1151]. The mechanism is abnormal automaticity in partially depolarised cells, characterised by EADs and DADs.

2.1.2 Phase II arrhythmias

Following the acute rhythm disturbances of phase Ia and Ib the heart mostly shows normal sinus rhythm for a period of up to 3-6 hrs. By 8 hrs numerous ventricular ectopic beats coexist with sinus beats. After 12-24 hrs most of the beats are of ventricular origin, originating in the subendocardial Purkinje system [108,520].

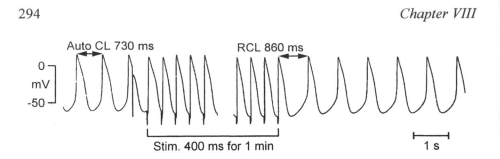

Figure VIII.11. Spontaneous activity in a Purkinje fibre in a 24-hr infarcted canine preparation and effect of overdrive stimulation. CL: cycle length. RCL: recovery cycle length. Modified from [624].

Short salvos of ventricular tachycardia are frequently precipitated by the excessive sympathetic tone and can be prevented by β -receptor blockade. The frequency of the tachycardia usually increases with time. The abnormal pulses start most often late in diastole following a long cycle; early coupled extrasystoles are rather seldom. These characteristics suggest idioventricular rhythm, involving abnormal impulse formation rather than triggered activity or abnormal conduction. Diastolic depolarisation probably starts from a reduced membrane potential in the Purkinje fibres overlying the surviving subendocardium of transmural infarcts; overdrive reduces the frequency and causes some hyperpolarisation (Fig. VIII.11) but the effect is much less pronounced compared to control conditions. The delayed arrhythmias may persist for 24 to 72 hrs. A discussion of possible changes in ionic currents is presented in Chapter IX on remodeling.

2.1.3   Phase III arrhythmias

The incidence of arrhythmias increases again after more than 5 days following an infarct. In many patients only premature ventricular beats are seen and they occur irregularly, while in others short runs of tachycardia are present. Survival is reduced as the incidence and severity of the arrhythmias increases. Sustained ventricular tachycardias are inducible by electrical stimulation, a finding strongly indicating that the arrhythmias are due to reentry. The arrhythmias originate in the surviving cells overlying the infarct or in the border zone, where viable excitable cells form a network within inexcitable scar tissue.

The dispersion of ERP with postrepolarisation refractoriness and the enhanced anisotropic properties of the tissue in the infarcts are likely to cause both block and slow conduction. Block of conduction in an anisotropic structure, even without gross anatomical abnormalities, can occur in the longitudinal or the transverse direction.

The safety factor for conduction in an anisotropic tissue is lower in the longitudinal direction of rapid conduction than in the transverse direction of slow conduction [1080]. The low safety factor in the longitudinal direction is due to the relatively large current load. When the current produced by the depolarisation is critically lowered due to insufficient Na^+ current, longitudinal conduction is blocked. The line of block then is perpendicular to the axis of the fibres.

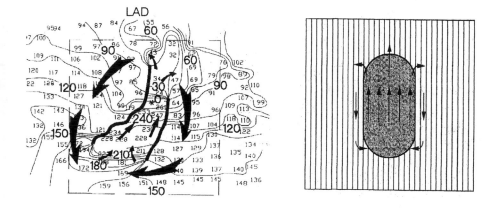

Figure VIII.12. Left: Activation map of a stable reentrant circuit in a 4-day old canine infarct. Numbers indicate activation times. Thick lines: lines of functional block. Arrows point out activation pattern. The common central pathway corresponds to the area in which full-thickness disturbance of gap junctions was demonstrated using connexin-labelling. Right: Diagram showing how an area of myocardium with enhanced anisotropy due to impaired transverse coupling (shaded area) may form a common central conduction pathway and determine lines of functional block at its longitudinal interface with surrounding myocardium. The impulse spreads laterally when it arrives in an area where transverse propagation becomes possible and from there it can return. Due to the large curvature, propagation around the corners of functional block is extremely slow. Modified from [859].

Block in the transverse direction is possible when the coupling resistance becomes too elevated. This has been typically described under conditions where the gap junctional changes occurred throughout the entire thickness of the surviving epicardial fibres. Block is parallel to the long axis; the surviving central cells form the common pathway of the figure 8 reentry circuit (Fig. VIII.12).

2.2 Atrial fibrillation

Atrial fibrillation (AF) is a frequent chronic arrhythmia in the human species, increasing in probability with age. At an age older than 65 years the prevalence becomes 5% among the population [1268]. AF is very often associated with thrombo-embolic complications, irregular ventricular rate and impairment of the ventricular contractile function. Multiple etiological factors can play a role: elevation of intra-atrial pressure, inflammation, intoxicants, increased tone of sympathetic and/or parasympathetic system, hyperthyroidism.

Distinction should be made between paroxysmal, persistent and permanent AF. Paroxysmal AF is characterised by episodes of AF that terminate spontaneously. In persistent AF long episodes of arrhythmia can be ended by application of an electric shock or pharmacological intervention. Permanent AF is a form that cannot be ended by shock or pharmaca. During recent years it has become evident that the existence of AF creates the functional and anatomical substrate in which the arrhythmia becomes stable: "AF begets AF" [1279]. Chemical or electrical defibrillation has a higher success rate when the AF has existed only for a short time. An analysis of changes in ionic currents and in the expression of channel and transporter proteins underlying these adaptive processes is given in Chapter IX on remodeling.

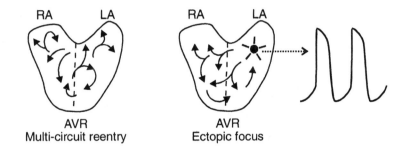

Figure VIII.13. Schematic representation of concepts of atrial-fibrillation mechanisms. Left: multiple, simultaneous reentry circuits. Right: Ectopic focus in left atrium, rapidly discharging and maintaining the arrhythmia. LA: left atrial appendage; RA right atrial appendage; AVR: atrioventricular ring. Atria are represented in an unfolded manner, with dashed line indicating the position of the septum.

Different models and mechanisms have been proposed for the generation of AF [791] with as extremes multiple circuit reentry and ectopic foci (Fig. VIII.13). In chronic AF the arrhythmia is mostly of the multiple micro-reentry type, but at the beginning it is often due to macro-reentry or abnormal automatism. In human paroxysmal AF resistant to drug therapy, ectopic impulses originating from the orifice of the pulmonary veins have been shown to invade and activate the atria at high rate (350/min) [411,512] (Fig. VIII.14). Cardiac muscle cells are found deep into the veins as a layer overlying the other structures and are at the origin of spontaneous bursting activity. At the cellular level they show spontaneous diastolic depolarisation (Fig. VIII.15). It is interesting to note that embryologically these cells have the same origin as SAN cells. Pacemaker activity can also originate from other loci. One of the substrate currents, the i_f current has been found in human atrial appendages [883] and its activation is facilitated by noradrenaline and serotonin [867]. In cat right atrium, diastolic depolarisation has been described which is caused by activation of i_{CaT} and Na^+/Ca^{2+} exchanger current secondary to the release of Ca^{2+} [484]. In dilated atria and in conditions of enhanced tone of the sympathetic system, atrial cells may become Ca^{2+} overloaded and secondarily develop DADs [59].

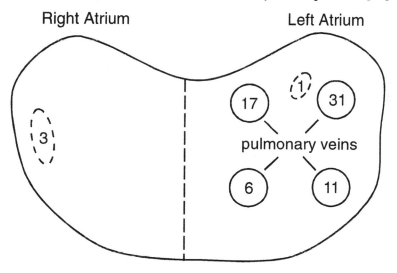

Figure VIII.14. Diagram of the sites of 69 foci triggering atrial fibrillation in 45 patients. Note clustering in the orifices of the pulmonary veins [411].

Conditions for reentry are present in the atria. Atrial action potentials are characterised by a marked heterogeneity, and especially the repolarisation phase is different between right and left, between appendage, roof and crista terminalis [326] (Fig. VIII.16). Differences in configuration and duration become more pronounced during high frequency pacing. Frequent activation causes shortening of ERP and fall in conduction velocity and augment temporal and spatial heterogeneity [365]. If increased vagal tone is present, the ERP and wavelength show an excess shortening, increasing the probability of reentry. Reentry as such can occur in a relatively fixed closed circuit (e.g. orifice of veins, coronary sinus, vena cava) or be of functional nature, as in the leading circle reentry concept of Allessie [16] or the spiral-wave concept of Jalife [855]. In many cases the arrhythmia starts as a tachycardia, but a typical fibrillation is born with multiple wavelets when the reentry waves split and multiply.

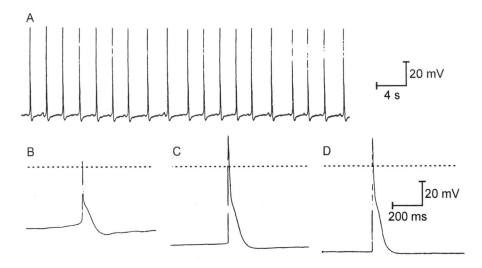

Figure VIII.15. A: Spontaneous electrical activity of the guinea pig isolated pulmonary vein. B, C and D show action potentials in three different locations. Note spontaneous diastolic depolarisation in B. Modified from [176].

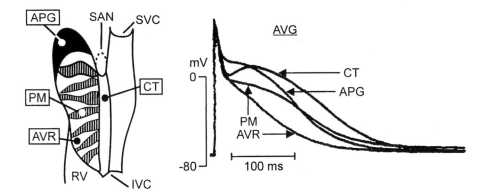

Figure VIII.16. Heterogeneity of action potentials in atrial tissue. Left: schematic diagram of canine right atrium: APG: appendage; PM: pectinate muscle; AVR: atrioventricular ring; CT: crista terminalis; SAN: sinoatrial node; SVC: superior vena cava; RV: right ventricle; IVC: inferior vena cava. Right: superimposed average (AVG) action potentials from the different locations indicated in the diagram. Modified from [326].

2.3   Long QT and Brugada syndrome

2.3.1   Congenital LQT syndrome

Torsade de pointes arrhythmia, first described by Dessertenne [244], a French cardiologist, is a ventricular arrhythmia, with a very typical ECG signature (Fig. VIII.17). The ventricular complexes are polymorphous in nature and show characteristic undulating peaks, forming a torsade. In most cases the start of the arrhythmia is pause-related with a succession of "short, long, short" complexes. The pause is either due to a sinus node slowing or a postextrasystolic compensatory pause (which is the most frequent situation) [1217]. The extrasystole however mostly occurs on the basis of slow sinus rate and abnormal prolongation of the QT.

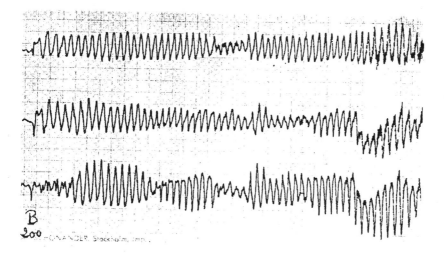

Figure VIII.17. ECG recordings by Dessertenne in derivations I, II and III during a torsade de pointes arrhythmia in a 80-year old patient (rate 200/min). In his description the author asks special attention for the "pointes en haut", followed by "pointes en bas" and finally again upwards that can be seen in derivation III. Modified from [244].

Congenital LQTs is rather rare, but frequency of syncopes and sudden death is high. Recently the relation has been made between LQT syndromes and cot death and in one case the presence of a mutation in the Na^+ channel causing one of the LQTs (LQT3), has been demonstrated [993,996]. Clinically two inherited LQT syndromes are known [see 924]. The Jervell, Lange-Nielsen syndrome was first described for an Norvegian family with 6 children. The ECG of the parents was normal; 4 children were born deaf-mute, had an ECG with prolonged QT, frequent syncopes and in 3 cases these were lethal before the age of ten. Heredity is autosomal recessive. The second syndrome, known as Romano-Ward syndrome is also characterised by a long QT and sudden death but no deaf-mutism; heredity is autosomal dominant.

The Romano-Ward syndrome corresponds to mutations on 5 different genes [995]. In four of these syndromes (LQT 1, 2 ,5 and 6) mutations are present in K^+ channels and are accompanied by a decrease of their function (fall in i_{Kr} and i_{Ks} current). Mutations in the Na^+ channel result in an augmentation or gain of function (LQT3). Information on LQT4 is still missing. The K^+ channel mutations affect the *HERG*- or *KCNH2*-gene (LQT2) and the *MiRP1*- or *KCNE2*-gene (LQT6) for the i_{Kr} current, the K_vLQT1- or *KCNQ1*-gene (LQT1) and the *MinK*- or *KCNE1*-gene (LQT5) for the i_{Ks} current; the *SCN5A* is mutated in the LQT3 syndrome. In the Jervell, Lange-Nielsen syndrome mutations of the K_vLQT1 and *MinK* are present in both alleles.

The decrease in outward current or the increase in inward current are responsible for the prolongation of the action potential duration in LQTs [552,1023]. Prolongation of APD is especially pronounced at low rates and is accompanied by an increased occurrence of EADs. Conditions favouring the genesis of EADs involve the enhancement of Na^+/Ca^{2+} exchange current and reactivation of L-type Ca^{2+} current. Pause-induced EADs have been implicated in the initiation of these arrhythmias. Experimental as well as modeling studies [1218] have shown that pause-induced EADs develop preferentially in M cells. Not only EADs but also DADs may be the initiators of TdP. Prolongation of the action potential indeed leads to increased levels of $[Ca^{2+}]_i$ and enhanced propensity to generate DADs [1300,1301]. Lengthening of the action potential is also accompanied by an increased dispersion, a longer vulnerable period and a greater probability of unidirectional conduction.

The majority of the cardiac events (62%) [995] in LQT1 patients occur during exercise when sympathetic tone is elevated, only 3% during rest or sleep. Swimming as a trigger is particularly frequent (33%). These patients benefit from β-blocker therapy [995]. Intravenous injection of epinephrine on the other hand, markedly prolongs the QT interval in LQT1 patients [804]. In animal cellular models of LQT1 it has been shown that dispersion is sensibly increased in the presence of isoproterenol, the effect being due to prolongation of the action potential in M cells while shortening occurs in subepicardial and subendocardial cells. The disparate effects on subepicardial cells and M cells cause increased dispersion and enhanced probability of unidirectional conduction [1021,1024]. An explanation can be found in the fact that sympathetic stimulation stimulates i_{Ks} and thus exerts a shortening effect on the action potential duration. This last effect however, only occurs when i_{Ks} is sufficiently present. When i_{Ks} is less expressed (as in LQT1 and LQT5), the repolarisation reserve will be much less, especially in M cells. In these cells a stimulatory effect on the i_{CaL} causes instead prolongation of the action potential.

The association of deafness in the Jervell, Lange-Nielsen syndrome has found an explanation in the fact that the i_{Ks} current plays an important role in the formation of the endolymph in the middle ear. Studies with transgenic mice with knockout for the *KCNE1* [277] or *KCNQ1* [151], have shown deficient production of endolymph, a solution which normally contains an elevated K^+ concentration. In these mice, auditory cells undergo a secondary degeneration caused by the absence of the secretion of endolymph, resulting in deafness.

In LQT2 patients most of the cardiac events (43%) occur during emotional stress, with 26% elicited by auditory stimuli [995]. Intravenous injection of epinephrine causes a transient prolongation of the QT interval [804]. Also in animal cellular models, in which i_{Kr} is blocked by E-4031 or dofetilide, isoproterenol transiently prolongs the action potential [889] and increases dispersion [1024]. An elevated sympathetic tone is thus proarrhythmic in the LQT2 syndrome.

The syncopes in the LQT3 (Na^+ channel mutations) occur for 39% of the genotypic patients during the night or at rest when cardiac frequency is very low. LQT3 patients show clear lengthening of the QT interval during the night [1106]. Excessive prolongation of the action potential is accompanied by an increased probability to develop EADs. This has been confirmed in a LQT3 transgenic mouse model, with deletion of KPQ aminoacids in the linker between domain 3 and 4 of the channel protein. The cardiac Na^+ current in these mice is characterised by the existence of a slowly inactivating component which persists during the plateau of the action potential [815].

Pacing in LQT3 patients to avoid slow rates is a therefore a useful therapeutic intervention. Rapid pacing not only prevents excessive slowing but has been shown to shorten the action potential more in LQT3 patients [994] and cellular models [889] than in LQT2.

In vivo sinus rate is modulated by sympathetic tone. Since β-blockers cause slowing of the heart rate (which should be avoided) their usefulness in LQT3 may be questioned. The effect of sympathetic stimulation, however, is not restricted to a change in sinus rate. In patients [804] and in cellular models [889,1024] β-receptor stimulation indeed causes prolongation of APD and dispersion in LQT1 and LQT2 but shortening in LQT3, independent of the rate. Propranolol, on the other hand, facilitated the occurrence of arrhythmias in a cellular model of LQT3 [1023]. β -receptor stimulation thus exerts antiarrhythmic activity in LQT3.

A non-negligible fraction of cardiac events in the LQT3 occurs also during exercise or stress (in 32% of the cases) [14,995]. Recent in vitro experiments on heterozygotic mice with ΔKPQ mutation provide a possible explanation. Sudden acceleration of the rate in these preparations causes a transient lengthening of the action potential (Fig. VIII.18) In some cases this paradoxical lengthening is accompanied by appearance of EADs and generation of TdP arrhythmias. Possible underlying mechanisms for the prolongation and EAD generation are a potentiation of the persistent Na^+ current [182], facilitation of i_{CaL}, and enhancement of the Na^+/Ca^{2+} exchange current [1300,1301]. Summarizing, it can be concluded that in LQT3 a continuous tone of sympathetic activity is antiarrhythmic and favourable, but a sudden surge of sympathetic activity may be dangerous by causing an abrupt acceleration of the rate.

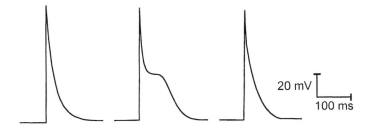

Figure VIII.18. Acceleration-induced transient prolongation of the action potential duration (APD) in a mouse ventricular preparation with a ΔKPQ mutation in the *SCNA5A* gene (LQT3). The cycle length (CL) of stimulation was changed from 500 ms to 200 ms. Examples of action potentials at steady-state CL of 500ms (left), at the maximum of APD prolongation (middle), which was obtained at the 20th beat following the change in CL and at the 50th beat (right). Note the development of a typical plateau; in 30% of the cases the transient prolongation was accompanied by EADs. Unpublished records. The transgenic mouse model was developed by D. Nuyens (Centre for Transgene Technology and Gene Therapy, K.U.Leuven) and the micro-electrode measurements were made by M. Stengl (CARIM, Cardiology, Univ. Maastricht).

From a therapeutic point of view it is important to note that the late (persistent) Na^+ current of the LQT3 mutant channel (ΔKPQ) for instance is more sensitive to flecainide block than the peak Na^+ current (normal and mutant channel) [775]. Mutations in the Na^+ channel also cause important changes in the sensitivity to drugs. In patients with a D1790G mutation, flecainide was highly effective while lidocaine was not [72]. In another LQT3 mutant (R1623Q) however, an unusual high sensitivity to inactivated state block by lidocaine has been demonstrated [540].

2.3.2   The Brugada syndrome

The Brugada syndrome is caused by mutations in the *SCN5A* gene [406]. It is especially prominent in the populations of East Asia and frequently leads to sudden death. Electrocardiographically it is characterised by ST elevation in precordial leads V1 to V3, and right bundle branch block, without prolongation of the QT [117]. In some cases the existence of a real bundle branch block has been verified. ST elevation becomes prominent by administration of class Ic antiarrhythmics (Fig. VIII.19) [118,406,932].

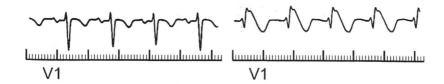

Figure VIII.19. ST elevation in precordial lead V1 in a patient with a Brugada-type mutation in the *SCN5A* gene, which became manifest (right recording) only after administration of a Na$^+$ channel blocker (ajmaline). Modified from [118].

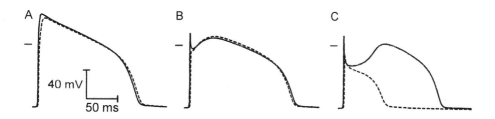

Figure VIII.20. Effect of accelerated inactivation of the Na$^+$ current on the simulated propagating endocardial (A), left ventricular epicardial (B) and right ventricular epicardial action potentials (C). Full lines: normal inactivation, dashed lines simulation with doubled rates of inactivation. Note marked shortening of the right ventricular epicardial action potential. Modified from [291].

At the channel level different changes have been found: faster inactivation (T1620M) [291], slower recovery from inactivation (T1620M) [291], (R1512W) [932], loss of Na$^+$ current (R4132 mutation), a larger proportion of Na$^+$ channels entering the inactivated state ("intermediate state" [1234]). The loss of function or smaller inward current results in faster repolarisation especially in those cells where i$_{to}$ is most pronounced (subepicardial cells). The faster repolarisation especially in the subepicardial cells of the right ventricle generates ST segment elevation in the right precordial leads (Fig. VIII.19 and Fig. VIII.20) [15,927]. The concomitant marked dispersion is most likely the reason for the increased propensity of reentry (see phase 2 reentry) [686].

Although patients with the Brugada syndrome have no prolonged QT, some patients with prolonged QT show ST denivellation upon administration of flecainide [890]. The close relationship between the two syndromes is further emphasized by the observation that LQT3 and Brugada symptoms can occur in the same patient through one single mutation [1204]. The mutation results in a disturbed fast inactivation so that persistent current is generated; at the same time slow recovery from inactivation is induced.

2.3.3   Acquired LQT syndrome

The congenital LQT syndrome is rather rare, but frequency of syncopes and sudden death is high. Of higher frequency is the occurrence of TdP arrhythmias induced by drugs, with or without accompanying electrolyte disturbances (hypokalaemia, hypomagnesaemia) or other pathologic conditions (stretch, hypertrophy). The drugs responsible belong to different groups but have the common effect of blocking K^+ currents (i_{Kr}, i_{Ks} and i_{to}). Among the antiarrhythmics, drugs of class Ia and III should be mentioned: procainamide, quinidine, disopyramide, sotalol, dofetilide, ibutilide. Others belong to the antihistamines (e.g. terfenadine, astemizole), antimicrobials (e.g. erythromycine, ketoconazole), gastrointestinal drugs (e.g. cisapride), and psychotropic drugs (e.g. haloperidol). Chemically, they all have at least one aromatic ring, they block i_{Kr} by entering the channel and are trapped when the activation gate closes [141,142,743].

Excessive prolongation of the action potential and increased tendency for EADs is the main mechanism for the initiation of the arrhythmia. Increased risk occurs when electrolyte disturbances reduce the repolarisation reserve by blocking K^+ current or when K^+ currents become less expressed as in hypertrophy or with stretch. The hypothesis has been formulated that mild mutations might be present in the LQT genes among the general population which predispose these persons to drug-induced arrhythmias [1001].

2.4   Arrhythmias in hypertrophy and heart failure

The hypertrophic and failing heart undergoes a number of modifications in the myocytes and in the extracellular matrix, which are predisposing to arrhythmias (for an analysis of remodeling processes involved see Chapter IX). Ventricular ectopy and arrhythmias are a frequent complication, which not only have a negative effect on the pump function but may result in sudden death.

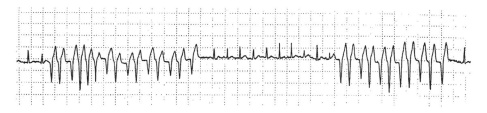

Figure VIII.21. Spontaneous ventricular arrhythmias in a conscious rabbit with heart failure. Lead II ECG. Modified from [881].

The mechanisms involved are enhanced tendency to automatism and triggered activity on one hand, and favourable conditions for reentry on the other hand.

i) Extrasystoles are initiated either by diastolic depolarisation or by EADs. Diastolic depolarisation has been recorded in ventricular myocytes [813] and is possible by the enhanced expression of i_f and shift of its activation curve in the depolarised direction, as shown in animal models [158]. The simultaneous fall in different K^+ currents and electrogenic pump current and an increased Na^+/Ca^{2+} exchange current shift net background current in the inward direction and slow repolarisation. The occurrence of EADs is favoured by the prolongation of the action potential especially at low frequencies of stimulation and in the presence of class III drugs [1223]. Increased Na^+/Ca^{2+} exchange current again plays a conditioning role and facilitates reactivation of i_{CaL} [1052].

ii) Favourable conditions for reentry are generated by disturbed conduction and enhanced dispersion of the action potential duration. Conduction disturbances are caused by changes in the myocytes and in the extracellular matrix. Conductance of gap junctions is decreased: elevated $[Ca^{2+}]_i$ (especially in heart failure), reduced phosphorylation of connexins, incorporation of amphiphiles and effect of radicals are possible mechanisms. Gap junctions furthermore undergo an important redistribution and shift to the lateral side of the cells [308,858]. Some of these lateral junctions are found in cell membrane invaginations and thus are not functional [719]. Together with the development of fibrosis in the extracellular matrix these changes are responsible for enhancement of anisotropic conduction. Prolongation of the action potential is accompanied by enhanced dispersion. The duration of the vulnerable period is prolonged, creating ideal conditions for an extra stimulus to generate unidirectional propagation and reentry.

Chapter IX

Remodeling

Remodeling in general can be defined as the long-term functional and morphological adaptation of cardiac cells to chronic stimuli, such as mechanical overload, ischaemia, arrhythmia, hormonal imbalance [1116]. In this section we discuss the changes in electrophysiological properties induced with a delay of hours to days in specific pathophysiological entities, such as hypertrophy and heart failure, atrial fibrillation, myocardial infarct, preconditioning and T wave memory.

1.   HYPERTROPHY AND HEART FAILURE

1.1   Introduction

Three compensatory mechanisms are initiated in the presence of an imbalance between cardiac workload and work output: i) the Frank-Starling mechanism, ii) stimulation of the sympathetic system and iii) myocardial cell hypertrophy. Each of these compensatory mechanisms however has a limited potential. If pressure or volume overload further increase, the pumping capacity of the ventricle may become insufficient. This fall in contraction and cardiac output is accompanied by neuroendocrine responses such as endothelin and angiotensin secretion, leading to vasoconstriction and water and salt retention. To a certain extent this is counteracted by secretion of atrial natriuretic peptide by the atria causing vasodilatation and natriuresis. Later the situation can deteriorate and evolve into a decompensated state of heart failure.

Hypertrophy and arrhythmogenesis
- APD lengthening leading to EADs
- Automatism: diastolic depolarisation
- Fall in conduction velocity
- gap junction conductance
- microfibrosis

Electrophysiologically hypertrophy is characterised by prolongation of the action potential with tendency to EADs and increased automaticity. This is accompanied by a fall in conduction velocity due to reduced expression of gap connexins and increased formation of microfibrosis, all resulting in an enhanced tendency to arrhythmias. These electrophysiological changes are conditioned by alterations in the density and function of channels, ion transporters and receptors in cardiac myocytes, accompanied eventually by maladaptive cell death and apoptosis and hyperplasia of the extracellular matrix. In failure, Ca^{2+}_i transients are reduced in amplitude, slowed in time course and accompanied by a marked disturbance of the excitation-contraction coupling.

1.2 Prolongation of action potential duration, slowing of conduction and increased arrhythmogenesis

1.2.1 Prolongation of the action potential

Prolongation of the action potential duration (APD) is one of the initial electrophysiological manifestations of hypertrophy. It is far from uniform and shows spatial heterogeneity. Heterogeneity over the wall of the ventricle with more pronounced prolongation in the subepicardial myocytes has been documented and results in changes of the T wave (rat, guinea pig) [120,1032]. In the dog AVN-block model of hypertrophy, heterogeneity in the prolongation exists between right and left ventricle with prolongation more pronounced in the left than in the right ventricle and thus amplification of interventricular dispersion. This type of dispersion becomes extra magnified in the presence of class III drugs [1223,1224] (Fig. IX.1).

The frequency-dependence of APD is steeper, with action potential prolongation especially pronounced at low frequencies. At the same time dispersion is increased. Such prolongation results frequently in EADs and arrhythmias of the torsade de pointes type, with an increased risk of sudden death. Similar changes occur in the human [1150].

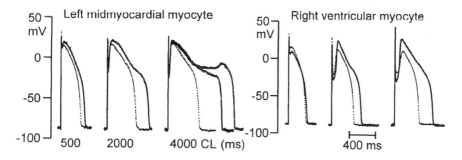

Figure IX.1. Action potential prolongation and hypertrophy. Increased sensitivity to block of i_{Kr} by a class III agent, almokalant, in a canine left and right ventricular myocyte at three different cycle lengths (thick line presence of almokalant). Hypertrophy was caused by volume overload in the presence of chronic AVN block. Action potential prolongation is most pronounced at long cycle lengths and more in left than in right ventricle. Left: example of EAD development. Modified from [1223].

The mechanisms underlying the prolongation of the action potential are reduction of K^+ currents, diminution of active Na^+ pump current, and increase in Na$^+$/Ca^{2+} exchange current. Changes in i$_{CaL}$ are of minor importance.

> **Lengthening of action potential duration**
> - Reduction in K$^+$ currents
> - Diminution of Na$^+$/K$^+$ pump current
> - Increased Na$^+$/Ca^{2+} exchange current

Different K$^+$ currents undergo downregulation: i$_{to}$, i$_{Kr}$, i$_{Ks}$ and i$_{K1}$. In small animals, where the action potential is characterised by a pronounced initial spike, the fall in i$_{to}$ provides an explanation for the prolongation of the APD. In larger animals with a relatively long plateau a reduction in delayed K$^+$ current is of more importance.

i$_{to}$ expression at the mRNA and protein level is reduced in humans and in many experimental hypertrophy models (rat, dog). The reduction is especially pronounced in the subepicardial cells [772] and is accompanied by a switch from K$_V$4.3 to K$_V$1.4. Such a change in the expression fits with the notion of a return to the fetal type of protein expression. A switch but in the reversed direction occurs during normal development [405] and can be induced in cultured newborn rat ventricular cells by α-receptor stimulation or by triiodothyronine (T3) treatment [404].

Reduction of i$_{Kr}$ density with minor changes in the kinetics is observed in feline hearts (pressure overload) and is accompanied by a diminution in the sensitivity to quinidine [1333]. In the volume-overloaded dog model rather i$_{Ks}$ and less i$_{Kr}$ undergo downregulation [1224]. Changes in i$_{K1}$ are minor during the compensatory phase of hypertrophy but become pronounced in failure.

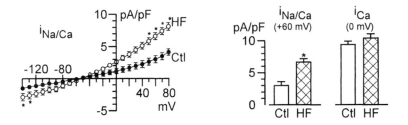

Figure IX.2. Left: Current-voltage relationship for i$_{Na/Ca}$ in control and in heart failure. Right: Comparison of mean values for i$_{Na/Ca}$ and i$_{CaL}$ in control and heart failure. Rabbit ventricular myocytes. Modified from [881].

The density of Na$^+$/K$^+$ ATPase protein is reduced; at the same time there exists a change in the expression of isoform type which results in a smaller sensitivity to Na$^+$ but increased block by ouabain [997]. The Na$^+$/Ca^{2+} exchange current, in contrast to the decreased Na$^+$/K$^+$ ATPase, is upregulated and increased in density [1052] (Fig. IX.2). When acting in the forward mode the exchanger generates inward current and causes prolongation of the action potential. In the reversed mode it facilitates greater Ca^{2+} influx and can trigger repetitive Ca^{2+} release from the SR [1052]. The changes in both pump and exchange current favour prolongation of the action potential plateau.

The L-type Ca^{2+} current and DHP binding sites are not changed in density or even slightly increased as long as there is compensatory hypertrophy. In the decompensatory state with manifestation of failure, the Ca^{2+} current may diminish with slower inactivation and reduced Ca^{2+} release from SR (see excitation-contraction coupling). Under those conditions the action potential is markedly prolonged and the Ca^{2+}_i transient shows a reduced peak and slow relaxation (Fig. IX.3).

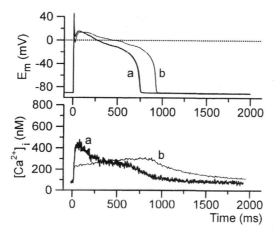

Figure IX.3. Action potentials and Ca^{2+}_i transients in cardiomyocytes from failing canine hearts. Two examples of moderate (a) and severe failure (b) are shown. Action potentials are prolonged, peak Ca^{2+}_i transients depressed and prolonged. Modified from [834].

1.2.2 Conduction is slowed

Slowing of conduction is not caused by changes in the active properties of the membrane such as the upstroke velocity of the action potential, but is due to increase in cellular and extracellular longitudinal resistance: gap junction conductance goes down, while later an extensive microfibrosis process develops in the extracellular space [958].

Slowing of conduction
- fall in gap junction conductance
- development of microfibrosis

In the acute hypertrophic response conduction is not expected to be negatively affected since Cx expression in experimental models of hypertension is rather enhanced [60]. Acute exposure of neonatal cells to cAMP [230] or angiotensin [268] causes an increase in Cx expression and in the number of gap junctions, via less degradation (cAMP) and more synthesis (angiotensin).

In the chronic stage of hypertrophy, however, connexin expression is diminished and gap junction number and size are reduced [955]. Cx43 staining may decrease to 60% of the control [60,858]. The ratio of gap junctional area to total intercalated disk area goes down to 70% of the normal value [308,1172], a phenomenon which is accompanied by a reduction of conduction velocity in the longitudinal direction by 30% (Fig. IX.4). Similarly to what occurs in the healing infarct, a shift of gap junctions to the lateral sides of the cell is manifest [1172]. Contrary to expectation this shift is not accompanied by an improved transverse conduction. Apparently some of these junctions are not functional because they are located in cell membrane invaginations [719,1172]. The overall effect of changes in longitudinal and transverse conduction is a fall in anisotropic ratio (Fig. IX.4).

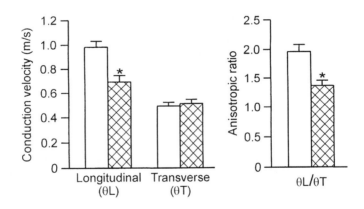

Figure IX.4. Changes in anisotropic conduction properties in rat hypertrophied right ventricle. Longitudinal conduction is slowed due to gap junction disorganisation. Anisotropic ratio is down to 1.38 from the normal value of 1.98. White bars: control; hatched bars: hypertrophy. Modified from [1172].

At an advanced stage of heart failure in cardiomyopathic hamsters, junctional conductance between pairs of cells is decreased to very low values, ranging between 3 and 30% of normal [236]. Such a situation causes pronounced dispersion of APD, non-uniform anisotropic conduction and alteration in the safety factor. Apart from a fall in gap junction conductance there exists also an enhanced tendency to produce fibrosis, at least in the pressure-induced hypertrophy. This again will cause a larger reduction of conduction velocity in the transverse direction and anisotropic conduction will be further enhanced.

1.2.3 Enhanced automatism and increased arrhythmogenesis

Fifty percent of deaths among patients with HF are due to the occurrence of severe arrhythmias. Increased automatism, triggered activity and slowing of conduction form the substrate for the propensity to arrhythmias.

Increased arrhythmogenesis	
Altered impulse formation automatism EAD	Altered impulse conduction gap junction, microfibrosis APD dispersion

Favourable conditions for enhanced automatism are created by changes in the expression and function of i_f, i_{CaT}, $i_{Na/Ca}$ and i_{K1} currents. The i_f current has been shown to be present in plain ventricular myocytes and to become activated at normal diastolic membrane potentials as a consequence of the shift of the activation curve to less negative potentials [157]. Increased expression and expression of different isoforms of the *HCN* gene could be the reason for this positive shift [1015]. The i_{CaT}, which promotes diastolic depolarisation in the SAN, also is upregulated. Other changes such as increased expression of Na^+/Ca^{2+} exchanger and downregulation of i_{K1} [588] favour a less negative maximum diastolic potential and initiation of automatism. Spontaneous depolarisations independent of previous action potential and thus different in mechanism from EADs or DADs have been observed in pacing-induced HF in dogs [813].

The probability to generate triggered activity also is increased due to the prolongation of the action potential. EADs are especially prominent at low frequencies where the action potential may be abnormally lengthened.

Conditions conducive to reentry are generated by changes in gap junction and dispersion of APD. The fall in gap junction conductance, the redistribution of gap junctions, and the development of extracellular microfibrosis are responsible for a substantial fall in conduction velocity and an amplification of anisotropic conduction. The dispersion of the action potential duration prolongs the duration of the vulnerable period and thus increases the probability to generate unidirectional conduction and reentry.

1.3   Excitation-contraction coupling

Depending on the state (compensatory or decompensatory hypertrophy) excitation-contraction coupling is improved or decreased. In the compensatory state contraction as well as Ca^{2+}_i transients are increased especially at low frequencies of stimulation (AVB dog model [1052] (Fig. IX.5) and spontaneous hypertensive rat [159]). Upregulation of the Na^+/Ca^{2+} exchanger, acting in the reverse mode may have a positive effect on Ca^{2+} release during the peak of the action potential and on the Ca^{2+} loading of the SR. The higher density of the exchanger thus preserves systolic function [1052]. By improving Ca^{2+} removal from the cell it preserves also the diastolic function or relaxation of the hypertrophic heart.

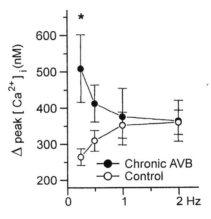

Figure IX.5. Frequency-dependence of the peak amplitude of Ca^{2+}_i transients in cells from control dogs (open symbols) and from cells of dogs with chronic AVN block (volume hypertrophy) (closed symbols). Note compensatory increase of the amplitude of Ca^{2+}_i transient at low frequency. Modified from [1052].

When the hypertrophied state becomes decompensatory the coupling is reduced, and Ca^{2+}_i transients as well as contraction become smaller, delayed and slower (Fig. IX.3). Distinction can be made between a phasic (SR-dependent) and tonic component (possibly due to reverse Na^+/Ca^{2+} exchange component [265]) in the Ca^{2+}_i transient. i_{CaL} and the number of ryanodine receptors however are still within normal limits [382], but Ca^{2+} ATPase and phospholamban are decreased. Initially only the function of the Ca^{2+} ATPase is disturbed: the affinity for Ca^{2+} and the V_{max} are reduced. Later a siginificant decline in the density of SR Ca^{2+} pump is observed [1120].

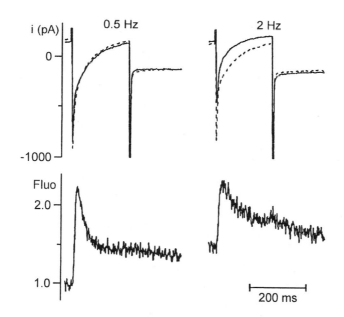

Figure IX.6. i_{CaL} current and Ca^{2+}_i transients during voltage clamp depolarisations in human ventricular cardiomyocytes in end-stage failure. Peak Ca^{2+}_i transient is decreased and diastolic Ca^{2+}_i increased at elevated frequency. Currents in steady-state are indicated in full lines, dashed lines indicate initial values at the start of the frequency change. At 2 Hz the i_{CaL} current shows a marked use-dependent decline. Modified from [1051].

In heart failure the frequency relation for contraction and Ca^{2+}_i transient are reversed with reduced contraction and Ca^{2+}_i transients at elevated frequencies [1051] (Fig. IX.6). Under those conditions modulation of i_{CaL} by β-receptor stimulation is attenuated. The failure of β-receptor modulation is the consequence of a prolonged elevation of the sympathetic tone during the compensatory phase. The result is a diminished expression of β-receptors [246] and a desensitisation of the remaining receptors by phosphorylation through the β-adrenergic receptor kinase [910]. The deficiency of modulatory phenomena may be critical in the evolution from compensatory hypertrophy to heart failure.

2. ATRIAL FIBRILLATION

2.1 Different types of remodeling

Depending on the etiology or the model used to induce atrial fibrillation (AF) the electrophysiological changes are different. At present one distinguishes two models: AF induced by rapid atrial pacing or repeated induction of fibrillation and AF induced by rapid ventricular pacing and consequent failure and dilatation.

2.1.1   Atrial pacing model

In models in which chronic AF is generated by repeated electrical induction (goat) [1279] or in which the atria are continuously paced at elevated frequency (dog) [1335], the arrhythmia is characterised by a pronounced shortening of the atrial action potential and of the effective refractory period (ERP). These changes already reach a maximum after 12 to 24 hrs of AF or rapid pacing. Paradoxically the shortening of ERP (measured when sinus rate is restored) is especially pronounced at lower rates and is accompanied by a loss of rate adaptation or further shortening at elevated rates (Fig. IX.7, right and Fig. IX.8). In the dog model, there exists a marked spatial heterogeneity of the ERP, as judged from the variability in cycle length of AF in different locations. This may be related to exaggerated local differences in sympathetic innervation. Experimentally it has been shown that rapid rates of atrial pacing indeed produce an heterogeneous increase in atrial sympathetic innervation and NA content [523].

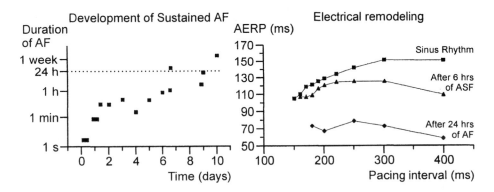

Figure IX.7. The goat model of sustained atrial fibrillation. Left: A representative example of the development of sustained atrial fibrillation. As the pacemaker was switched on (day one), the induced episodes of AF lasted only for a couple of seconds. However, the duration of AF induced by 1s burst at 50 Hz became longer the more frequent AF was reinduced. After one week, AF became sustained (more than 24 hrs). "Atrial fibrillation begets atrial fibrillation". Right: Example of the change in atrial ERP (AERP) with time the atrium was in the fibrillatory state. In sinus rhythm the AERP was 150 ms at a pacing interval of 400 ms and shortened upon stimulation at higher frequencies. After 24 hrs of AF the AERP became very short and did not change anymore with frequency. Modified from [1279].

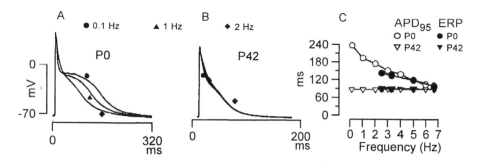

Figure IX.8. Action potential and ERP changes in atrial cells from dogs subjected to atrial pacing at 400/min for zero (control P0) and 42 days (P42). A and B show superimposed action potentials at 0.1, 1 and 2 Hz.; C: Action potential duration and ERP at different frequencies in control and after 42 days of repetitive pacing. At 42 days the frequency-dependence of APD and ERP became flat. Modified from [1335].

Inducibility of AF, i.e. the percentage of animals in which AF can be induced by a premature stimulation, follows a similar time course as the change in ERP and is constant at 100% after 24 hrs of AF [1279]. It takes more time for the duration of the arrhythmia to become stable (Fig. IX.7, left). In the dog model but not in the goat, this second period of stabilisation during which the induced AF becomes sustained (longer than 24 hrs) is accompanied by a slowing of conduction [365]. Shortening of the ERP is attended by an abbreviation of the wavelength and sets the conditions for a greater number of reentrant wavelets. Slowing of the conduction eventually amplifies the probability to generate reentry and makes the arrhythmia more stable.

On electrical reversion the ERP remains short but with continuing sinus rhythm, returns to normal values after 24 to 48 hrs. This is the case even when AF has persisted for weeks or months. Reversibility of electrical parameters has also been shown in humans and the extent of reversibility depends on the duration in sinus rate [458]. Inducibility however remains increased and is due to the fact that structural changes, that develop after days of AF (microfibrosis), do not reverse or reverse more slowly [316].

2.1.2   Ventricular pacing model

A different type of remodeling is present when AF complicates congestive heart failure or is induced in animals with rapid ventricular pacing. In the ECG the overall frequency of atrial complexes is smaller and the rhythm is less irregular. Reentry is of the macro-reentry type. The duration of atrial action potential and refractoriness is not changed at low frequencies and lengthened, instead of shortened, at high frequencies [642,643] (Fig. IX.9).

A marked change occurs in conduction, becoming slower and very heterogeneous.

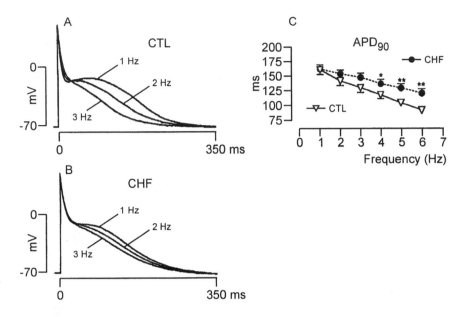

Figure IX.9. Examples of atrial action potentials at 1, 2 and 3 Hz stimulation in control (A) and in animals with congestive heart failure (CHF) in which AF is present as a complication (B). C: graph showing mean values for APD in control (open symbols) and in CHF (closed symbols) as a function of frequency. Action potentials in CHF are prolonged at all, but especially at high frequencies, in contrast to the marked shortening of the action potential in atrial pacing-induced fibrillation. Modified from [643].

2.2 Mechanism of remodeling. Changes in ionic currents and in structure

2.2.1 Ion currents

2.2.1.1 Atrial pacing model

In the atrial pacing model [791] the shortening of atrial ERP and APD can entirely be explained by a marked decrease in i_{CaL}. The change in current is due to a decrease in the number of channels, while time-dependence, voltage-dependence and frequency-dependence are not modified. Concomitantly with the reduction in i_{CaL}, the Ca^{2+}_i transients are diminished and show a marked negative staircase. Initial changes during the induction of AF however may be very different. High frequency stimulation leads to Ca^{2+} overload and post-tachycardia contractile dysfunction, correlated with reduced Ca storage in the SR [1112]. It is highly likely that this Ca^{2+}

overload during the induction period plays an important role in the remodeling process. In accord with this hypothesis it has been shown that verapamil or mibefradil, blockers of the i_{CaL} and i_{CaT} respectively, can prevent electrical remodeling.

The change in i_{CaL} is accompanied by an equally important decrease in i_{to}. In patients also i_{Kur} current and $K_v1.5$ mRNA are reduced [1186]. No changes have been found in i_{K1}, i_{Kr}, i_{Ks}, i_{Cl}, i_{CaT} or $i_{K.ATP}$. Although an increased vagal tone *in vivo* promotes the induction of AF, $i_{K.ACh}$ has not been found to be affected.

In the dog, i_{Na} is reduced, an effect that develops with a slower time course than that of i_{CaL} and is partly responsible for the fall in conduction velocity. In the goat model macroscopic conduction is not changed but the distribution of Cx40 is disturbed in a patchy way with small areas of low density [1176].

2.2.1.2   Heart failure model

In AF accompanying ventricular failure, the changes in atrial ionic currents are different from those in AF models induced by atrial pacing, but they are comparable to those occurring in the ventricle during hypertrophy and failure [316,642]. i_{CaL} and i_{Ks} are reduced by 30%, i_{to} by 50%, while the Na^+/Ca^{2+} exchange current is increased by 45% [643,1185]. i_{K1}, i_{Kur}, i_{Kr} or i_{CaT} are not changed. The changes in ionic currents thus resemble the modulation occurring in the ventricle itself. The difference in current changes between the two models of AF is reflected in the types of reentry, which for the congestive heart model is of the macroreentry type whereas it is of the multiple wavelet type in the rapid pacing model [641]. From a therapeutic point of view it is important to notice that blocking of outward K^+ current e.g. by dofetilide [641] may be useful in AF accompanying ventricular hypertrophy or failure but not in AF with marked shortening of the AP due to the absence of i_{Ca}.

2.2.2   Structural changes

In both types of AF structural changes occur in the myocytes as well as in the extracellular matrix. In the atrial pacing model cellular changes are comparable to "hibernation" and include loss of myofibrils, increase of glycogen, abnormal mitochondria and loss of SR [39]. To a certain extent these changes make atrial cells more like Purkinje cells. Development of microfibrosis and separation of cells by connective tissue plays an additional role in the stabilisation of AF, by favouring non-uniform anisotropic conduction [1075]. Heterogeneous conduction owing to an excessive increase of interstitial fibrosis is especially pronounced in the CHF model [316,642]; it is also characteristic for human AF and increases with age.

3.   INFARCT

Ventricular myocytes surviving an acute period of ischaemia undergo a number of adaptations, that reflect in electrophysiological changes [see 108]. Important changes also occur in the extracellular matrix. Adaptation is not restricted to the infarct zone but involves peri-infarct myocytes and cells remote from the infarct zone. When the infarct is in the left ventricle, important changes also occur in the right ventricle [549]. This is not unexpected since neurohumoral activation produces modulating factors that appear in the circulation and influence the whole heart. Arrhythmias are a frequent complication of healing (hrs to 2 weeks) and healed (weeks to months) infarct. Knowledge about the adaptive electrophysiological changes that occur may be useful for planning an efficient treatment.

3.1   Healing infarct (hours to 2 weeks)

Information on the electrophysiological changes during the healing process following an infarct is available for subepicardial myocytes and subendocardial Purkinje cells adjacent to the infarct border [108,869].

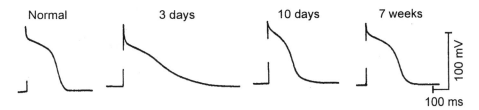

Figure IX.10. Changes in action potential of Purkinje fibres in the subendocardial border zone of a canine infarct 3, 10 days and 7 weeks after coronary occlusion. Unpublished records by Friedman and Wit. Modified from [1288].

Subendocardial Purkinje fibres often show a reduced maximum diastolic potential accompanied by diastolic depolarisation and spontaneous activity. The repolarisation phase is gradual, of triangular shape and mostly prolonged (Fig. IX.10). A typical plateau is absent and the final repolarisation is markedly slowed, causing an enhanced difference between APD50 and APD90. The prolongation of the action potential is often accompanied by secondary depolarisations or early afterdepolarisations especially at low rates [524]. Stimulation at high rates may result in partial depolarisation. dV/dt_{max} is markedly reduced. With time, mostly after 2 weeks, diastolic membrane potential, action potential amplitude and maximum rate of depolarisation return to normal values [108].

The fall in maximum diastolic potential is caused by a reduction of i_{K1} conductance and the depolarisation as such is responsible for the diminution of dV/dt_{max}. Changes in action potential configuration can be related to a reduction of i_{CaL}, i_{to} and i_{K1} and a slowing of the recovery of i_{to}.

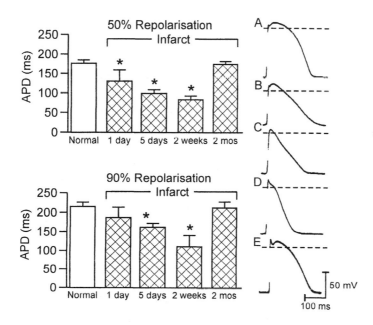

Figure IX.11. Changes in action potential duration of subepicardial cells measured at 50% (upper left) and 90% repolarisation (lower left) with increasing time after coronary occlusion. Asterisks denote values significantly different from control. At right: examples of action potential configuration for control (A), 1 day (B), 5 days (C), 2 weeks (D) and 2 months (E). Modified from [1171].

In subepicardial cells the resting potential is less affected than in endocardial Purkinje fibres. In contrast to the prolongation in subendocardial cells the action potential duration is not changed or even slightly shortened [684]. The change in configuration however is comparable (Fig. IX.11). Phase 1 is less expressed and the slope of the final repolarisation is much reduced. The amplitude and rate of rise of the upstroke are diminished and the action potential is followed by prolonged postrepolarisation refractoriness [274]. The action potential is relatively insensitive to β-receptor stimulation, i.e. there is no increase in plateau level or no shortening of the action potential.

Changes in dV/dt_{max} and the existence of postrepolarisation refractoriness can be explained by the observed decrease in the density of the Na^+ current, with the availability curve shifted in the negative direction and recovery from inactivation slowed [892]. The shift in inactivation also explains the presence of a larger tonic block by lidocaine. The changes in repolarisation can be correlated with a downregulation of i_{to}, i_{CaL} and i_{K1} currents. The smaller response to β-receptor stimulation is caused by a fall in receptor density, an increased desensitisation and change in G protein coupling [100].

Conduction is slowed in subepicardial cells overlaying the necrotic cells, especially in the transverse direction; the ECG shows pronounced delays of activation and a fractionated QRS complex. Anisotropy thus is more pronounced [263,1359]. Important changes are found in cell connections and gap junctions. They involve a redistribution of gap junctions from the intercalated disc to lateral sides of the cell. Multiple small and short junctions become uniformly dispersed over the whole surface of the cell in a pattern strikingly similar to early development. The normal intercalated disk loses its characteristic long gap junctions at its periphery [857,859]. The redistribution of junctions to the lateral sides is, contrary to expectation, not accompanied by an improved transversal conduction. Many of these junctions seem to be not functional because they are located in invaginations of the sarcolemma [719]. The gap junction conductance may also be lowered because of relative ischaemic conditions with acidosis and elevated $[Ca^{2+}]_i$. At 3-5 days post-infarct inducibility of tachycardias was closely related to the disorganisation of the gap junctions extending through the entire thickness of the subepicardial layer and these locations corresponded to the central common pathway of figure-of-8 reentrant circuits [857] (see Fig. VIII.12).

3.2   Healed stage (2 weeks to months)

Between 2 weeks and several months, adaptive processes are not limited to cells in the infarct zone or to cells close to the scar. Changes also occur in cells remote to the scar (4 to 6 mm) and these changes are different from the alterations in the adjacent cells (< 2 mm). Hypertrophic changes also occur in the right ventricle when the infarct is located in the left ventricle.

3.2.1   Infarct- and peri-infarct cells

After 2 weeks to months, cells in the border zone show normalisation of the resting membrane potential, the action potential amplitude and dV/dt_{max}. The resting potential in ischaemic cells remains more sensitive to external K^+: the cells depolarise in the presence of low $[K^+]_e$, suggesting that i_{K1} is still reduced [766] (Fig. IX.12). The action potential stays short in the beginning but normalises at a later period (2 months) [871]. Marked regional differences remain however. In general, subepicardial cells show shorter action potentials while subendocardial show a continued tendency of prolonged action potentials. Following repolarisation an extended period of diminished excitability or postrepolarisation refractoriness still exists. The duration of refractoriness shows a marked dispersion. In subendocardial Purkinje fibres transmembrane action potentials and diastolic depolarisation were not different from normal cells after 2-4 months recovery, but still showed an enhanced triggered activity especially after stimulation of β - or α-receptors [576].

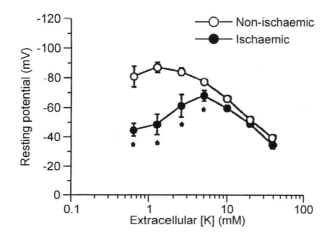

Figure IX.12. Effect of $[K^+]_e$ on resting membrane potential in human non-ischaemic and ischaemic ventricular muscles. At $[K^+]_e$ concentrations below 5.4 mM, "ischaemic" preparations depolarised due to lowered i_{K1} conductance. Modified from [766].

Information on changes of ionic current in the plasma membrane based on direct measurements is scarce [943]. i_{Kr} and i_{Ks} have been reported to fall, but the significance of this finding is not clear. The Ca^{2+}_i transient is smaller and shows a prolonged relaxation phase. The Na^+/Ca^{2+} exchange current as such is not changed as long as there is no failure.

Changes in gap junctions, which started already during the healing phase become more pronounced. The number of gap junctions per unit length of disc membrane, as well as the gap junction size are decreased. There is also a fall in the number of intercalated disc contacts per myocyte [687]. Normally each ventricular cell is, on the average, connected to 11.2 other cells; this value is reduced to 6.5 and is associated with a greater reduction of side-to-side connections than end-to-end connections (by 75% and 22% respectively) [687,1056]. The final result is a reduction of junctional conductance between cell pairs. The expected fall in conduction velocity remains limited however. Theoretical analysis demonstrates that longitudinal conduction is very insensitive to gap junctional conductance and only decreases by 13% when halving the conductance. The transversal conduction velocity is more sensitive and falls by 36% for the same relative change [533] (Fig. IX.13). It is therefore not unexpected to see that reentry develops as a consequence of transversal block in the subepicardial fibres [857].

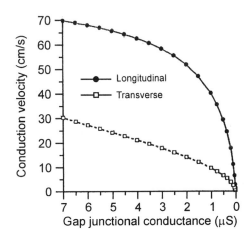

Figure IX.13. Computer simulation of conduction velocity for the longitudinal and transverse direction as a function of gap junctional conductance. Conduction velocity in the longitudinal direction is much less sensitive to changes in gap conductance than the transverse conduction. Modified from [533].

Concomitantly with reduction in gap junction coupling between the cells other fundamental changes occur in the extracellular space with development of microfibrosis between the cells. Interstitial bundles of collagen oriented parallel to the long axis of myocytes accumulate between groups of cells, a process which is promoted by Ang II and antagonised by bradykinin [1291]. Propagation is impaired and may follow a zig-zag pattern, especially when an extrasystole is generated [857]. The reported changes in gap junction, in their regional distribution and the development of extracellular fibrosis have important consequences for the inducibility and persistence of arrhythmias.

3.2.2   Remote cells

Cells at a distance of 4-6 mm from the scar are characterised by a marked hypertrophy, as shown by morphometric and membrane capacitance indexes [219] [for references see 146]. Hypertrophy is not homogeneously distributed, but a gradient exists from the scar to the more distant cells. The action potential is considerably prolonged and, depending on experimental conditions, early afterdepolarisations are present and may lead to extrasystoles [894]. The prolongation of the action potential can be correlated to the smaller i_{to} (in rodents) and to the reduction of i_{Kr} (cat) or/and i_{Ks} (dog) in larger mammals [1333]. Changes are not restricted to the number of channels. Also their function is affected, as for instance the sensitivity to drugs; in the cat i_{Kr} has been shown to become more sensitive to block by quinidine [1333].

4. PRECONDITIONING

4.1 Description

Preconditioning is a phenomenon whereby an endogenous protection against ischaemia in heart cells is activated [see 396]. The original finding [770] consisted in the observation that serial brief periods (e.g. 5 min) of ischaemia followed by reperfusion (e.g. 10 min) could delay the onset and the extent of necrosis which normally is the result of a longer (e.g. 30 min) coronary occlusion. Cardiomyocytes, as well as endothelial tissue and nerves were conserved. High energy phosphates were better preserved and the rise in lactate was slower during the ischaemic insult following a preconditioning period [771]. The protection offered by preconditioning shows two time-dependent phenomena. First, it depends on the duration of the ischaemic insult: protection is lost when the ischaemic insult lasts longer than 60-90 min. Second, protection also depends on the delay between the preconditioning stimulus and the ischaemic insult. In this respect two different protection intervals have to be distinguished: an early and a late window of protection. Early protection is seen when the insult ischaemia occurs within the first 1-2 hrs following the conditioning short ischaemic periods. Thereafter the protection disappears. However when an ischaemic insult is delayed until 24 hrs or up to 3-4 days, protection is again seen. This second period of protection has been called the second window [1324].

Indirect evidence has been provided in the human for the existence of the first window of protection. Patients suffering angina before a myocardial infarction have a better in-hospital prognosis [587]. Electrocardiographic signs of silent ischaemia (ST denivellation) are reduced by preceding exercise. Anginal symptoms are worse in the morning and diminish with repetition, a phenomenon known as the warm-up angina [820]. Aortic clamping preceding the ischaemia during surgical interventions reduces the fall in ATP, and repeated inflations of an intracoronary balloon induce some tolerance against following inflations [619]. The existence of a second window of protection in the human has been confirmed by using nitroglycerin as a pharmacological inducer [630]. The protection, tested after 24 hrs by balloon inflation of a coronary artery, was not limited to a reduction in infarct size but also involved a decrease in stunning.

4.2   Possible mechanisms

To understand possible mechanisms involved in preconditioning it is important to realise that protection not only is generated by preceding ischaemia but also by pacing or exercise, or by activation of certain membrane receptors, such as AT1, opoid, M2 or B2. The cardioprotective effects of preconditioning apparently involve the release of mediators such as adenosine, bradykinin, acetylcholine, NO, prostacyclines and endothelin. Other evidence strongly suggests the activation of mitochondrial K.ATP channels and the release of radicals as intermediates [see 102,275,653].

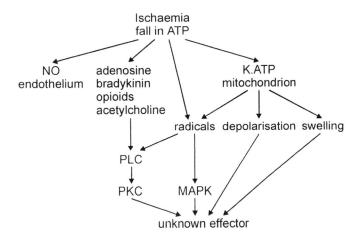

Figure IX.14. Possible sequence of signaling reactions during the preconditioning process. Scheme based on Fig. 7 in ref. [839].

Fig. IX.14 gives a summary of possible signaling reactions in endothelial, neuronal and cardiac cells, related to the induction of preconditioning. In cardiac myocytes ischaemia causes a substantial fall in ATP with formation of adenosine, activation of K.ATP and enhanced oxygen radical generation in the mitochondria. NO, bradykinin, endothelin are released from endothelial cells, while neuronal cells secrete acetylcholine and noradrenaline. Stimulation of membrane receptors and oxygen radicals activate PLC, PKC, PTK and MAPK. Although many intermediate reactions have been analysed the final effector(s) remain still unknown.

Opening of K.ATP channels in mitochondria is considered one of the important triggers and mediators. Although its intervention in preconditioning has been amply demonstrated, it is far from clear how it leads to protection. Three possible mechanisms have been proposed [833]:

i) Opening of the channel leads to a massive influx of K^+ ions into the mitochondrial matrix. This is possible because the K^+ distribution between the cytoplasm (120 mM) and the mitochondrial matrix (180-200 mM) is far from equilibrium. Under normal conditions K^+ ions are continuously extruded from the mitochondrion via the K^+/H^+ exchanger [362] (Fig. IX.15), while influx remains small because of a low K^+ permeability (K.ATP channels closed). K^+ influx upon activation of K.ATP channels should cause a fall in electrical gradient. The magnitude of depolarisation depends on the concomitant influx of anions. If anion influx is appreciable the depolarisation is limited; the influx of salt is then accompanied by water and swelling of the mitochondrial matrix. This osmotic challenge has been shown to cause activation of FA oxidation and ATP synthesis in isolated mitochondria [412] [see also 363]. Controversy exists on the topic of optimisation of mitochondrial respiration; and instead of an increase, a reduction of ATP synthesis by K.ATP openers has also been reported [465]. According to Garlid [363] this latter effect occurs because of the use of too elevated concentrations of K.ATP openers.

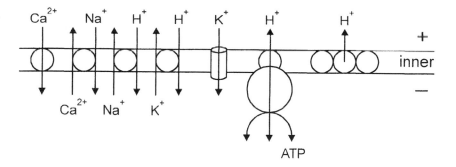

Figure IX.15. Opening of K.ATP channels causes K^+ influx in the mitochondrial matrix. When accompanied by anion influx also water will enter, which will increase mitochondrial volume. If influx of anions is restricted, the inner mitochondrial membrane will depolarise.

ii) According to a second hypothesis the depolarisation as a consequence of the K^+ influx causes a net loss of Ca^{2+} ions from the mitochondria (actually less influx from the cytoplasm). In this way the danger of ischaemic activation of the permeability transition pore is avoided, which normally would result in irreversible loss of the cell [225].

iii) A third possibility is facilitation of radical production and consequent activation of kinases [839].

Although a vast amount of information has been collected on intermediate steps, the end-effectors of preconditioning remain unknown. Some mechanisms have been excluded. Activation of the plasma membrane K.ATP channels seems to be of minor importance. Preconditioning can be obtained by selective pharmacologic activation of the mitochondrial channel by diazoxide [670]. Activation of K.ATP channels in the plasma membrane causes shortening of the APD and stabilisation of the membrane potential and could avoid Ca^{2+} overload. Preconditioning however is not dependent on APD shortening or hyperpolarisation [397]. Reduced contractility of stunned myocardium also is not required.

The question whether early and late protection depend on an entirely different set of triggers and signaling pathways is not solved. Both phenomena are multifactorial [102]. The second window protection is probably more dependent on activation of genes and modulated expression of proteins.

5.   T WAVE MEMORY

The T wave is a component of the ECG which is more sensitive than the QRS complex to electrolyte abnormalities, metabolic changes (ischaemia) and drugs. Changes in the permeation or kinetics of channels and transporters responsible for the repolarisation process are more sensitive to metabolic interference than the processes responsible for the rapid depolarisation. These changes are called primary T wave abnormalities in contrast to those that are secondary to variations in the QRS complex following alteration of the activation sequence [556]. Apart from the "metabolic" modulation of channels, a change in the gene expression of channel and transporters also can cause primary T wave abnormalities: they are slower in development, but especially slower in disappearance and have been called "cardiac memory".

Cardiac memory as described by Rosenbaum [935] refers to long-term changes in the T wave when sinus rhythm is restored after prolonged abnormal activation as occurs with artificial pacing, bundle branch block or arrhythmia (Fig. IX.16 and Fig. IX.17).

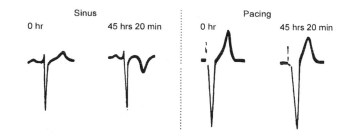

Figure IX.16. Effects of long-term right ventricular pacing on the V2 electrocardiogram in a patient. Left: V2 electrograms during sinus rhythm before pacing (0 hr), and directly following the arrest of pacing during 45 hrs and 20 min. Note the inversion of the T wave. The depolarisation process (QRS) instantaneously returns to normal while repolarisation remains disturbed. Right: V2 electrograms during pacing at the start of the procedure (0 hr) and after 45 hrs and 20 min. The changes in the repolarisation, seen during sinus rhythm, are present in a "hidden" form during pacing. Modified from [935].

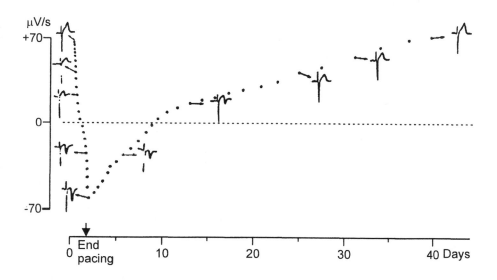

Figure IX.17. Progression and regression of the T wave changes (lead V2) induced by right ventricular pacing (120/min) in a patient. The QRS-T complexes were recorded during brief interruptions of the pacing. Note the rapid changes during pacing and the slower return to normal during sinus rhythm. Modified from [935].

These changes should be distinguished from the classic T wave change (e.g. for an extrasystole) that occurs and disappears instantaneously, and is proportional in magnitude to the change of the QRS complex but opposite in direction. In cardiac memory, the direction of the T wave vector changes

progressively during pacing and approaches that of the paced or arrhythmic
QRS complex (Fig. IX.18).

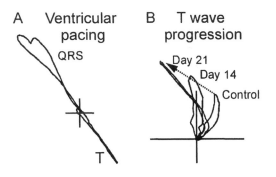

Figure IX.18. Frontal plane vectocardiographic depiction of cardiac memory in a dog heart.
A: control recording of the QRS-T vectors, before onset of pacing, B: recording of the T wave
vector during pacing, and its evolution from control to day 21. Modified from [1038].

This directional change of the T wave vector develops and dissipates
slowly [934,935]. Two periods can be distinguished. Short memory takes
minutes to develop and hours to disappear [914]; long-term memory [1038]
takes days to be induced or to vanish. Short-term memory of the
repolarisation process has recently been shown to exist also in the atrium
[441].

In the dog the change in T wave vector is associated with significant
changes in the epicardial and subendocardial action potentials, not in the
midmyocardial ones. Both epicardial and endocardial action potentials are
lengthened especially at low rates. The relationship between APD and cycle
length becomes steeper, with more overlapping between epicardial and
endocardial action potentials at elevated rates [1038]. The lengthening at
lower rates is accompanied by a change in configuration, more specifically a
much less pronounced phase 1. The reduction in phase 1 is correlated with a
decrease in i_{to} density, a positive shift of the activation curve, and a slower
recovery from inactivation. The changes in current are conditioned by a fall
in $K_v.4.3$ messenger RNA and protein expression [1331]. One of the
initiating signals is probably the alteration in contraction and mechanical
stretch which then activates the angiotensin pathway [914]. All these
changes result in adaptation of the transmural electrical gradient of
repolarisation and are responsible for the vector change.

References

1. (2001). Handbook of Fluorescent Probes and Research Products. Molecular Probes.
2. Abbott GW, Sesti F, Splawski I, Buck ME, Lehmann MH, Timothy KW, Keating MT, Goldstein SA (1999). MiRP1 forms IKr potassium channels with HERG and is associated with cardiac arrhythmia. *Cell, 97*: 175-187.
3. Accili EA, Redaelli G, DiFrancesco D (1996). Activation of the hyperpolarization-activated current (i_f) in sino-atrial node myocytes of the rabbit by vasoactive intestinal peptide. *Pflügers Archiv, 431*: 803-805.
4. Accili EA, Redaelli G, DiFrancesco D (1997). Differential control of the hyperpolarization-activated current (i_f) by cAMP gating and phosphatase inhibition in rabbit sino-atrial node myocytes. *J Physiol (Lond), 500*: 643-651.
5. Accili EA, Redaelli G, DiFrancesco D (1998). Two distinct pathways of muscarinic current responses in rabbit sino-atrial node myocytes. *Pflügers Archiv, 437*: 164-167.
6. Accili EA, Robinson RB, DiFrancesco D (1997). Properties and modulation of I_f in newborn versus adult cardiac SA node. *Am J Physiol, 272*: H1549-1552.
7. Aggarwal R, Shorofsky SR, Goldman L, Balke CW (1997). Tetrodotoxin-blockable calcium currents in rat ventricular myocytes; a third type of cardiac cell sodium current. *J Physiol (Lond), 505*: 353-369.
8. Aguilar Bryan L, Nichols CG, Wechsler SW, Clement JPt, Boyd AEr, Gonzalez G, Herrera Sosa H, Nguy K, Bryan J, Nelson DA (1995). Cloning of the beta cell high-affinity sulfonylurea receptor: a regulator of insulin secretion. *Science, 268*: 423-426.
9. Aiello EA, Jabr RI, Cole WC (1995). Arrhythmia and delayed recovery of cardiac action potential during reperfusion after ischemia. Role of oxygen radical-induced no-reflow phenomenon. *Circ Res, 77*: 153-162.
10. Aimond F, Rauzier JM, Bony C, Vassort G (2000). Simultaneous activation of p38 MAPK and p42/44 MAPK by ATP stimulates the K^+ current ITREK in cardiomyocytes. *J Biol Chem, 275*: 39110-39116.
11. Aksnes G, Ellingsen O, Rutlen DL, Ilebekk A (1989). Myocardial K^+ repletion and rise in contractility after brief ischemic periods in the pig. *J Mol Cell Cardiol, 21*: 681-690.
12. Albitz R, Droogmans G, Nilius B, Casteels R (1992). Thrombin stimulates L-type calcium channels of guinea pig cardiomyocytes in cell-attached patches but not after intracellular dialysis. *Cell Calcium, 13*: 203-210.

13. Alcolea S, Theveniau-Ruissy M, Jarry-Guichard T, Marics I, Tzouanacou E, Chauvin J-P, Briand J-P, Moorman AFM, Lamers WH, Gros DB (1999). Downregulation of connexin 45 gene products during mouse heart development. *Circ Res*, *84*: 1365-1379.

14. Ali RH, Zareba W, Moss AJ, Schwartz PJ, Benhorin J, Vincent GM, Locati EH, Priori S, Napolitano C, Towbin JA, Hall WJ, Robinson JL, Andrews ML, Zhang L, Timothy K, Medina A (2000). Clinical and genetic variables associated with acute arousal and nonarousal-related cardiac events among subjects with long QT syndrome. *Am J Cardiol*, *85*: 457-461.

15. Alings M, Wilde A (1999). "Brugada" syndrome: clinical data and suggested pathophysiological mechanism. *Circulation*, *99*: 666-673.

16. Allessie MA, Bonke FI, Schopman FJ (1977). Circus movement in rabbit atrial muscle as a mechanism of tachycardia. III. The "leading circle" concept: a new model of circus movement in cardiac tissue without the involvement of an anatomical obstacle. *Circ Res*, *41*: 9-18.

17. Altomare C, Bucchi A, Camatini E, Baruscotti M, Viscomi C, Moroni A, DiFrancesco D (2001). Integrated allosteric model of voltage gating of HCN channels. *J Gen Physiol*, *117*: 519-518.

18. Amos GJ, Wettwer E, Metzger F, Li Q, Himmel HM, Ravens U (1996). Differences between outward currents of human atrial and subepicardial ventricular myocytes. *J Physiol (Lond)*, *491.1*: 31-50.

19. An WF, Bowlby MR, Betty M, Cao J, Ling HP, Mendoza G, Hinson JW, Mattsson KI, Strassle BW, Trimmer JS, Rhodes KJ (2000). Modulation of A-type potassium channels by a family of calcium sensors. *Nature*, *403*: 553-556.

20. Angst BD, Khan LUR, Severs NJ, Whitely K, Rothery S, Thompson RP, Magee AI, Gourdie RG (1997). Dissociated spatial patterning of gap junctions and cell adhesion junctions during postnatal differentiation of ventricular myocardium. *Circ Res*, *80*: 88-94.

21. Antzelevitch C (2000). Electrical heterogeneity, cardiac arrhythmias, and the sodium channel. *Circ Res*, *87*: 964-965.

22. Antzelevitch C, Burashnikov A (2001). Cardiac arrhythmias: reentry and triggered activity. In: *Heart Physiology and Pathophysiology* (eds. N Sperelakis, Y Kurachi, A Terzic, MV Cohen), pp 1153-1179. Academic Press, San Diego.

23. Antzelevitch C, Jalife J, Moe GK (1980). Characteristics of reflection as a mechanism of reentrant arrhythmias and its relationship to parasystole. *Circulation*, *61*: 182-191.

24. Antzelevitch C, Litovsky SH, Lukas A (1990). Epicardium versus endocardium: electrophysiology and pharmacology. In: *Cardiac Electrophysiology From Cell to Bedside* (eds. DP Zipes, J J.). W.B. Saunders.

25. Antzelevitch C, Shimizu W, Yan GX, Sicouri S (1998). Cellular basis for QT dispersion. *J Electrocardiol*, *30 Suppl*: 168-175.

26. Antzelevitch C, Shimizu W, Yan GX, Sicouri S, Weissenburger J, Nesterenko VV, Burashnikov A, Di Diego J, Saffitz J, Thomas GP (1999). The M cell: its contribution to the ECG and to normal and abnormal electrical function of the heart. *J Cardiovasc Electrophysiol*, *10*: 1124-1152.

27. Antzelevitch C, Sicouri S, Litovsky SH, Lukas A, Krishnan SC, Di Diego JM, Gintant GA, Liu DW (1991). Heterogeneity within the ventricular wall. Electrophysiology and pharmacology of epicardial, endocardial, and M cells. *Circ Res*, *69*: 1427-1449.

28. Antzelevitch C, Yan GX, Shimizu W (1999). Transmural dispersion of repolarization and arrhythmogenicity: the Brugada syndrome versus the long QT syndrome. *J Electrocardiol*, *32 Suppl*: 158-165.

29. Anyukhovsky EP, Sosunov EA, Gainullin RZ, Rosen MR (1999). The controversial M cell. *J Cardiovasc Electrophysiol, 10*: 244-260.

30. Apell HJ, Karlish SJ (2001). Functional properties of Na,K-ATPase, and their structural implications, as detected with biophysical techniques. *J Membr Biol, 180*: 1-9.

31. Apkon M, Nerbonne JM (1991). Characterization of two distinct depolarization-activated K^+ currents in isolated adult rat ventricular myocytes. *J Gen Physiol, 97*: 973-1011.

32. Arai M, Matsui H, Periasamy M (1994). Sarcoplasmic reticulum gene expression in cardiac hypertrophy and heart failure. *Circ Res, 74*: 555-564.

33. Armstrong CM (1969). Inactivation of the potassium conductance and related phenomena caused by quaternary ammonium ion injection in squid axons. *J Gen Physiol, 54*: 553-575.

34. Arnsdorf MF, Makielski JC (2001). Excitability and impulse propagation. In: *Heart Physiology and Pathophysiology* (eds. N Sperelakis, Y Kurachi, A Terzic, MV Cohen), pp 99-132. Academic Press, San Diego.

35. Arrell DK, Neverova I, Van Eyk JE (2001). Cardiovascular proteomics: evolution and potential. *Circ Res, 88*: 763-773.

36. Ashcroft FM (2000). Ion Channels and Disease. Academic Press London.

37. Attwell D, Cohen I, Eisner D, Ohba M, Ojeda C (1979). The steady state TTX-sensitive ("window") sodium current in cardiac Purkinje fibres. *Pflügers Archiv, 379*: 137-142.

38. Aulbach F, Simm A, Maier S, Langenfeld H, Walter U, Kersting U, Kirstein M (1999). Insulin stimulates the L-type Ca^{2+} current in rat cardiac myocytes. *Cardiovasc Res, 42*: 113-120.

39. Ausma J, Wijffels M, van Eys G, Koide M, Ramaekers F, Allessie M, Borgers M (1997). Dedifferentiation of atrial cardiomyocytes as a result of chronic atrial fibrillation. *Am J Pathol, 151*: 985-997.

40. Axelsen KB, Palmgren MG (1998). Evolution of substrate specificities in the P-type ATPase superfamily. *J Mol Evol, 46*: 84-101.

41. Babenko A, Vassort G (1997). Enhancement of the ATP-sensitive K^+ current by extracellular ATP in rat ventricular myocytes. Involvement of adenylyl cyclase-induced subsarcolemmal ATP depletion. *Circ Res, 80*: 589-600.

42. Babenko AP, Samoilov VO, Kazantseva ST, Shevchenko YL (1992). ATP-sensitive $K(^+)$-channels in the human adult ventricular cardiomyocytes membrane. *FEBS Lett, 313*: 148-150.

43. Bahouth SW (1995). Thyroid hormone regulation of transmembrane signalling in neonatal rat ventricular myocytes by selective alteration of the expression and coupling of G-protein alpha-subunits. *Biochem J, 307*: 831-841.

44. Baker LC, London B, Choi B-R, Koren G, Salama G (2000). Enhanced dispersion of repolarization and refractoriness in transgenic mouse hearts promotes reentrant ventricular tachycardia. *Circ Res, 86*: 396-447.

45. Balati B, Varro A, Papp JG (1998). Comparison of the cellular electrophysiological characteristics of canine left ventricular epicardium, M cells, endocardium and Purkinje fibres. *Acta Physiol Scand, 164*: 181-190.

46. Balke CW, Kaplinsky E, Michelson EL, Naito M, Dreifus LS (1981). Reperfusion ventricular tachyarrhythmias: correlation with antecedent coronary artery occlusion tachyarrhythmias and duration of myocardial ischemia. *Am Heart J, 101*: 449-456.

47. Balser JR (1999). Structure and function of the cardiac sodium channels. *Cardiovasc Res*, *42*: 327-338.

48. Balser JR, Bennett PB, Roden DM (1990). Time-dependent outward current in guinea pig ventricular myocytes. Gating kinetics of the delayed rectifier. *J Gen Physiol*, *96*: 835-863.

49. Banach K, Weingart R (1996). Connexin43 gap junctions exhibit asymmetrical gating properties. *Pflügers Archiv*, *431*: 775-785.

50. Banach K, Weingart R (2000). Voltage gating of Cx43 gap junction channels involves fast and slow current transitions. *Pflügers Archiv*, *439*: 248-250.

51. Barhanin J, Lesage F, Guillemare E, Fink M, Lazdunski M, Romey G (1996). K$_v$LQT1 and IsK (minK) proteins associate to form the I_{Ks} cardiac potassium current. *Nature*, *384*: 78-79.

52. Baroudi G, Pouliot V, Denjoy I, Guicheney P, Shrier A, Chahine M (2001). Novel mechanism for Brugada syndrome: Defective surface localization of an SCN5A mutant (R1432G). *Circ Res*, *88*: 78e-83e.

53. Barr RC, Plonsey R (1984). Propagation of excitation in idealized anisotropic two-dimensional tissue. *Biophys J*, *45*: 1191-1202.

54. Barrere Lemaire S, Piot C, Leclercq F, Nargeot J, Richard S (2000). Facilitation of L-type calcium currents by diastolic depolarization in cardiac cells: impairment in heart failure. *Cardiovasc Res*, *47*: 336-349.

55. Barth W, Deten A, Bauer M, Reinohs M, Leicht M, Zimmer HG (2000). Differential remodeling of the left and right heart after norepinephrine treatment in rats: studies on cytokines and collagen. *J Mol Cell Cardiol*, *32*: 273-284.

56. Baruscotti M, DiFrancesco D, Robinson RB (2000). Na($^+$) current contribution to the diastolic depolarization in newborn rabbit SA node cells. *Am J Physiol*, *279*: H2303-2309.

57. Baruscotti M, DiFrancesco D, Robinson RB (2001). Single-channel properties of the sinoatrial node Na$^+$ current in the newborn rabbit. *Pflügers Archiv*, *442*: 192-196.

58. Bassani JW, Yuan W, Bers DM (1995). Fractional SR Ca release is regulated by trigger Ca and SR Ca content in cardiac myocytes. *Am J Physiol*, *268*: C1313-1319.

59. Bassani RA, Bassani JW, Lipsius SL, Bers DM (1997). Diastolic SR Ca efflux in atrial pacemaker cells and Ca-overloaded myocytes. *Am J Physiol*, *273*: H886-892.

60. Bastide B, Neyses L, Ganten D, Paul M, Willecke K, Traub O (1993). Gap junction protein connexin40 is preferentially expressed in vascular endothelium and conductive bundles of rat myocardium and is increased under hypertensive conditions. *Circ Res*, *73*: 1138-1149.

61. Batchvarov V, Malik M (2000). Measurement and interpretation of QT dispersion. *Prog Cardiovasc Dis*, *42*: 325-344.

62. Bates SE, Gurney AM (1999). Use-dependent facilitation and depression of L-type Ca^{2+} current in guinea-pig ventricular myocytes: modulation by Ca^{2+} and isoprenaline. *Cardiovasc Res*, *44*: 381-389.

63. Baukrowitz T, Tucker SJ, Schulte U, Benndorf K, Ruppersberg JP, Fakler B (1999). Inward rectification in KATP channels: a pH switch in the pore. *Embo J*, *18*: 847-853.

64. Baxter WT, Mironov SF, Zaitsev AV, Jalife J, Pertsov AM (2001). Visualizing excitation waves inside cardiac muscle using transillumination. *Biophys J*, *80*: 516-530.

65. Bazett HC (1920). An analysis of the time relationships of the heart. *Heart*, *7*: 353-370.

66. Bean BP (1985). Two kinds of calcium channels in canine atrial cells. Differences in kinetics, selectivity, and pharmacology. *J Gen Physiol*, *86*: 1-30.

67. Beardslee MA, Lerner DL, Tadros PN, Laing JG, Beyer EC, Yamada KA, Kléber AG, Schuessler RB, Saffitz JE (2000). Dephosphorylation and intracellular redistribution of ventricular connexin43 during electrical uncoupling induced by ischemia. *Circ Res, 87*: 656-662.

68. Beaulieu P, Cardinal R, Page P, Francoeur F, Tremblay J, Lambert C (1997). Positive chronotropic and inotropic effects of C-type natriuretic peptide in dogs. *Am J Physiol, 273*: H1933-1940.

69. Bechem M, Hoffmann H (1993). The molecular mode of action of the Ca agonist (-) BAY K 8644 on the cardiac Ca channel. *Pflügers Archiv, 424*: 343-353.

70. Beckman JS, Koppenol WH (1996). Nitric oxide, superoxide, and peroxynitrite: the good, the bad, and the ugly. *Am J Physiol, 271*: C1424-C1437.

71. Belardinelli L, Shryock JC, Song Y, Wang D, Srinivas M (1995). Ionic basis of the electrophysiological actions of adenosine on cardiomyocytes. *FASEB J, 9*: 359-365.

72. Benhorin J, Taub R, Goldmit M, Kerem B, Kass RS, Windman I, Medina A (2000). Effects of flecainide in patients with new SCN5A mutation: mutation-specific therapy for long-QT syndrome? *Circulation, 101*: 1698-1706.

73. Benitah JP, Vassort G (1999). Aldosterone upregulates Ca^{2+} current in adult rat cardiomyocytes. *Circ Res, 85*: 1139-1145.

74. Benndorf K, Friedrich M, Hirche H (1991). Anoxia opens ATP regulated K channels in isolated heart cells of the guinea pig. *Pflügers Archiv, 419*: 108-110.

75. Benndorf K, Nilius B (1988). Properties of an early outward current in single cells of the mouse ventricle. *Gen Physiol Biophys, 7*: 449-466.

76. Bennett PB, Yazawa K, Makita N, George AL, Jr. (1995). Molecular mechanism for an inherited cardiac arrhythmia. *Nature, 376*: 683-685.

77. Berger F, Borchard U, Hafner D, Putz I, Weis TM (1997). Effects of 17beta-estradiol on action potentials and ionic currents in male rat ventricular myocytes. *Naunyn Schmiedebergs Arch Pharmacol, 356*: 788-796.

78. Berger RD (2000). Repolarization alternans : toward a unifying theory of reentrant arrhythmia induction. *Circ Res, 87*: 1083-1084.

79. Berne RM, Sperelakis N, Geiger SR (1979). Handbook of Physiology. Section 2: The cardiovascular system. Vol I. The heart. American Physiological Society, Bethesda.

80. Berridge MJ (1993). Inositol trisphosphate and calcium signalling. *Nature, 361*: 315-325.

81. Bers D (1991). Excitation-contraction coupling and cardiac contractile force. Kluwer Academic Publishers, Dordrecht.

82. Bers DM (2000). Calcium fluxes involved in control of cardiac myocyte contraction. *Circ Res, 87*: 275-281.

83. Bers DM, Perez Reyes E (1999). Ca channels in cardiac myocytes: structure and function in Ca influx and intracellular Ca release. *Cardiovasc Res, 42*: 339-360.

84. Bett G, Noble D, Noble S, Earm Y, Ho WK, So IS (1992). Na-Ca exchange current during the cardiac action potential. *Adv Exp Med Biol, 311*: 453-454.

85. Beuckelmann DJ, Nabauer M, Erdmann E (1991). Characteristics of calcium-current in isolated human ventricular myocytes from patients with terminal heart failure. *J Mol Cell Cardiol, 23*: 929-937.

86. Beuckelmann DJ, Nabauer M, Erdmann E (1993). Alterations of K^+ currents in isolated human ventricular myocytes from patients with terminal heart failure. *Circ Res, 73*: 379-385.

87. Bezanilla F (2000). The voltage sensor in voltage-dependent ion channels. *Physiol Rev, 80*: 555-1372.

88.   Bezprozvanny I, Watras J, Ehrlich BE (1991). Bell-shaped calcium-response curves of Ins(1,4,5)P3- and calcium-gated channels from endoplasmic reticulum of cerebellum. *Nature, 351*: 751-754.
89.   Bezzina CR, Rook MB, Wilde AA (2001). Cardiac sodium channel and inherited arrhythmia syndromes. *Cardiovasc Res, 49*: 257-271.
90.   Bhatnagar A (1994). Biochemical mechanism of irreversible cell injury caused by free radical-initiated reactions. *Mol Cell Biochem, 137*: 9-16.
91.   Bhatnagar A, Srivastava SK, Szabo G (1990). Oxidative stress alters specific membrane currents in isolated cardiac myocytes. *Circ Res, 67*: 535-549.
92.   Biel M, Ludwig A, Zong X, Hofmann F (1999). Hyperpolarization-activated cation channels: a multi-gene family. *Rev Physiol Biochem Pharmacol, 136*: 165-181.
93.   Bielen FV, Glitsch HG, Verdonck F (1991). Dependence of Na$^+$ pump current on external monovalent cations and membrane potential in rabbit cardiac Purkinje cells. *J Physiol (Lond), 442*: 169-189.
94.   Bielen FV, Glitsch HG, Verdonck F (1992). The kinetics of the inhibition by dihydroouabain of the sodium pump current in single rabbit cardiac Purkinje cells. *Naunyn Schmiedebergs Arch Pharmacol, 345*: 100-107.
95.   Biggin PC, Roosild T, Choe S (2000). Potassium channel structure: domain by domain. *Curr Opin Struct Biol, 10*: 456-461.
96.   Blachly Dyson E, Zambronicz EB, Yu WH, Adams V, McCabe ER, Adelman J, Colombini M, Forte M (1993). Cloning and functional expression in yeast of two human isoforms of the outer mitochondrial membrane channel, the voltage-dependent anion channel. *J Biol Chem, 268*: 1835-1841.
97.   Blatter LA, Huser J, Rios E (1997). Sarcoplasmic reticulum Ca^{2+} release flux underlying Ca^{2+} sparks in cardiac muscle. *Proc Natl Acad Sci USA, 94*: 4176-4181.
98.   Blaustein MP, Lederer WJ (1999). Sodium/calcium exchange: its physiological implications. *Physiol Rev, 79*: 763-854.
99.   Bogdanov KY, Vinogradova TM, Lakatta EG (2001). Sinoatrial nodal cell ryanodine receptor and Na$^+$-Ca^{2+} exchanger : Molecular partners in pacemaker regulation. *Circ Res, 88*: 1254-1238.
100. Bohm M (1998). Catecholamine refractoriness and their mechanisms in cardiocirculatory shock and chronic heart failure. *Thorac Cardiovasc Surg, 46 Suppl 2*: 270-275.
101. Bohn G, Moosmang S, Conrad H, Ludwig A, Hofmann F, Klugbauer N (2000). Expression of T- and L-type calcium channel mRNA in murine sinoatrial node. *FEBS Lett, 481*: 73-76.
102. Bolli R (2000). The late phase of preconditioning. *Circ Res, 87*: 972-983.
103. Bond JM, Harper IS, Chacon E, Reece JM, Herman B, Lemasters JJ (1994). The pH paradox in the pathophysiology of reperfusion injury to rat neonatal cardiac myocytes. *Ann N Y Acad Sci, 723*: 25-37.
104. Borgnia M, Nielsen S, Engel A, Agre P (1999). Cellular and molecular biology of the aquaporin water channels. *Annu Rev Biochem, 68*: 425-458.
105. Bosch RF, Gaspo R, Busch AE, Lang HJ, Li GR, Nattel S (1998). Effects of the chromanol 293B, a selective blocker of the slow, component of the delayed rectifier K$^+$ current, on repolarization in human and guinea pig ventricular myocytes. *Cardiovasc Res, 38*: 441-450.
106. Bosch RF, Li GR, Gaspo R, Nattel S (1999). Electrophysiologic effects of chronic amiodarone therapy and hypothyroidism, alone and in combination, on guinea pig ventricular myocytes. *J Pharmacol Exp Ther, 289*: 156-165.

107. Bosch RF, Wang Z, Li GR, Nattel S (1999). Electrophysiological mechanisms by which hypothyroidism delays repolarization in guinea pig hearts. *Am J Physiol, 277*: H211-220.

108. Boyden PA, Jeck CD (1995). Ion channel function in disease. *Cardiovasc Res, 29*: 312-318.

109. Boyett MR, Honjo H, Harrison SM, Zang WJ, Kirby MS (1994). Ultra-slow voltage-dependent inactivation of the calcium current in guinea-pig and ferret ventricular myocytes. *Pflügers Archiv, 428*: 39-50.

110. Boyett MR, Jewell BR (1980). Analysis of the effects of changes in rate and rhythm upon electrical activity in the heart. *Prog Biophys Mol Biol, 36*: 1-52.

111. Boyle WA, Nerbonne JM (1992). Two functionally distinct 4-aminopyridine-sensitive outward K^+ currents in rat atrial myocytes. *J Gen Physiol, 100*: 1041-1067.

112. Brahmajothi MV, Campbell DL, Rasmusson RL, Morales MJ, Trimmer JS, Nerbonne JM, Strauss HC (1999). Distinct transient outward potassium current (Ito) phenotypes and distribution of fast-inactivating potassium channel alpha subunits in ferret left ventricular myocytes. *J Gen Physiol, 113*: 581-600.

113. Britton FC, Hatton WJ, Rossow CF, Duan D, Hume JR, Horowitz B (2000). Molecular distribution of volume-regulated chloride channels (ClC-2 and ClC-3) in cardiac tissues. *Am J Physiol, 279*: H2225-2233.

114. Brittsan AG, Kiss E, Edes I, Grupp IL, Grupp G, Kranias EG (1999). The effect of isoproterenol on phospholamban-deficient mouse hearts with altered thyroid conditions. *J Mol Cell Cardiol, 31*: 1725-1737.

115. Brosnihan KB, Li P, Ganten D, Ferrario CM (1997). Estrogen protects transgenic hypertensive rats by shifting the vasoconstrictor-vasodilator balance of RAS. *Am J Physiol, 273*: R1908-1915.

116. Brown HF, DiFrancesco D, Noble SJ (1979). How does adrenaline accelerate the heart? *Nature, 280*: 235-236.

117. Brugada P, Brugada J (1992). Right bundle branch block, persistent ST segment elevation and sudden cardiac death: a distinct clinical and electrocardiographic syndrome. A multicenter report. *J Am Coll Cardiol, 20*: 1391-1396.

118. Brugada R, Brugada J, Antzelevitch C, Kirsch GE, Potenza D, Towbin JA, Brugada P (2000). Sodium channel blockers identify risk for sudden death in patients with ST-segment elevation and right bundle branch block but structurally normal hearts. *Circulation, 101*: 510-515.

119. Brunner F, Kukovetz WR (1996). Postischemic antiarrhythmic effects of angiotensin-converting enzyme inhibitors. Role of suppression of endogenous endothelin secretion. *Circulation, 94*: 1752-1761.

120. Bryant SM, Shipsey SJ, Hart G (1997). Regional differences in electrical and mechanical properties of myocytes from guinea-pig hearts with mild left ventricular hypertrophy. *Cardiovasc Res, 35*: 315-323.

121. Bryant SM, Wan X, Shipsey SJ, Hart G (1998). Regional differences in the delayed rectifier current (IKr and IKs) contribute to the differences in action potential duration in basal left ventricular myocytes in guinea-pig. *Cardiovasc Res, 40*: 322-331.

122. Bukauskas FF, Bukauskiene A, Bennett MVL, Verselis VK (2001). Gating Properties of Gap Junction Channels Assembled from Connexin43 and Connexin43 Fused with Green Fluorescent Protein. *Biophys J, 81*: 137-152.

123. Bukauskas FF, Peracchia C (1997). Two distinct gating mechanisms in gap junction channels: CO2-sensitive and voltage-sensitive. *Biophys J, 72*: 2137-2142.

124.   Burashnikov A, Antzelevitch C (1998). Acceleration-induced action potential prolongation and early afterdepolarizations. *J Cardiovasc Electrophysiol*, 9: 934-948.

125.   Burashnikov A, Antzelevitch C (1999). Differences in the electrophysiologic response of four canine ventricular cell types to alpha 1-adrenergic agonists. *Cardiovasc Res*, 43: 901-908.

126.   Burnashev NA, Undrovinas AI, Fleidervish IA, Rosenshtraukh LV (1989). Ischemic poison lysophosphatidylcholine modifies heart sodium channels gating inducing long-lasting bursts of openings. *Pflügers Archiv*, 415: 124-126.

127.   Burt JM (1987). Block of intercellular communication: interaction of intracellular H^+ and Ca^{2+}. *Am J Physiol*, 253: C607-612.

128.   Burt JM, Spray DC (1988). Single-channel events and gating behavior of the cardiac gap junction channel. *Proc Natl Acad Sci USA*, 85: 3431-3434.

129.   Burton FL, Cobbe SM (2001). Dispersion of ventricular repolarization and refractory period. *Cardiovasc Res*, 50: 10-23.

130.   Calaghan SC, White E (1999). The role of calcium in the response of cardiac muscle to stretch. *Prog Biophys Mol Biol*, 71: 59-90.

131.   Caldwell RA, Baumgarten CM (1998). Plasmalogen-derived lysolipid induces a depolarizing cation current in rabbit ventricular myocytes. *Circ Res*, 83: 533-540.

132.   Callewaert G, Carmeliet E, Vereecke J (1984). Single cardiac Purkinje cells: general electrophysiology and voltage-clamp analysis of the pace-maker current. *J Physiol (Lond)*, 349: 643-661.

133.   Camacho SA, Figueredo VM, Brandes R, Weiner MW (1993). $Ca(^{2+})$-dependent fluorescence transients and phosphate metabolism during low-flow ischemia in rat hearts. *Am J Physiol*, 265: H114-122.

134.   Campbell DL, Rasmusson RL, Comer MB, Strauss HC (1995). The cardiac calcium-independent outward potassium current: kinetics, molecular properties, and role in ventricular repolarization. In: *Cardiac Electrophysiology From Cell to Bedside* (eds. DP Zipes, J Jalife), pp 83-96. Saunders Co, Philadelphia.

135.   Campbell DL, Rasmusson RL, Qu Y, Strauss HC (1993). The calcium-independent transient outward potassium current in isolated ferret right ventricular myocytes. I. Basic characterization and kinetic analysis. *J Gen Physiol*, 101: 571-601.

136.   Campbell DL, Rasmusson RL, Strauss HC (1992). Ionic current mechanisms generating vertebrate primary cardiac pacemaker activity at the single cell level: an integrative view. *Annu Rev Physiol*, 54: 279-302.

137.   Carmeliet E (1977). Repolarisation and frequency in cardiac cells. *J Physiol (Lond)*, 73: 903-923.

138.   Carmeliet E (1982). Induction and removal of inward-going rectification in sheep cardiac Purkinje fibres. *J Physiol (Lond)*, 327: 285-308.

139.   Carmeliet E (1987). Slow inactivation of the sodium current in rabbit cardiac Purkinje fibres. *Pflügers Archiv*, 408: 18-26.

140.   Carmeliet E (1992). A fuzzy subsarcolemmal space for intracellular Na^+ in cardiac cells? *Cardiovasc Res*, 26: 433-442.

141.   Carmeliet E (1992). Voltage- and time-dependent block of the delayed K^+ current in cardiac myocytes by dofetilide. *J Pharmacol Exp Ther*, 262: 809-817.

142.   Carmeliet E (1993). Use-dependent block and use-dependent unblock of the delayed rectifier K^+ current by almokalant in rabbit ventricular myocytes. *Circ Res*, 73: 857-868.

143.   Carmeliet E (1998). Effects of cetirizine on the delayed K^+ currents in cardiac cells: comparison with terfenadine. *Br J Pharmacol*, 124: 663-668.

144. Carmeliet E (1999). Antiarrhythmic drugs and ion channels: have we made the connection? *J Cardiovasc Electrophysiol, 10*: 755-759.
145. Carmeliet E (1999). Cardiac ionic currents and acute ischemia: from channels to arrhythmias. *Physiol Rev, 79*: 917-1017.
146. Carmeliet E (1999). Rapid delayed K^+ current and quinidine sensitivity are reduced in healed myocardial infarction. *J Cardiovasc Electrophysiol, 10*: 855-859.
147. Carmeliet E, Morad M, Van der Heyden G, Vereecke J (1986). Electrophysiological effects of tetracaine in single guinea-pig ventricular myocytes. *J Physiol (Lond), 376*: 143-161.
148. Carmeliet E, Mubagwa K (1998). Antiarrhythmic drugs and cardiac ion channels: mechanisms of action. *Prog Biophys Mol Biol, 70*: 1-72.
149. Carmeliet E, Vereecke J (1969). Adrenaline and the plateau phase of the cardiac action potential. Importance of Ca^{++}, Na^+ and K^+ conductance. *Pflügers Archiv, 313*: 300-315.
150. Carmeliet E, Vereecke J (1979). Electrogenesis of the action potential and automaticity. In: *Handbook of Physiology Section 3: The Cardiovascular System, Volume I, The Heart* (ed. NS R. M. Berne, S.R. Geiger), pp 269-334. American Physiological Society, Maryland.
151. Casimiro MC, Knollmann BC, Ebert SN, Vary JC, Jr., Greene AE, Franz MR, Grinberg A, Huang SP, Pfeifer K (2001). Targeted disruption of the Kcnq1 gene produces a mouse model of Jervell and Lange- Nielsen Syndrome. *Proc Natl Acad Sci USA, 98*: 2526-2531.
152. Catterall WA (2000). From ionic currents to molecular mechanisms: the structure and function of voltage-gated sodium channels. *Neuron, 26*: 13-25.
153. Catterall WA (2000). Structure and regulation of voltage-gated Ca^{2+} channels. *Annu Rev Cell Dev Biol, 16*: 521-555.
154. Catterall WA (2001). A 3D view of sodium channels. *Nature, 409*: 988-991.
155. Cavalié A, Pelzer D, Trautwein W (1986). Fast and slow gating behaviour of single calcium channels in cardiac cells. Relation to activation and inactivation of calcium-channel current. *Pflügers Archiv, 406*: 241-258.
156. Cerbai E, Amerini S, Mugelli A (1990). Histamine and abnormal automaticity in barium- and strophanthidin-treated sheep Purkinje fibers. *Agents Actions, 31*: 1-10.
157. Cerbai E, Barbieri M, Mugelli A (1994). Characterization of the hyperpolarization-activated current, I_f, in ventricular myocytes isolated from hypertensive rats. *J Physiol (Lond), 481*: 585-591.
158. Cerbai E, Barbieri M, Mugelli A (1996). Occurrence and properties of the hyperpolarization-activated current I_f in ventricular myocytes from normotensive and hypertensive rats during aging. *Circulation, 94*: 1674-1681.
159. Cerbai E, Crucitti A, Sartiani L, De Paoli P, Pino R, Rodriguez ML, Gensini G, Mugelli A (2000). Long-term treatment of spontaneously hypertensive rats with losartan and electrophysiological remodeling of cardiac myocytes. *Cardiovasc Res, 45*: 388-396.
160. Cerbai E, Pino R, Porciatti F, Sani G, Toscano M, Maccherini M, Giunti G, Mugelli A (1997). Characterization of the hyperpolarization-activated current, I_f, in ventricular myocytes from human failing heart. *Circulation, 95*: 568-571.
161. Cerbai E, Pino R, Sartiani L, Mugelli A (1999). Influence of postnatal-development on I_f occurrence and properties in neonatal rat ventricular myocytes. *Cardiovasc Res, 42*: 416-423.

162. Chan KW, Sui JL, Vivaudou M, Logothetis DE (1996). Control of channel activity through a unique amino acid residue of a G protein-gated inwardly rectifying K$^+$ channel subunit. *Proc Natl Acad Sci USA, 93*: 14193-14198.

163. Chandy KG (1991). Simplified gene nomenclature. *Nature, 352*: 26.

164. Chang F, Yu H, Cohen IS (1994). Actions of vasoactive intestinal peptide and neuropeptide Y on the pacemaker current in canine Purkinje fibers. *Circ Res, 74*: 157-162.

165. Charron P, Komajda M (2001). Are we ready for pharmacogenomics in heart failure? *Eur J Pharmacol, 417*: 1-9.

166. Chattou S, Diacono J, Feuvray D (1999). Decrease in sodium-calcium exchange and calcium currents in diabetic rat ventricular myocytes. *Acta Physiol Scand, 166*: 137-144.

167. Chen D, Xu L, Tripathy A, Meissner G, Eisenberg B (1997). Permeation through the calcium release channel of cardiac muscle. *Biophys J, 73*: 1337-1354.

168. Chen DP, Xu L, Tripathy A, Meissner G, Eisenberg B (1999). Selectivity and permeation in calcium release channel of cardiac muscle: alkali metal ions. *Biophys J, 76*: 1346-1366.

169. Chen H, Heinemann SH (2001). Interaction of Scorpion {alpha}-Toxins with Cardiac Sodium Channels: Binding Properties and Enhancement of Slow Inactivation. *J Gen Physiol, 117*: 505-518.

170. Chen Q, Kirsch GE, Zhang D, Brugada R, Brugada J, Brugada P, Potenza D, Moya A, Borggrefe M, Breithardt G, Ortiz Lopez R, Wang Z, Antzelevitch C, O'Brien RE, Schulze Bahr E, Keating MT, Towbin JA, Wang Q (1998). Genetic basis and molecular mechanism for idiopathic ventricular fibrillation. *Nature, 392*: 293-296.

171. Chen S, Wang J, Siegelbaum SA (2001). Properties of hyperpolarization-activated pacemaker current defined by coassembly of HCN1 and HCN2 subunits and basal modulation by cyclic nucleotide. *J Gen Physiol, 117*: 491-384.

172. Chen YJ, Lee SH, Hsieh MH, Hsiao CJ, Yu WC, Chiou CW, Chen SA (1999). Effects of 17beta-estradiol on tachycardia-induced changes of atrial refractoriness and cisapride-induced ventricular arrhythmia. *J Cardiovasc Electrophysiol, 10*: 587-598.

173. Cheng A, van Hoek AN, Yeager M, Verkman AS, Mitra AK (1997). Three-dimensional organization of a human water channel. *Nature, 387*: 627-630.

174. Cheng H, Lederer WJ, Cannell MB (1993). Calcium sparks: elementary events underlying excitation-contraction coupling in heart muscle. *Science, 262*: 740-744.

175. Cheng J, Kamiya K, Liu W, Tsuji Y, Toyama J, Kodama I (1999). Heterogeneous distribution of the two components of delayed rectifier K$^+$ current: a potential mechanism of the proarrhythmic effects of methanesulfonanilideclass III agents. *Cardiovasc Res, 43*: 135-147.

176. Cheung DW (1981). Electrical activity of the pulmonary vein and its interaction with the right atrium in the guinea-pig. *J Physiol (Lond), 314*: 445-456.

177. Chiang CE, Roden DM (2000). The long QT syndromes: genetic basis and clinical implications. *J Am Coll Cardiol, 36*: 1-12.

178. Chinn K (1993). Two delayed rectifiers in guinea pig ventricular myocytes distinguished by tail current kinetics. *J Pharmacol Exp Ther, 264*: 553-560.

179. Choi HS, Trafford AW, Eisner DA (2000). Measurement of calcium entry and exit in quiescent rat ventricular myocytes. *Pflügers Archiv, 440*: 600-608.

180. Chorvatova A, Gallo-Payet N, Casanova C, Payet MD (1996). Modulation of membrane potential and ionic currents by the AT1 and AT2 receptors of angiotensin II. *Cell Signal, 8*: 525-532.

181. Chutkow WA, Simon MC, Le Beau MM, Burant CF (1996). Cloning, tissue expression, and chromosomal localization of SUR2, the putative drug-binding subunit of cardiac, skeletal muscle, and vascular KATP channels. *Diabetes, 45*: 1439-1445.

182. Clancy CE, Rudy Y (1999). Linking a genetic defect to its cellular phenotype in a cardiac arrhythmia. *Nature, 400*: 566-569.

183. Clapham DE (1997). The molecular control of cardiac ion channels. *Heart Vessels, Suppl*: 168-169.

184. Clapham DE, Runnels LW, Strubing C (2001). The trp ion channel family. *Nat Rev Neurosci, 2*: 387-396.

185. Clark RB, Bouchard RA, Salinas Stefanon E, Sanchez Chapula J, Giles WR (1993). Heterogeneity of action potential waveforms and potassium currents in rat ventricle. *Cardiovasc Res, 27*: 1795-1799.

186. Clark RB, Giles WR, Imaizumi Y (1988). Properties of the transient outward current in rabbit atrial cells. *J Physiol (Lond), 405*: 147-168.

187. Clarke K, Stewart LC, Neubauer S, Balschi JA, Smith TW, Ingwall JS, Nedelec JF, Humphrey SM, Kléber AG, Springer CS, Jr. (1993). Extracellular volume and transsarcolemmal proton movement during ischemia and reperfusion: a 31P NMR spectroscopic study of the isovolumic rat heart. *NMR Biomed, 6*: 278-286.

188. Cleemann L, Wang W, Morad M (1998). Two-dimensional confocal images of organization, density, and gating of focal Ca^{2+} release sites in rat cardiac myocytes. *Proc Natl Acad Sci USA, 95*: 10984-10989.

189. Clemo HF, Baumgarten CM, Ellenbogen KA, Stambler BS (1996). Atrial natriuretic peptide and cardiac electrophysiology: autonomic and direct effects. *J Cardiovasc Electrophysiol, 7*: 149-162.

190. Clerc L (1976). Directional differences of impulse spread in trabecular muscle from mammalian heart. *J Physiol (Lond), 255*: 335-346.

191. Clozel JP, Ertel EA, Ertel SI (1999). Voltage-gated T-type Ca^{2+} channels and heart failure. *Proc Assoc Am Physicians, 111*: 429-437.

192. Coetzee WA (1992). Regulation of ATP sensitive potassium channel of isolated guinea pig ventricular myocytes by sarcolemmal monocarboxylate transport. *Cardiovasc Res, 26*: 1077-1086.

193. Coetzee WA, Amarillo Y, Chiu J, Chow A, Lau D, McCormack T, Moreno H, Nadal MS, Ozaita A, Pountney D, Saganich M, Vega-Saenz de Miera E, Rudy B (1999). Molecular diversity of K^+ channels. *Ann N Y Acad Sci, 868*: 233-285.

194. Cohen MV, Baines CP, Downey JM (2000). Ischemic preconditioning: from adenosine receptor of KATP channel. *Annu Rev Physiol, 62*: 79-109.

195. Colatsky JJ, Tsien RW (1979). Sodium channels in rabbit cardiac Purkinje fibres. *Nature, 278*: 265-268.

196. Colatsky TJ (1980). Voltage clamp measurements of sodium channel properties in rabbit cardiac Purkinje fibres. *J Physiol (Lond), 305*: 215-234.

197. Cole KC, Moore JW (1960). Ionic current measurements in the squid giant axon membrane. *J Gen Physiol, 44*: 649-670.

198. Cole WC, Picone JB, Sperelakis N (1988). Gap junction uncoupling and discontinuous propagation in the heart. A comparison of experimental data with computer simulations. *Biophys J, 53*: 809-818.

199. Collier ML, Levesque PC, Kenyon JL, Hume JR (1996). Unitary Cl⁻ channels activated by cytoplasmic Ca^{2+} in canine ventricular myocytes. *Circ Res, 78*: 936-944.

200. Colombini M (1987). Regulation of the mitochondrial outer membrane channel, VDAC. *J Bioenerg Biomembr, 19*: 309-320.

201. Colquhoun D, Hawkes AG (1977). Relaxation and fluctuations of membrane currents that flow through drug-operated channels. *Proc R Soc Lond B Biol Sci, 199*: 231-262.

202. Colquhoun D, Hawkes AG (1981). On the stochastic properties of single ion channels. *Proc R Soc Lond B Biol Sci, 211*: 205-235.

203. Colquhoun D, Hawkes AG (1982). On the stochastic properties of bursts of single ion channel openings and of clusters of bursts. *Philos Trans R Soc Lond B Biol Sci, 300*: 1-59.

204. Colquhoun D, Neher E, Reuter H, Stevens CF (1981). Inward current channels activated by intracellular Ca in cultured cardiac cells. *Nature, 294*: 752-754.

205. Connolly DL, Shanahan CM, Weissberg PL (1998). The aquaporins. A family of water channel proteins. *Int J Biochem Cell Biol, 30*: 169-172.

206. Cook SJ, Chamunorwa JP, Lancaster MK, O'Neill SC (1997). Regional differences in the regulation of intracellular sodium and in action potential configuration in rabbit left ventricle. *Pflügers Archiv, 433*: 515-522.

207. Coppen SR, Severs NJ, Gourdie RG (1999). Connexin45 (alpha 6) expression delineates an extended conduction system in the embryonic and mature rodent heart. *Dev Genet, 24*: 82-90.

208. Coraboeuf E, Carmeliet E (1982). Existence of two transient outward currents in sheep cardiac Purkinje fibers. *Pflügers Archiv, 392*: 352-359.

209. Coraboeuf E, Weidmann S (1949). Potentiels d'action du muscle cardiaque obtenus à l'aide de microéléctrodes intracellulaires. Présence d'une inversion de potentiel. *CR Soc Biol, Paris, 143*: 1360-1361.

210. Coronel R, Fiolet JW, Wilms Schopman JG, Opthof T, Schaapherder AF, Janse MJ (1989). Distribution of extracellular potassium and electrophysiologic changes during two-stage coronary ligation in the isolated, perfused canine heart. *Circulation, 80*: 165-177.

211. Coronel R, Wilms Schopman FJ, Janse MJ (1997). Profibrillatory effects of intracoronary thrombus in acute regional ischemia of the in situ porcine heart. *Circulation, 96*: 3985-3991.

212. Coronel R, Wilms Schopman FJ, Opthof T, Cinca J, Fiolet JW, Janse MJ (1992). Reperfusion arrhythmias in isolated perfused pig hearts. Inhomogeneities in extracellular potassium, ST and TQ potentials, and transmembrane action potentials. *Circ Res, 71*: 1131-1142.

213. Coronel R, Wilms Schopman FJ, Opthof T, van Capelle FJ, Janse MJ (1991). Injury current and gradients of diastolic stimulation threshold, TQ potential, and extracellular potassium concentration during acute regional ischemia in the isolated perfused pig heart. *Circ Res, 68*: 1241-1249.

214. Corr PB, Yamada KA, DaTorre SD (1990). Modulation of alpha-adrenergic receptors and their intracellular coupling in the ischemic heart. *Basic Res Cardiol, 1*: 31-45.

215. Coughlin SR (1999). How the protease thrombin talks to cells. *Proc Natl Acad Sci USA, 96*: 11023-11027.

216. Coulombe A, Lefevre IA, Baro I, Coraboeuf E (1989). Barium- and calcium-permeable channels open at negative membrane potentials in rat ventricular myocytes. *J Membr Biol, 111*: 57-67.

217. Courtemanche M, Ramirez RJ, Nattel S (1998). Ionic mechanisms underlying human atrial action potential properties: insights from a mathematical model. *Am J Physiol, 275*: H301-321.

218. Courtemanche M, Ramirez RJ, Nattel S (1999). Ionic targets for drug therapy and atrial fibrillation-induced electrical remodeling: insights from a mathematical model. *Cardiovasc Res, 42*: 477-489.

219. Cox MM, Berman I, Myerburg RJ, Smets MJ, Kozlovskis PL (1991). Morphometric mapping of regional myocyte diameters after healing of myocardial infarction in cats. *J Mol Cell Cardiol, 23*: 127-135.

220. Craelius W, Chen V, el Sherif N (1988). Stretch activated ion channels in ventricular myocytes. *Biosci Rep, 8*: 407-414.

221. Cranefield PF (1977). Action potentials, afterpotentials, and arrhythmias. *Circ Res, 41*: 415-423.

222. Cranefield PF, Aronson RS (1974). Initiation of sustained rhythmic activity by single propagated action potentials in canine cardiac Purkinje fibers exposed to sodium-free solution or to ouabain. *Circ Res, 34*: 477-481.

223. Cribbs LL, Lee J-H, Yang J, Satin J, Zhang Y, Daud A, Barclay J, Williamson MP, Fox M, Rees M, Perez-Reyes E (1998). Cloning and Characterization of {alpha}1H From Human Heart, a Member of the T-Type Ca^{2+} Channel Gene Family. *Circ Res, 83*: 103-109.

224. Cribbs LL, Martin BL, Schroder EA, Keller BB, Delisle BP, Satin J (2001). Identification of the T-Type calcium channel (CaV3.1d) in developing mouse heart. *Circ Res, 88*: 403-407.

225. Crompton M, Andreeva L (1993). On the involvement of a mitochondrial pore in reperfusion injury. *Basic Res Cardiol, 88*: 513-523.

226. Crumb WJ, Jr., Pigott JD, Clarkson CW (1995). Comparison of Ito in young and adult human atrial myocytes: evidence for developmental changes. *Am J Physiol, 268*: H1335-1342.

227. Cui J, Kagan A, Qin D, Mathew J, Melman YF, McDonald TV (2001). Analysis of the cyclic nucleotide binding domain of the herg potassium channel and interactions with kcne2. *J Biol Chem, 276*: 17244-17251.

228. Cui J, Melman Y, Palma E, Fishman GI, McDonald TV (2000). Cyclic AMP regulates the HERG K^+ channel by dual pathways. *Curr Biol, 10*: 671-674.

229. Curran ME, Splawski I, Timothy KW, Vincent GM, Green ED, Keating MT (1995). A molecular basis for cardiac arrhythmia: HERG mutations cause long QT syndrome. *Cell, 80*: 795-803.

230. Darrow BJ, Fast VG, Kléber AG, Beyer EC, Saffitz JE (1996). Functional and structural assessment of intercellular communication: Increased conduction velocity and enhanced connexin expression in dibutyryl cAMP-treated cultured cardiac myocytes. *Circ Res, 79*: 174-183.

231. Davidenko JM, Kent PF, Chialvo DR, Michaels DC, Jalife J (1990). Sustained vortex-like waves in normal isolated ventricular muscle. *Proc Natl Acad Sci USA, 87*: 8785-8789.

232. Davidenko JM, Pertsov AM, Salomonsz R, Baxter WP, Jalife J (1992). Spatiotemporal irregularities of spiral wave activity in isolated ventricular muscle. *J Electrocardiol, 24 Suppl*: 113-122.

233. Davidenko JM, Pertsov AV, Salomonsz R, Baxter W, Jalife J (1992). Stationary and drifting spiral waves of excitation in isolated cardiac muscle. *Nature, 355*: 349-351.

234. de Gasparo M, Catt KJ, Inagami T, Wright JW, Unger T (2000). International union of pharmacology. XXIII. The angiotensin II receptors. *Pharmacol Rev, 52*: 415-472.

235. De Mello WC (1999). Cell coupling and impulse propagation in the failing heart. *J Cardiovasc Electrophysiol, 10*: 1409-1420.

236. De Mello WC (1999). Gap junctional conductance in cardiomyopathic hamsters: the role of c-Src. *Circ Res*, *85*: 661-662.
237. De Mello WC, Motta GE (1969). The effect of aldosterone on membrane potential of cardiac muscle fibers. *J Pharmacol Exp Ther*, *167*: 166-172.
238. De Smedt H, Missiaen L, Parys JB, Henning RH, Sienaert I, Vanlingen S, Gijsens A, Himpens B, Casteels R (1997). Isoform diversity of the inositol trisphosphate receptor in cell types of mouse origin. *Biochem J*, *322*: 575-583.
239. Deal KK, England SK, Tamkun MM (1996). Molecular physiology of cardiac potassium channels. *Physiol Rev*, *76*: 49-67.
240. Decking UK, Schlieper G, Kroll K, Schrader J (1997). Hypoxia-induced inhibition of adenosine kinase potentiates cardiac adenosine release. *Circ Res*, *81*: 154-164.
241. Demir SS, Clark JW, Murphey CR, Giles WR (1994). A mathematical model of a rabbit sinoatrial node cell. *Am J Physiol*, *266*: C832-852.
242. Denyer JC, Brown HF (1990). Pacemaking in rabbit isolated sino-atrial node cells during Cs^+ block of the hyperpolarization-activated current i_f. *J Physiol (Lond)*, *429*: 401-409.
243. Denyer JC, Brown HF (1990). Rabbit sino-atrial node cells: isolation and electrophysiological properties. *J Physiol (Lond)*, *428*: 405-424.
244. Dessertenne F (1966). La tachycardie ventriculaire à deux foyers opposés variables. *Arch Mal Coeur Vaiss*, *59*: 263-272.
245. D'Hahan N, Moreau C, Prost AL, Jacquet H, Alekseev AE, Terzic A, Vivaudou M (1999). Pharmacological plasticity of cardiac ATP-sensitive potassium channels toward diazoxide revealed by ADP. *Proc Natl Acad Sci USA*, *96*: 12162-12167.
246. Dhalla NS, Dixon IM, Suzuki S, Kaneko M, Kobayashi A, Beamish RE (1992). Changes in adrenergic receptors during the development of heart failure. *Mol Cell Biochem*, *114*: 91-95.
247. Dhein S (1998). Gap junction channels in the cardiovascular system: pharmacological and physiological modulation. *Trends Pharmacol Sci*, *19*: 229-241.
248. Di Diego JM, Sun ZQ, Antzelevitch C (1996). I_{to} and action potential notch are smaller in left vs. right canine ventricular epicardium. *Am J Physiol*, *271*: H548-561.
249. Di Lisa F, Blank PS, Colonna R, Gambassi G, Silverman HS, Stern MD, Hansford RG (1995). Mitochondrial membrane potential in single living adult rat cardiac myocytes exposed to anoxia or metabolic inhibition. *J Physiol (Lond)*, *486*: 1-13.
250. Diaz PJ, Rudy Y, Plonsey R (1983). Intercalated discs as a cause for discontinuous propagation in cardiac muscle: a theoretical simulation. *Ann Biomed Eng*, *11*: 177-189.
251. DiFrancesco D (1981). A new interpretation of the pace-maker current in calf Purkinje fibres. *J Physiol (Lond)*, *314*: 359-376.
252. DiFrancesco D (1982). Block and activation of the pace-maker channel in calf purkinje fibres: effects of potassium, caesium and rubidium. *J Physiol (Lond)*, *329*: 485-507.
253. DiFrancesco D (1986). Characterization of single pacemaker channels in cardiac sino-atrial node cells. *Nature*, *324*: 470-473.
254. DiFrancesco D (1993). Pacemaker mechanisms in cardiac tissue. *Annu Rev Physiol*, *55*: 455-472.
255. DiFrancesco D (1995). The pacemaker current (I_f) plays an important role in regulating SA node pacemaker activity. *Cardiovasc Res*, *30*: 307-308.
256. DiFrancesco D (1996). The hyperpolarization-activated (i_f) current: Autonomic regulation and the control of pacing. In: *Molecular physiology and pharmacology of cardiac ion channels and transporters* (ed. SE M Morad, W Trautwein, Y Kurachi), pp 31-37. Kluwer Academic Publishers, Dordrecht.

257. DiFrancesco D, Ducouret P, Robinson RB (1989). Muscarinic modulation of cardiac rate at low acetylcholine concentrations. *Science, 243*: 669-671.

258. DiFrancesco D, Ferroni A, Mazzanti M, Tromba C (1986). Properties of the hyperpolarizing-activated current (i_f) in cells isolated from the rabbit sino-atrial node. *J Physiol (Lond), 377*: 61-88.

259. DiFrancesco D, Moroni A, Baruscotti M, Accili EA (2001). Cardiac pacemaker currents. In: *Heart Physiology and Pathophysiology* (eds. N Sperelakis, Y Kurachi, A Terzic, MV Cohen), pp 357-372. Academic Press, San Diego.

260. DiFrancesco D, Noble D (1985). A model of cardiac electrical activity incorporating ionic pumps and concentration changes. *Philos Trans R Soc Lond B Biol Sci, 307*: 353-398.

261. DiFrancesco D, Tortora P (1991). Direct activation of cardiac pacemaker channels by intracellular cyclic AMP. *Nature, 351*: 145-147.

262. DiFrancesco D, Tromba C (1987). Acetylcholine inhibits activation of the cardiac hyperpolarizing-activated current, i_f. *Pflügers Archiv, 410*: 139-142.

263. Dillon SM, Allessie MA, Ursell PC, Wit AL (1988). Influences of anisotropic tissue structure on reentrant circuits in the epicardial border zone of subacute canine infarcts. *Circ Res, 63*: 182-206.

264. DiMarco JP, Sellers TD, Berne RM, West GA, Belardinelli L (1983). Adenosine: electrophysiologic effects and therapeutic use for terminating paroxysmal supraventricular tachycardia. *Circulation, 68*: 1254-1263.

265. Dipla K, Mattiello JA, Margulies KB, Jeevanandam V, Houser SR (1999). The sarcoplasmic reticulum and the Na^+/Ca^{2+} exchanger both contribute to the Ca^{2+} transient of failing human ventricular myocytes. *Circ Res, 84*: 435-444.

266. Doble BW, Ping P, Kardami E (2000). The {epsilon} subtype of protein kinase C Is required for cardiomyocyte connexin-43 phosphorylation. *Circ Res, 86*: 293-301.

267. Dobrev D, Wettwer E, Himmel HM, Kortner A, Kuhlisch E, Schuler S, Siffert W, Ravens U (2000). G-Protein beta(3)-subunit 825T allele is associated with enhanced human atrial inward rectifier potassium currents. *Circulation, 102*: 692-697.

268. Dodge SM, Beardslee MA, Darrow BJ, Green KG, Beyer EC, Saffitz JE (1998). Effects of angiotensin II on expression of the gap junction channel protein connexin43 in neonatal rat ventricular myocytes. *J Am Coll Cardiol, 32*: 800-807.

269. Doering AE, Lederer WJ (1993). The mechanism by which cytoplasmic protons inhibit the sodium-calcium exchanger in guinea-pig heart cells. *J Physiol (Lond), 466*: 481-499.

270. Doerr T, Denger R, Trautwein W (1989). Calcium currents in single SA nodal cells of the rabbit heart studied with action potential clamp. *Pflügers Archiv, 413*: 599-603.

271. Dominguez G, Fozzard HA (1970). Influence of extracellular K^+ concentration on cable properties and excitability of sheep cardiac Purkinje fibers. *Circ Res, 26*: 565-574.

272. Donoso P, Mill JG, O'Neill SC, Eisner DA (1992). Fluorescence measurements of cytoplasmic and mitochondrial sodium concentration in rat ventricular myocytes. *J Physiol (Lond), 448*: 493-509.

273. Downar E, Janse MJ, Durrer D (1977). The effect of acute coronary artery occlusion on subepicardial transmembrane potentials in the intact porcine heart. *Circulation, 56*: 217-224.

274. Downar E, Janse MJ, Durrer D (1977). The effect of "ischemic" blood on transmembrane potentials of normal porcine ventricular myocardium. *Circulation, 55*: 455-462.

275. Downey JM, Cohen MV (2000). Do mitochondrial K(ATP) channels serve as triggers rather than end-effectors of ischemic preconditioning's protection? *Basic Res Cardiol*, *95*: 272-274.

276. Doyle DA, Morais Cabral J, Pfuetzner RA, Kuo A, Gulbis JM, Cohen SL, Chait BT, MacKinnon R (1998). The structure of the potassium channel: molecular basis of K^+ conduction and selectivity. *Science*, *280*: 69-77.

277. Drici MD, Arrighi I, Chouabe C, Mann JR, Lazdunski M, Romey G, Barhanin J (1998). Involvement of IsK-associated K^+ channel in heart rate control of repolarization in a murine engineered model of Jervell and Lange- Nielsen syndrome. *Circ Res*, *83*: 95-102.

278. Droogmans G, Nilius B (1989). Kinetic properties of the cardiac T-type calcium channel in the guinea-pig. *J Physiol (Lond)*, *419*: 627-650.

279. Drouin E, Charpentier F, Gauthier C (1996). alpha1-adrenergic stimulation induces early afterdepolarizations in ferret Purkinje fibers. *J Cardiovasc Pharmacol*, *27*: 320-326.

280. Drouin E, Charpentier F, Gauthier C, Laurent K, Le Marec H (1995). Electrophysiologic characteristics of cells spanning the left ventricular wall of human heart: evidence for presence of M cells. *J Am Coll Cardiol*, *26*: 185-192.

281. Du XJ, Cox HS, Dart AM, Esler MD (1998). Depression of efferent parasympathetic control of heart rate in rats with myocardial infarction: effect of losartan. *J Cardiovasc Pharmacol*, *31*: 937-944.

282. Du XY, Sorota S (1997). Cardiac swelling-induced chloride current depolarizes canine atrial myocytes. *Am J Physiol*, *272*: H1904-1916.

283. Duan D, Winter C, Cowley S, Hume JR, Horowitz B (1997). Molecular identification of a volume-regulated chloride channel. *Nature*, *390*: 417-421.

284. Duan D, Ye L, Britton F, Horowitz B, Hume JR (2000). A novel anionic inward rectifier in native cardiac myocytes. *Circ Res*, *86*: E63-71.

285. Duan D, Zhong J, Hermoso M, Satterwhite CM, Rossow CF, Hatton WJ, Yamboliev I, Horowitz B, Hume JR (2001). Functional inhibition of native volume-sensitive outwardly rectifying anion channels in muscle cells and Xenopus oocytes by anti-ClC-3 antibody. *J Physiol (Lond)*, *531*: 437-444.

286. Dubey RK, Gillespie DG, Jackson EK, Keller PJ (1998). 17Beta-estradiol, its metabolites, and progesterone inhibit cardiac fibroblast growth. *Hypertension*, *31*: 522-528.

287. Duchen MR (2000). Mitochondria and calcium: from cell signalling to cell death. *J Physiol (Lond)*, *529 Pt 1*: 57-68.

288. Duchen MR, McGuinness O, Brown LA, Crompton M (1993). On the involvement of a cyclosporin A sensitive mitochondrial pore in myocardial reperfusion injury. *Cardiovasc Res*, *27*: 1790-1794.

289. Duff HJ, Feng ZP, Wang L, Sheldon RS (1997). Regulation of expression of the [3H]-dofetilide binding site associated with the delayed rectifier K^+ channel by dexamethasone in neonatal mouse ventricle. *J Mol Cell Cardiol*, *29*: 1959-1965.

290. Duggal P, Vesely MR, Wattanasirichaigoon D, Villafane J, Kaushik V, Beggs AH (1998). Mutation of the gene for IsK associated with both Jervell and Lange- Nielsen and Romano-Ward forms of Long-QT syndrome. *Circulation*, *97*: 142-146.

291. Dumaine R, Towbin JA, Brugada P, Vatta M, Nesterenko DV, Nesterenko VV, Brugada J, Brugada R, Antzelevitch C (1999). Ionic mechanisms responsible for the electrocardiographic phenotype of the Brugada syndrome are temperature dependent. *Circ Res*, *85*: 803-809.

292. Dupont E, Matsushita T, Kaba RA, Vozzi C, Coppen SR, Khan N, Kaprielian R, Yacoub MH, Severs NJ (2001). Altered connexin expression in human congestive heart failure. *J Mol Cell Cardiol, 33*: 359-371.

293. Duprat F, Lesage F, Fink M, Reyes R, Heurteaux C, Lazdunski M (1997). TASK, a human background K$^+$ channel to sense external pH variations near physiological pH. *Embo J, 16*: 5464-5471.

294. Durrer D, Van Dam RT, Freud GE, Janse MJ, Meijler FL, Arzbaecher RC (1970). Total excitation of the isolated human heart. *Circulation, 41*: 899-912.

295. Duru F, Barton M, Luscher TF, Candinas R (2001). Endothelin and cardiac arrhythmias: do endothelin antagonists have a therapeutic potential as antiarrhythmic drugs? *Cardiovasc Res, 49*: 272-280.

296. Earm YE, Noble D (1990). A model of the single atrial cell: relation between calcium current and calcium release. *Proc R Soc Lond B Biol Sci, 240*: 83-96.

297. Earm YE, Shimoni Y, Spindler AJ (1983). A pace-maker-like current in the sheep atrium and its modulation by catecholamines. *J Physiol (Lond), 342*: 569-590.

298. Echevarria M, Ilundain AA (1998). Aquaporins. *J Physiol Biochem, 54*: 107-118.

299. Egan TM, Noble D, Noble SJ, Powell T, Spindler AJ, Twist VW (1989). Sodium-calcium exchange during the action potential in guinea-pig ventricular cells. *J Physiol (Lond), 411*: 639-661.

300. Egger M, Niggli E (1999). Regulatory function of Na-Ca exchange in the heart: milestones and outlook. *J Membr Biol, 168*: 107-130.

301. Ehara T, Iyadomi I, Hirahara K (1994). Regulation of cyclic AMP-dependent Cl⁻ channel in heart. *Jpn J Physiol, 44*: S173-176.

302. Ehara T, Noma A, Ono K (1988). Calcium-activated non-selective cation channel in ventricular cells isolated from adult guinea-pig hearts. *J Physiol (Lond), 403*: 117-133.

303. Einthoven W, Fahr G, de Waart A (1913). Uber die Richtung und die manifeste Grosse der Potential-Schwankungen im menschlichen Herzen und uber die Einfluss der Herzlage auf die Form des Elektrokardiogramms. *Pflügers Archiv, 150*: 275.

304. Eisner DA, Choi HS, Diaz ME, O'Neill SC, Trafford AW (2000). Integrative analysis of calcium cycling in cardiac muscle. *Circ Res, 87*: 1087-1094.

305. Elenes S, Rubart M, Moreno AP (1999). Junctional communication between isolated pairs of canine atrial cells is mediated by homogeneous and heterogeneous gap junction channels. *J Cardiovasc Electrophysiol, 10*: 990-1004.

306. Elharrar V, Foster PR, Jirak TL, Gaum WE, Zipes DP (1977). Alterations in canine myocardial excitability during ischemia. *Circ Res, 40*: 98-105.

307. Emanueli C, Maestri R, Corradi D, Marchione R, Minasi A, Tozzi MG, Salis MB, Straino S, Capogrossi MC, Olivetti G, Madeddu P (1999). Dilated and failing cardiomyopathy in bradykinin B(2) receptor knockout mice. *Circulation, 100*: 2359-2365.

308. Emdad L, Uzzaman M, Takagishi Y, Honjo H, Uchida T, Severs NJ, Kodama I, Murata Y (2001). Gap Junction Remodeling in Hypertrophied Left Ventricles of Aortic-banded Rats: Prevention by Angiotensin II Type 1 Receptor Blockade. *J Mol Cell Cardiol, 33*: 219-231.

309. Ertel EA, Campbell KP, Harpold MM, Hofmann F, Mori Y, Perez-Reyes E, Schwartz A, Snutch TP, Tanabe T, Birnbaumer L, Tsien RW, Catterall WA (2000). Nomenclature of voltage-gated calcium channels. *Neuron, 25*: 533-535.

310. Ertel SI, Ertel EA, Clozel JP (1997). T-type Ca^{2+} channels and pharmacological blockade: potential pathophysiological relevance. *Cardiovasc Drugs Ther, 11*: 723-739.

311. Ertl R, Jahnel U, Nawrath H, Carmeliet E, Vereecke J (1991). Differential electrophysiologic and inotropic effects of phenylephrine in atrial and ventricular heart muscle preparations from rats. *Naunyn Schmiedebergs Arch Pharmacol, 344*: 574-581.

312. Escande D, Coulombe A, Faivre JF, Coraboeuf E (1986). Characteristics of the time-dependent slow inward current in adult human atrial single myocytes. *J Mol Cell Cardiol, 18*: 547-551.

313. Escande D, Coulombe A, Faivre JF, Deroubaix E, Coraboeuf E (1987). Two types of transient outward currents in adult human atrial cells. *Am J Physiol, 252*: H142-148.

314. Escande D, Loisance D, Planche C, Coraboeuf E (1985). Age-related changes of action potential plateau shape in isolated human atrial fibers. *Am J Physiol, 249*: H843-850.

315. Evans AM, Cannell MB (1997). The role of L-type Ca^{2+} current and Na^+ current-stimulated Na/Ca exchange in triggering SR calcium release in guinea-pig cardiac ventricular myocytes. *Cardiovasc Res, 35*: 294-302.

316. Everett TH, Li H, Mangrum JM, McRury ID, Mitchell MA, Redick JA, Haines DE (2000). Electrical, morphological, and ultrastructural remodeling and reverse remodeling in a canine model of chronic atrial fibrillation. *Circulation, 102*: 1454-1460.

317. Fabiato A (1985). Time and calcium dependence of activation and inactivation of calcium-induced release of calcium from the sarcoplasmic reticulum of a skinned canine cardiac Purkinje cell. *J Gen Physiol, 85*: 247-289.

318. Fareh S, Benardeau A, Nattel S (2001). Differential efficacy of L- and T-type calcium channel blockers in preventing tachycardia-induced atrial remodeling in dogs. *Cardiovasc Res, 49*: 762-770.

319. Fares N, Bois P, Lenfant J, Potreau D (1998). Characterization of a hyperpolarization-activated current in dedifferentiated adult rat ventricular cells in primary culture. *J Physiol (Lond), 506*: 73-82.

320. Fast VG, Kléber AG (1994). Anisotropic conduction in monolayers of neonatal rat heart cells cultured on collagen substrate. *Circ Res, 75*: 591-595.

321. Fearon IM, Palmer AC, Balmforth AJ, Ball SG, Varadi G, Peers C (1999). Modulation of recombinant human cardiac L-type Ca^{2+} channel alpha1C subunits by redox agents and hypoxia. *J Physiol (Lond), 514*: 629-637.

322. Fearon IM, Varadi G, Koch S, Isaacsohn I, Ball SG, Peers C (2000). Splice variants reveal the region involved in oxygen sensing by recombinant human L-Type Ca^{2+} channels. *Circ Res, 87*: 537-539.

323. Fedida D, Braun AP, Giles WR (1993). Alpha 1-adrenoceptors in myocardium: functional aspects and transmembrane signaling mechanisms. *Physiol Rev, 73*: 469-487.

324. Fedida D, Giles WR (1991). Regional variations in action potentials and transient outward current in myocytes isolated from rabbit left ventricle. *J Physiol (Lond), 442*: 191-209.

325. Fedida D, Wible B, Wang Z, Fermini B, Faust F, Nattel S, Brown AM (1993). Identity of a novel delayed rectifier current from human heart with a cloned K^+ channel current. *Circ Res, 73*: 210-216.

326. Feng J, Yue L, Wang Z, Nattel S (1998). Ionic mechanisms of regional action potential heterogeneity in the canine right atrium. *Circ Res, 83*: 541-551.

327. Fermini B, Wang Z, Duan D, Nattel S (1992). Differences in rate dependence of transient outward current in rabbit and human atrium. *Am J Physiol, 263*: H1747-1754.

328. Ferrari R (1997). Angiotensin converting enzyme inhibitor-calcium antagonist combination: an alliance for cardioprotection? *J Hypertens Suppl, 15*: S109-117.

329. Ferrari R, Bachetti T, Agnoletti L, Comini L, Curello S (1998). Endothelial function and dysfunction in heart failure. *Eur Heart J, 19 Suppl G*: G41-47.

330. Ferrier GR, Carmeliet E (1990). Effects of alpha-adrenergic agents on transient inward current in rabbit Purkinje fibers. *J Mol Cell Cardiol, 22*: 191-200.

331. Ferrier GR, Howlett SE (2001). Cardiac excitation-contraction coupling: role of membrane potential in regulation of contraction. *Am J Physiol, 280*: H1928-1944.

332. Ferrier GR, Saunders JH, Mendez C (1973). A cellular mechanism for the generation of ventricular arrhythmias by acetylstrophanthidin. *Circ Res, 32*: 600-609.

333. Fill M, Zahradnikova A, Villalba-Galea CA, Zahradnik I, Escobar AL, Györke S (2000). Ryanodine receptor adaptation. *J Gen Physiol, 116*: 873-882.

334. Findlay I (1987). ATP-sensitive K^+ channels in rat ventricular myocytes are blocked and inactivated by internal divalent cations. *Pflügers Archiv, 410*: 313-320.

335. Findlay I, Faivre JF (1991). ATP-sensitive K channels in heart muscle. Spare channels. *FEBS Lett, 279*: 95-97.

336. Fink M, Lesage F, Duprat F, Heurteaux C, Reyes R, Fosset M, Lazdunski M (1998). A neuronal two P domain K^+ channel stimulated by arachidonic acid and polyunsaturated fatty acids. *EMBO J, 17*: 3297-3308.

337. Fiolet JW, Baartscheer A, Schumacher CA, Coronel R, ter Welle HF (1984). The change of the free energy of ATP hydrolysis during global ischemia and anoxia in the rat heart. Its possible role in the regulation of transsarcolemmal sodium and potassium gradients. *J Mol Cell Cardiol, 16*: 1023-1036.

338. Firek L, Giles WR (1995). Outward currents underlying repolarization in human atrial myocytes. *Cardiovasc Res, 30*: 31-38.

339. Fozzard HA (1979). Conduction of the action potential. In: *Handbook of Physiology Section 2: The cardiovascular system Vol I The heart* (eds. RM Berne, N Sperelakis, SR Geiger), pp 334-356. American Physiological Society, Bethesda.

340. Fozzard HA, Hanck DA (1996). Structure and function of voltage-dependent sodium channels: comparison of brain II and cardiac isoforms. *Physiol Rev, 76*: 887-926.

341. Fozzard HA, Lipkind G (1995). Ion channels and pumps in cardiac function. *Adv Exp Med Biol, 382*: 3-10.

342. Fozzard HA, Schoenberg M (1972). Strength-duration curves in cardiac Purkinje fibres: effects of liminal length and charge distribution. *J Physiol (Lond), 226*: 593-618.

343. Frace AM, Maruoka F, Noma A (1992). External K^+ increases Na^+ conductance of the hyperpolarization-activated current in rabbit cardiac pacemaker cells. *Pflügers Archiv, 421*: 97-99.

344. Frankenhaeuser B, Hodgkin AL (1957). The action of calcium on the the electrical properties of squid axons. *J Physiol (Lond), 137*: 218-244.

345. Franz MR (1999). Current status of monophasic action potential recording: theories, measurements and interpretations. *Cardiovasc Res, 41*: 25-40.

346. Franz MR, Swerdlow CD, Liem LB, Schaefer J (1988). Cycle length dependence of human action potential duration in vivo. Effects of single extrastimuli, sudden sustained rate acceleration and deceleration, and different steady-state frequencies. *J Clin Invest, 82*: 972-979.

347. Franz MR, Zabel M (2000). Electrophysiological basis of QT dispersion measurements. *Prog Cardiovasc Dis, 42*: 311-324.

348. Frazier DW, Krassowska W, Chen PS, Wolf PD, Danieley ND, Smith WM, Idcker RE (1988). Transmural activations and stimulus potentials in three-dimensional anisotropic canine myocardium. *Circ Res, 63*: 135-146.

349. Freer RJ, Pappano AJ, Peach MJ, Bing KT, McLean MJ, Vogel S, Sperelakis N (1976). Mechanism for the postive inotropic effect of angiotensin II on isolated cardiac muscle. *Circ Res, 39*: 178-183.

350. Friel DD, Bean BP (1988). Two ATP-activated conductances in bullfrog atrial cells. *J Gen Physiol, 91*: 1-27.

351. Fujioka Y, Komeda M, Matsuoka S (2000). Stoichiometry of Na^+-Ca^{2+} exchange in inside-out patches excised from guinea-pig ventricular myocytes. *J Physiol (Lond), 523 Pt 2*: 339-351.

352. Fujita A, Kurachi Y (2000). Molecular aspects of ATP-sensitive K^+ channels in the cardiovascular system and K^+ channel openers. *Pharmacol Ther, 85*: 39-53.

353. Furukawa T, Kimura S, Furukawa N, Bassett AL, Myerburg RJ (1992). Potassium rectifier currents differ in myocytes of endocardial and epicardial origin. *Circ Res, 70*: 91-103.

354. Furukawa T, Myerburg RJ, Furukawa N, Bassett AL, Kimura S (1990). Differences in transient outward currents of feline endocardial and epicardial myocytes. *Circ Res, 67*: 1287-1291.

355. Gadsby DC, Nagel G, Hwang TC (1995). The CFTR chloride channel of mammalian heart. *Annu Rev Physiol, 57*: 387-416.

356. Gadsby DC, Nairn AC (1999). Control of CFTR channel gating by phosphorylation and nucleotide hydrolysis. *Physiol Rev, 79*: 77-1372.

357. Gallo MP, Malan D, Bedendi I, Biasin C, Alloatti G, Levi RC (2001). Regulation of cardiac calcium current by NO and cGMP-modulating agents. *Pflügers Archiv, 441*: 621-628.

358. Gambassi G, Hansford RG, Sollott SJ, Hogue BA, Lakatta EG, Capogrossi MC (1993). Effects of acidosis on resting cytosolic and mitochondrial Ca^{2+} in mammalian myocardium. *J Gen Physiol, 102*: 575-597.

359. Gao J, Cohen IS, Mathias RT, Baldo GJ (1994). Regulation of the beta-stimulation of the Na^+-K^+ pump current in guinea-pig ventricular myocytes by a cAMP-dependent PKA pathway. *J Physiol (Lond), 477*: 373-380.

360. Gao J, Mathias RT, Cohen IS, Shi J, Baldo GJ (1996). The effects of ß-stimulation on the Na^+-K^+ pump current-voltage relationship in guinea-pig ventricular myocytes. *J Physiol (Lond), 494.3*: 697-708.

361. Gao J, Mathias RT, Cohen IS, Wang Y, Sun X, Baldo GJ (1999). Activation of PKC increases Na^+-K^+ pump current in ventricular myocytes from guinea pig heart. *Pflügers Archiv, 437*: 643-651.

362. Garlid KD (1978). Unmasking the mitochondrial K/H exchanger: swelling-induced K^+-loss. *Biochem Biophys Res Commun, 83*: 1450-1455.

363. Garlid KD (2000). Opening mitochondrial K(ATP) in the heart--what happens, and what does not happen. *Basic Res Cardiol, 95*: 275-279.

364. Garlid KD, Beavis AD (1986). Evidence for the existence of an inner membrane anion channel in mitochondria. *Biochim Biophys Acta, 853*: 187-204.

365. Gaspo R, Bosch RF, Talajic M, Nattel S (1997). Functional mechanisms underlying tachycardia-induced sustained atrial fibrillation in a chronic dog model. *Circulation, 96*: 4027-4035.

366. Gauss R, Seifert R, Kaupp UB (1998). Molecular identification of a hyperpolarization-activated channel in sea urchin sperm. *Nature, 393*: 583-587.

367. Geller L, Merkely B, Lang V, Szabo T, Fazekas L, Kekesi V, Kiss O, Horkay F, Schaldach M, Toth M, Juhasz-Nagy A (1998). Increased monophasic action potential

dispersion in endothelin-1-induced ventricular arrhythmias. *J Cardiovasc Pharmacol*, *31*: S434-436.

368. Gidh-Jain M, Huang B, Jain P, Gick G, El-Sherif N (1998). Alterations in cardiac gene expression during ventricular remodeling following experimental myocardial infarction. *J Mol Cell Cardiol*, *30*: 627-637.

369. Gilbert JC, Shirayama T, Pappano AJ (1991). Inositol trisphosphate promotes Na-Ca exchange current by releasing calcium from sarcoplasmic reticulum in cardiac myocytes. *Circ Res*, *69*: 1632-1639.

370. Gilmour RF, Jr., Zipes DP (1980). Different electrophysiological responses of canine endocardium and epicardium to combined hyperkalemia, hypoxia, and acidosis. *Circ Res*, *46*: 814-825.

371. Gintant GA (1996). Two components of delayed rectifier current in canine atrium and ventricle. Does IKs play a role in the reverse rate dependence of class III agents? *Circ Res*, *78*: 26-37.

372. Gintant GA, Datyner NB, Cohen IS (1984). Slow inactivation of a tetrodotoxin-sensitive current in canine cardiac Purkinje fibers. *Biophys J*, *45*: 509-512.

373. Glitsch HG, Tappe A (1995). Change of Na^+ pump current reversal potential in sheep cardiac Purkinje cells with varying free energy of ATP hydrolysis. *J Physiol (Lond)*, *484*: 605-616.

374. Goethals M, Raes A, van Bogaert PP (1993). Use-dependent block of the pacemaker current I_f in rabbit sinoatrial node cells by zatebradine (UL-FS 49). On the mode of action of sinus node inhibitors. *Circulation*, *88*: 2389-2401.

375. Goette A, Arndt M, Rocken C, Spiess A, Staack T, Geller JC, Huth C, Ansorge S, Klein HU, Lendeckel U (2000). Regulation of angiotensin II receptor subtypes during atrial fibrillation in humans. *Circulation*, *101*: 2678-2681.

376. Gögelein H, Hartung J, Englert HC (1999). Molecular basis, pharmacology and physiological role of cardiac K(ATP) channels. *Cell Physiol Biochem*, *9*: 227-241.

377. Goldin AL (2001). Resurgence of sodium channel research. *Annu Rev Physiol*, *63*: 871-894.

378. Goldin AL, Barchi RL, Caldwell JH, Hofmann F, Howe JR, Hunter JC, Kallen RG, Mandel G, Meisler MH, Netter YB, Noda M, Tamkun MM, Waxman SG, Wood JN, Catterall WA (2002). Nomenclature of voltage-gated sodium channels. *Neuron*, *28*: 365-368.

379. Goldstein JA, Butterfield MC, Ohnishi Y, Shelton TJ, Corr PB (1994). Arrhythmogenic influence of intracoronary thrombosis during acute myocardial ischemia. *Circulation*, *90*: 139-147.

380. Goldstein SA, Bockenhauer D, O'Kelly I, Zilberberg N (2001). Potassium leak channels and the KCNK family of two-P-domain subunits. *Nat Rev Neurosci*, *2*: 175-184.

381. Gomez AM, Benitah JP, Henzel D, Vinet A, Lorente P, Delgado C (1997). Modulation of electrical heterogeneity by compensated hypertrophy in rat left ventricle. *Am J Physiol*, *272*: H1078-1086.

382. Gomez AM, Valdivia HH, Cheng H, Lederer MR, Santana LF, Cannell MB, McCune SA, Altschuld RA, Lederer WJ (1997). Defective excitation-contraction coupling in experimental cardiac hypertrophy and heart failure. *Science*, *276*: 800-806.

383. Gondo N, Kumagai K, Nakashima H, Saku K (2001). Angiotensin II provokes cesium-induced ventricular tachyarrhythmias. *Cardiovasc Res*, *49*: 381-390.

384. Gorza L, Schiaffino S, Volpe P (1993). Inositol 1,4,5-trisphosphate receptor in heart: evidence for its concentration in Purkinje myocytes of the conduction system. *J Cell Biol, 121*: 345-353.

385. Gouin L, Cardinal R, Adam A, Drapeau G, Nadeau R (1996). Kinin-induced prolongation of action-potential duration in right ventricular muscle from rat: involvement of B1 and B2 receptors. *J Cardiovasc Pharmacol, 28*: 337-343.

386. Grammer JB, Bosch RF, Kuhlkamp V, Seipel L (2000). Molecular remodeling of Kv4.3 potassium channels in human atrial fibrillation. *J Cardiovasc Electrophysiol, 11*: 626-633.

387. Green LS, Fuller MP, Lux RL (1997). Three-dimensional distribution of ST-T wave alternans during acute ischemia. *J Cardiovasc Electrophysiol, 8*: 1413-1419.

388. Greenstein JL, Wu R, Po S, Tomaselli GF, Winslow RL (2000). Role of the calcium-independent transient outward current Ito1 in shaping action potential morphology and duration. *Circ Res, 87*: 1026-1033.

389. Gribble FM, Ashfield R, Ammala C, Ashcroft FM (1997). Properties of cloned ATP-sensitive K^+ currents expressed in Xenopus oocytes. *J Physiol (Lond), 498*: 87-98.

390. Griese M, Perlitz V, Jungling E, Kammermeier H (1988). Myocardial performance and free energy of ATP-hydrolysis in isolated rat hearts during graded hypoxia, reoxygenation and high K_e^+-perfusion. *J Mol Cell Cardiol, 20*: 1189-1201.

391. Griffiths EJ (1999). Reversal of mitochondrial Na/Ca exchange during metabolic inhibition in rat cardiomyocytes. *FEBS Lett, 453*: 400-404.

392. Griffiths EJ (2000). Mitochondria--potential role in cell life and death. *Cardiovasc Res, 46*: 24-27.

393. Griffiths EJ, Halestrap AP (1995). Mitochondrial non-specific pores remain closed during cardiac ischaemia, but open upon reperfusion. *Biochem J, 307*: 93-98.

394. Gros DB, Jongsma HJ (1996). Connexins in mammalian heart function. *Bioessays, 18*: 719-730.

395. Gross GJ, Burke RP, Castle NA (1995). Characterisation of transient outward current in young human atrial myocytes. *Cardiovasc Res, 29*: 112-117.

396. Gross GJ, Fryer RM (1999). Sarcolemmal versus mitochondrial ATP-sensitive K^+ channels and myocardial preconditioning. *Circ Res, 84*: 973-979.

397. Grover GJ, D'Alonzo AJ, Parham CS, Darbenzio RB (1995). Cardioprotection with the KATP opener cromakalim is not correlated with ischemic myocardial action potential duration. *J Cardiovasc Pharmacol, 26*: 145-152.

398. Gruver C, Pappano AJ (1993). Effect of membrane incorporation of 1-palmitoylcarnitine on surface charge of human erythrocytes. *J Mol Cell Cardiol, 25*: 1275-1284.

399. Gu H, Ek-Vitorin JF, Taffet SM, Delmar M (2000). Coexpression of Connexins 40 and 43 Enhances the pH Sensitivity of Gap Junctions : A Model for Synergistic Interactions Among Connexins. *Circ Res, 86*: 98e-103e.

400. Guatimosim S, Sobie EA, dos Santos Cruz J, Martin LA, Lederer WJ (2001). Molecular identification of a TTX-sensitive Ca^{2+} current. *Am J Physiol, 280*: C1327-1339.

401. Guerrero PA, Schuessler RB, Davis LM, Beyer EC, Johnson CM, Yamada KA, Saffitz JE (1997). Slow ventricular conduction in mice heterozygous for a connexin43 null mutation. *J Clin Invest, 99*: 1991-1998.

402. Guia A, Stern MD, Lakatta EG, Josephson IR (2001). Ion Concentration-Dependence of Rat Cardiac Unitary L-Type Calcium Channel Conductance. *Biophys J, 80*: 2742-2714.

403. Guo J, Ono K, Noma A (1995). A sustained inward current activated at the diastolic potential range in rabbit sino-atrial node cells. *J Physiol (Lond)*, *483*: 1-13.
404. Guo W, Kamiya K, Toyama J (1997). Evidences of antagonism between amiodarone and triiodothyronine on the K^+ channel activities of cultured rat cardiomyocytes. *J Mol Cell Cardiol*, *29*: 617-627.
405. Guo W, Kamiya K, Toyama J (1997). Roles of the voltage-gated K^+ channel subunits, Kv 1.5 and Kv 1.4, in the developmental changes of K^+ currents in cultured neonatal rat ventricular cells. *Pflügers Archiv*, *434*: 206-208.
406. Gussak I, Antzelevitch C, Bjerregaard P, Towbin JA, Chaitman BR (1999). The Brugada syndrome: clinical, electrophysiologic and genetic aspects. *J Am Coll Cardiol*, *33*: 5-15.
407. Györke S, Fill M (1993). Ryanodine receptor adaptation: control mechanism of Ca^{2+}-induced Ca^{2+} release in heart. *Science*, *260*: 807-809.
408. Hagiwara N, Irisawa H, Kameyama M (1988). Contribution of two types of calcium currents to the pacemaker potentials of rabbit sino-atrial node cells. *J Physiol (Lond)*, *395*: 233-253.
409. Hagiwara N, Irisawa H, Kasanuki H, Hosoda S (1992). Background current in sino-atrial node cells of the rabbit heart. *J Physiol (Lond)*, *448*: 53-72.
410. Haigney MC, Lakatta EG, Stern MD, Silverman HS (1994). Sodium channel blockade reduces hypoxic sodium loading and sodium-dependent calcium loading. *Circulation*, *90*: 391-399.
411. Haissaguerre M, Jais P, Shah DC, Takahashi A, Hocini M, Quiniou G, Garrigue S, Le Mouroux A, Le Metayer P, Clementy J (1998). Spontaneous initiation of atrial fibrillation by ectopic beats originating in the pulmonary veins. *N Engl J Med*, *339*: 659-666.
412. Halestrap AP (1989). The regulation of the matrix volume of mammalian mitochondria in vivo and in vitro and its role in the control of mitochondrial metabolism. *Biochim Biophys Acta*, *973*: 355-382.
413. Halimi F, Piot O, Guize L, Le Heuzey JY (1997). Electrophysiological effects of vasoactive intestinal peptide in rabbit atrium: a modulation of acetylcholine activity. *J Mol Cell Cardiol*, *29*: 37-44.
414. Hamill OP, Marty A, Neher E, Sakmann B, Sigworth FJ (1981). Improved patch-clamp techniques for high-resolution current. *Pflügers Archiv*, *391*: 85-100.
415. Han J, Leem C, So I, Kim E, Hong S, Ho W, Sung H, Earm YE (1994). Effects of thyroid hormone on the calcium current and isoprenaline-induced background current in rabbit ventricular myocytes. *J Mol Cell Cardiol*, *26*: 925-935.
416. Han W, Wang Z, Nattel S (2000). A comparison of transient outward currents in canine cardiac Purkinje cells and ventricular myocytes. *Am J Physiol*, *279*: H466-474.
417. Han X, Ferrier GR (1992). Ionic mechanisms of transient inward current in the absence of Na^+-Ca^{2+} exchange in rabbit cardiac Purkinje fibres. *J Physiol (Lond)*, *456*: 19-38.
418. Hanck DA, Makielski JC, Sheets MF (2000). Lidocaine alters activation gating of cardiac Na channels. *Pflügers Archiv*, *439*: 814-821.
419. Hancox JC, Levi AJ (1994). L-type calcium current in rod- and spindle-shaped myocytes isolated from rabbit atrioventricular node. *Am J Physiol*, *267*: H1670-1680.
420. Hancox JC, Mitcheson JS (1997). Ion channel and exchange currents in single myocytes isolated from the rabbit atrioventricular node. *Can J Cardiol*, *13*: 1175-1182.
421. Hansen CA, Joseph SK, Robishaw JD (1994). Ins 1,4,5-P3 and Ca^{2+} signaling in quiescent neonatal cardiac myocytes. *Biochim Biophys Acta*, *1224*: 517-526.

422. Hara M, Danilo P, Jr., Rosen MR (1998). Effects of gonadal steroids on ventricular repolarization and on the response to E4031. *J Pharmacol Exp Ther*, *285*: 1068-1072.

423. Hara M, Matsumori A, Ono K, Kido H, Hwang MW, Miyamoto T, Iwasaki A, Okada M, Nakatani K, Sasayama S (1999). Mast cells cause apoptosis of cardiomyocytes and proliferation of other intramyocardial cells in vitro. *Circulation*, *100*: 1443-1449.

424. Hara M, Shvilkin A, Rosen MR, Danilo P, Boyden PA (1999). Steady-state and nonsteady-state action potentials in fibrillating canine atrium: abnormal rate adaptation and its possible mechanisms. *Cardiovasc Res*, *42*: 455-469.

425. Harvey RD, Clark CD, Hume JR (1990). Chloride current in mammalian cardiac myocytes. Novel mechanism for autonomic regulation of action potential duration and resting membrane potential. *J Gen Physiol*, *95*: 1077-1102.

426. Harvey RD, Hume JR (2001). Chloride channels in heart. In: *Heart Physiology and Pathophysiology* (eds. N Sperelakis, Y Kurachi, A Terzic, MV Cohen), pp 373-388. Academic Press, San Diego.

427. Hasenfuss G (1998). Alterations of calcium-regulatory proteins in heart failure. *Cardiovasc Res*, *37*: 279-289.

428. Hasenfuss G, Meyer M, Schillinger W, Preuss M, Pieske B, Just H (1997). Calcium handling proteins in the failing human heart. *Basic Res Cardiol*, *1*: 87-93.

429. Hasenfuss G, Schillinger W, Lehnart SE, Preuss M, Pieske B, Maier LS, Prestle J, Minami K, Just H (1999). Relationship between Na^+-Ca^{2+}-exchanger protein levels and diastolic function of failing human myocardium. *Circulation*, *99*: 641-648.

430. Hatem SN, A.Bénardeau, Rücker-Martin C, Samuel J-L, Coraboeuf E, Mercadier J-J (1996). Differential regulation of voltage-activated potassium currents in cultured human atrial myocytes. *Am J Physiol*, *271*: H1609-H1619.

431. Hattori Y, Atsushi S, Hiroaki F, Toyama J (1997). Effects of cilazapril on ventricular arrhythmia in patients with congestive heart failure. *Clin Ther*, *19*: 481-486.

432. Hattori Y, Matsuda N, Kimura J, Ishitani T, Tamada A, Gando S, Kemmotsu O, Kanno M (2000). Diminished function and expression of the cardiac Na^+-Ca^{2+} exchanger in diabetic rats: implication in Ca^{2+} overload. *J Physiol (Lond)*, *527 Pt 1*: 85-94.

433. He DS, Burt JM (2000). Mechanism and selectivity of the effects of halothane on gap junction channel function. *Circ Res*, *86*: E104-109.

434. Heath BM, Terrar DA (2000). Protein kinase C enhances the rapidly activating delayed rectifier potassium current, IKr, through a reduction in C-type inactivation in guinea-pig ventricular myocytes. *J Physiol (Lond)*, *522 Pt 3*: 391-402.

435. Heathers GP, Evers AS, Corr PB (1989). Enhanced inositol trisphosphate response to alpha 1-adrenergic stimulation in cardiac myocytes exposed to hypoxia. *J Clin Invest*, *83*: 1409-1413.

436. Heidbüchel H, Vereecke J, Carmeliet E (1987). The electrophysiological effects of acetylcholine in single human atrial cells. *J Mol Cell Cardiol*, *19*: 1207-1219.

437. Heidbüchel H, Vereecke J, Carmeliet E (1989). Different K^+ channels in human atrial cells. *Pflügers Archiv*, *414*: S171-172.

438. Heidbüchel H, Vereecke J, Carmeliet E (1990). Three different potassium channels in human atrium. Contribution to the basal potassium conductance. *Circ Res*, *66*: 1277-1286.

439. Hellgren I, Mustafa A, Riazi M, Suliman I, Sylven C, Adem A (2000). Muscarinic M3 receptor subtype gene expression in the human heart. *Cell Mol Life Sci*, *57*: 175-180.

440. Hering S, Berjukow S, Sokolov S, Marksteiner R, Weiss RG, Kraus R, Timin EN (2000). Molecular determinants of inactivation in voltage-gated Ca^{2+} channels. *J Physiol (Lond)*, *528 Pt 2*: 237-249.

441. Herweg B, Chang F, Chandra P, Danilo P, Rosen MR (2001). Cardiac memory in canine atrium : Identification and Implications. *Circulation, 103*: 455-461.

442. Hess P, Lansman JB, Tsien RW (1984). Different modes of Ca channel gating behaviour favoured by dihydropyridine Ca agonists and antagonists. *Nature, 311*: 538-544.

443. Heubach JF, Kohler A, Wettwer E, Ravens U (2000). T-Type and tetrodotoxin-sensitive Ca^{2+} currents coexist in guinea pig ventricular myocytes and are both blocked by mibefradil. *Circ Res, 86*: 628-635.

444. Heusch G, Rose J, Ehring T (1997). Cardioprotection by ACE inhibitors in myocardial ischaemia/reperfusion. The importance of bradykinin. *Drugs, 54*: 31-41.

445. Hilgemann DW, Noble D (1987). Excitation-contraction coupling and extracellular calcium transients in rabbit atrium: reconstruction of basic cellular mechanisms. *Proc R Soc Lond B Biol Sci, 230*: 163-205.

446. Hill JA, Jr., Coronado R, Strauss HC (1988). Reconstitution and characterization of a calcium-activated channel from heart. *Circ Res, 62*: 411-415.

447. Hill MR, Wallick DW, Martin PJ, Levy MN (1995). Effects of repetitive vagal stimulation on heart rate and on cardiac vasoactive intestinal polypeptide efflux. *Am J Physiol, 268*: H1939-1946.

448. Hille B (1977). Local anesthetics: hydrophilic and hydrophobic pathways for the drug-receptor reaction. *J Gen Physiol, 69*: 497-515.

449. Hille B (1992). Ionic channels of excitable cells. Sinauer Associates Inc. Sunderland, Massachusetts.

450. Himmel HM, Wettwer E, Li Q, Ravens U (1999). Four different components contribute to outward current in rat ventricular myocytes. *Am J Physiol, 277*: H107-118.

451. Hirano Y, Fozzard HA, January CT (1989). Characteristics of L- and T-type Ca^{2+} currents in canine cardiac Purkinje cells. *Am J Physiol, 256*: H1478-1492.

452. Hirano Y, Moscucci A, January CT (1992). Direct measurement of L-type Ca^{2+} window current in heart cells. *Circ Res, 70*: 445-455.

453. Hiraoka M, Kawano S, Hirano Y, Furukawa T (1998). Role of cardiac chloride currents in changes in action potential characteristics and arrhythmias. *Cardiovasc Res, 40*: 23-33.

454. Ho W-K, Brown HF, Noble D (1994). High selectivity of the i_f channel to Na^+ and K^+ in rabbit isolated sinoatrial node cells. *Pflügers Archiv, 426*: 68-74.

455. Ho W-K, Earm YE, Lee SH, Brown HF, Noble D (1996). Voltage- and time-dependent block of delayed rectifier K^+ current in rabbit sino-atrial node cells by external Ca^{2+} and Mg^{2+}. *J Physiol (Lond), 494.3*: 727-742.

456. Ho W-K, Kim I, Lee CO, Earm YE (1998). Voltage-dependent blockade of HERG channels expressed in Xenopus oocytes by external Ca^{2+} and Mg^{2+}. *J Physiol (Lond), 507*: 631-638.

457. Hobai IA, O'Rourke B (2000). Enhanced Ca^{2+}-activated Na^+-Ca^{2+} exchange activity in canine pacing-induced heart failure. *Circ Res, 87*: 690-709.

458. Hobbs WJ, Fynn S, Todd DM, Wolfson P, Galloway M, Garratt CJ (2000). Reversal of atrial electrical remodeling after cardioversion of persistent atrial fibrillation in humans. *Circulation, 101*: 1145-1151.

459. Hockerman GH, Peterson BZ, Johnson BD, Catterall WA (1997). Molecular determinants of drug binding and action on L-type calcium channels. *Annu Rev Pharmacol Toxicol, 37*: 361-396.

460.   Hodgkin AL, Huxley AF (1952). Currents carried by sodium and potassium ions through the membrane of the giant axon of Loligo. *J Physiol (Lond)*, *116*: 449-472.

461.   Hodgkin AL, Huxley AF (1952). A quantitative description of membrane current and its application to conduction and excitation in nerve. *J Physiol (Lond)*, *117*: 500-544.

462.   Hodgkin AL, Rushton WAH (1946). The electrical constants of a crustacean nerve fibre. *Proc R Soc Lond B Biol Sci*, *133*: 444-479.

463.   Hofmann F, Lacinova L, Klugbauer N (1999). Voltage-dependent calcium channels: from structure to function. *Rev Physiol Biochem Pharmacol*, *139*: 33-87.

464.   Hojo Y, Ikeda U, Tsuruya Y, Ebata H, Murata M, Okada K, Saito T, Shimada K (1997). Thyroid hormone stimulates Na^+-Ca^{2+} exchanger expression in rat cardiac myocytes. *J Cardiovasc Pharmacol*, *29*: 75-80.

465.   Holmuhamedov EL, Jovanovic S, Dzeja PP, Jovanovic A, Terzic A (1998). Mitochondrial ATP-sensitive K+ channels modulate cardiac mitochondrial function. *Am J Physiol*, *275*: H1567-1576.

466.   Holtz J (1998). Role of ACE inhibition or AT1 blockade in the remodeling following myocardial infarction. *Basic Res Cardiol*, *93*: 92-100.

467.   Hondeghem LM (1991). Ideal antiarrhythmic agents: Chemical defribrillators. *J Cardiovasc Electrophysiol*, *2*: S169-S177.

468.   Hondeghem LM, Katzung BG (1977). Time- and voltage-dependent interactions of antiarrhythmic drugs with cardiac sodium channels. *Biochim Biophys Acta*, *472*: 373-398.

469.   Hondeghem LM, Snyders DJ (1990). Class III antiarrhythmic agents have a lot of potential but a long way to go. Reduced effectiveness and dangers of reverse use dependence. *Circulation*, *81*: 686-690.

470.   Hool LC (2001). Hypoxia alters the sensitivity of the L-Type Ca^{2+} channel to {alpha}-adrenergic receptor stimulation in the presence of {beta}-adrenergic receptor stimulation. *Circ Res*, *88*: 1036-1043.

471.   Hoppe UC, Beuckelmann DJ (1998). Modulation of the hyperpolarization-activated inward current (I_f) by antiarrhythmic agents in isolated human atrial myocytes. *Naunyn Schmiedebergs Arch Pharmacol*, *358*: 635-640.

472.   Horie M, Hayashi S, Kawai C (1990). Two types of delayed rectifying K^+ channels in atrial cells of guinea pig heart. *Jpn J Physiol*, *40*: 479-490.

473.   Horie M, Watanuki M, Tsuchiya K, Hayashi S, Obayashi K, Xie L-H, Yuzuki Y, Takahashi A, Sasayama S (1996). Autonomic regulation of cardiac ATP-sensitive K^+ channel activation. CRC Press, Tokyo.

474.   Hu K, Mochly-Rosen D, Boutjdir M (2000). Evidence for functional role of epsilon PKC isozyme in the regulation of cardiac Ca^{2+} channels. *Am J Physiol*, *279*: H2658-3088.

475.   Huang B, Qin D, Deng L, Boutjdir M, N E-S (2000). Reexpression of T-type Ca^{2+} channel gene and current in post-infarction remodeled rat left ventricle. *Cardiovasc Res*, *46*: 442-449.

476.   Huang CL, Feng S, Hilgemann DW (1998). Direct activation of inward rectifier potassium channels by PIP2 and its stabilization by Gbetagamma. *Nature*, *391*: 803-806.

477.   Huang JM, Xian H, Bacaner M (1992). Long-chain fatty acids activate calcium channels in ventricular myocytes. *Proc Natl Acad Sci USA*, *89*: 6452-6456.

478.   Hume JR, Duan D, Collier ML, Yamazaki J, Horowitz B (2000). Anion transport in heart. *Physiol Rev*, *80*: 31-81.

479. Hume JR, Uehara A (1985). Ionic basis of the different action potential configurations of single guinea-pig atrial and ventricular myocytes. *J Physiol (Lond)*, *368*: 525-544.

480. Hund TJ, Rudy Y (2000). Determinants of excitability in cardiac myocytes: mechanistic investigation of memory effect. *Biophys J*, *79*: 3095-3104.

481. Hunter PJ, McNaughton PA, Noble D (1975). Analytical models of propagation in excitable cells. *Prog Biophys Mol Biol*, *30*: 99-144.

482. Hunter PJ, Smaill BH (1988). The analysis of cardiac function: a continuum approach. *Prog Biophys Mol Biol*, *52*: 101-164.

483. Hurst JW (1998). Naming of the waves in the ECG, with a brief account of their genesis. *Circulation*, *98*: 1937-1942.

484. Huser J, Blatter LA, Lipsius SL (2000). Intracellular Ca^{2+} release contributes to automaticity in cat atrial pacemaker cells. *J Physiol (Lond)*, *524 Pt 2*: 415-422.

485. Hwang TC, Horie M, Nairn AC, Gadsby DC (1992). Role of GTP-binding proteins in the regulation of mammalian cardiac chloride conductance. *J Gen Physiol*, *99*: 465-489.

486. Hwang TC, Nagel G, Nairn AC, Gadsby DC (1994). Regulation of the gating of cystic fibrosis transmembrane conductance regulator Cl channels by phosphorylation and ATP hydrolysis. *Proc Natl Acad Sci USA*, *91*: 4698-4702.

487. Ichas F, Jouaville LS, Mazat JP (1997). Mitochondria are excitable organelles capable of generating and conveying electrical and calcium signals. *Cell*, *89*: 1145-1153.

488. Iino M (1996). Functional properties of inositol 1,4,5-trisphosphate receptor and Ca^{2+} signaling. In: *Organellar ion channels and transporters* (eds. DE Clapham, BE Ehrlich), pp 67-73. The Rockefeller University Press, New-York.

489. Ikeda T, Uchida T, Hough D, Lee JJ, Fishbein MC, Mandel WJ, Chen PS, Karagueuzian HS (1996). Mechanism of spontaneous termination of functional reentry in isolated canine right atrium. Evidence for the presence of an excitable but nonexcited core. *Circulation*, *94*: 1962-1973.

490. Imahashi K, Kusuoka H, Hashimoto K, Yoshioka J, Yamaguchi H, Nishimura T (1999). Intracellular sodium accumulation during ischemia as the substrate for reperfusion injury. *Circ Res*, *84*: 1401-1406.

491. Inagaki N, Gonoi T, Clement JPt, Namba N, Inazawa J, Gonzalez G, Aguilar Bryan L, Seino S, Bryan J (1995). Reconstitution of IKATP: an inward rectifier subunit plus the sulfonylurea receptor. *Science*, *270*: 1166-1170.

492. Inoue I, Nagase H, Kishi K, Higuti T (1991). ATP-sensitive K^+ channel in the mitochondrial inner membrane. *Nature*, *352*: 244-247.

493. Investigators TCAST (1989). Preliminary report: effect of encainide and flecainide on mortality in a randomized trial of arrhythmia suppression after myocardial infarction. The Cardiac Arrhythmia Suppression Trial (CAST) Investigators. *N Engl J Med*, *321*: 406-412.

494. Iost N, Virag L, Opincariu M, Szecsi J, Varro A, Papp JG (1998). Delayed rectifier potassium current in undiseased human ventricular myocytes. *Cardiovasc Res*, *40*: 508-515.

495. Irisawa H, Brown HF, Giles W (1993). Cardiac pacemaking in the sinoatrial node. *Physiol Rev*, *73*: 197-227.

496. Isenberg G (1976). Cardiac Purkinje fibers: cesium as a tool to block inward rectifying potassium currents. *Pflügers Archiv*, *365*: 99-106.

497. Isenberg G (2001). How can overexpression of Na^+,Ca^{2+}-exchanger compensate the negative inotropic effects of downregulated SERCA? *Cardiovasc Res*, *49*: 1-6.

498. Isenberg G, Han S, Schiefer A, Wendt Gallitelli MF (1993). Changes in mitochondrial calcium concentration during the cardiac contraction cycle. *Cardiovasc Res, 27*: 1800-1809.

499. Isenberg G, Vereecke J, van der Heyden G, Carmeliet E (1983). The shortening of the action potential by DNP in guinea-pig ventricular myocytes is mediated by an increase of a time-independent K conductance. *Pflügers Archiv, 397*: 251-259.

500. Ishibashi K, Kuwahara M, Sasaki S (2000). Molecular biology of aquaporins. *Rev Physiol Biochem Pharmacol, 141*: 1-32.

501. Ishii TM, Takano M, Xie LH, Noma A, Ohmori H (1999). Molecular characterization of the hyperpolarization-activated cation channel in rabbit heart sinoatrial node. *J Biol Chem, 274*: 12835-12839.

502. Isomoto S, Kurachi Y (1997). Function, regulation, pharmacology, and molecular structure of ATP-sensitive K^+ channels in the cardiovascular system. *J Cardiovasc Electrophysiol, 8*: 1431-1446.

503. Ito H, Sugimoto T, Kobayashi I, Takahashi K, Katada T, Ui M, Kurachi Y (1991). On the mechanism of basal and agonist-induced activation of the G protein-gated muscarinic K^+ channel in atrial myocytes of guinea pig heart. *J Gen Physiol, 98*: 517-533.

504. Ito H, Vereecke J, Carmeliet E (1992). Intracellular protons inhibit inward rectifier K^+ channel of guinea-pig ventricular cell membrane. *Pflügers Archiv, 422*: 280-286.

505. Izrailtyan I, Kresh JY (1997). Bradykinin modulation of isolated rabbit heart function is mediated by intrinsic cardiac neurons. *Cardiovasc Res, 33*: 641-649.

506. Jabr RI, Cole WC (1995). Oxygen-derived free radical stress activates nonselective cation current in guinea pig ventricular myocytes. Role of sulfhydryl groups. *Circ Res, 76*: 812-824.

507. Jack JJB, Noble D, Tsien RW (1975). Electric current flow in excitable cells. Clarendon pPress, Oxford.

508. Jackson PS, Strange K (1993). Volume-sensitive anion channels mediate swelling-activated inositol and taurine efflux. *Am J Physiol, 265*: C1489-1500.

509. Jacobsen AN, Du XJ, Lambert KA, Dart AM, Woodcock EA (1996). Arrhythmogenic action of thrombin during myocardial reperfusion via release of inositol 1,4,5-triphosphate. *Circulation, 93*: 23-26.

510. Jahnel U, Nawrath H, Carmeliet E, Vereecke J (1991). Depolarization-induced influx of sodium in response to phenylephrine in rat atrial heart muscle. *J Physiol (Lond), 432*: 621-637.

511. Jahnel U, Nawrath H, Rupp J, Ochi R (1993). L-type calcium channel activity in human atrial myocytes as influenced by 5-HT. *Naunyn Schmiedebergs Arch Pharmacol, 348*: 396-402.

512. Jais P, Haissaguerre M, Shah DC, Chouairi S, Gencel L, Hocini M, Clementy J (1997). A focal source of atrial fibrillation treated by discrete radiofrequency ablation. *Circulation, 95*: 572-576.

513. Jalife J (1999). Spatial and temporal organization in ventricular fibrillation. *Trends Cardiovasc Med, 9*: 119-127.

514. Jalife J (2000). Ventricular fibrillation: mechanisms of initiation and maintenance. *Annu Rev Physiol, 62*: 25-50.

515. Jalife J, Delmar M (2000). Propagation through cardiac muscle. In: *An introduction to Cardiac Cellular Electrophysiology* (eds. A Zaza, MR Rosen), pp 83-135. Harwood Academic Publishers.

516. Jalife J, Gray R (1996). Drifting vortices of electrical waves underlie ventricular fibrillation in the rabbit heart. *Acta Physiol Scand, 157*: 123-131.

517. Jalife J, Sicouri S, Delmar M, Michaels DC (1989). Electrical uncoupling and impulse propagation in isolated sheep Purkinje fibers. *Am J Physiol, 257*: H179-189.

518. Jalife JJ, Delmar M, Davidenko JM, Anumonwo J (1999). Basic Cardiac Electrophysiology for the Clinician. Futura Publ Cy, Armonk.

519. Janse MJ (1986). Electrophysiology and electrocardiology of acute myocardial ischemia. *Can J Cardiol*: 46a-52a.

520. Janse MJ, Wit AL (1989). Electrophysiological mechanisms of ventricular arrhythmias resulting from myocardial ischemia and infarction. *Physiol Rev, 69*: 1049-1169.

521. January CT, Riddle JM (1989). Early afterdepolarizations: mechanism of induction and block. A role for L-type Ca^{2+} current. *Circ Res, 64*: 977-990.

522. Janvier NC, McMorn SO, Harrison SM, Taggart P, Boyett MR (1997). The role of Na^+-Ca^{2+} exchange current in electrical restitution in ferret ventricular cells. *J Physiol (Lond), 504*: 301-314.

523. Jayachandran JV, Sih HJ, Winkle W, Zipes DP, Hutchins GD, Olgin JE (2000). Atrial fibrillation produced by prolonged rapid atrial pacing is associated with heterogeneous changes in atrial sympathetic innervation. *Circulation, 101*: 1185-1191.

524. Jeck C, Pinto J, Boyden P (1995). Transient outward currents in subendocardial Purkinje myocytes surviving in the infarcted heart. *Circulation, 92*: 465-473.

525. Jeck CD, Boyden PA (1992). Age-related appearance of outward currents may contribute to developmental differences in ventricular repolarization. *Circ Res, 71*: 1390-1403.

526. Jentsch TJ, Friedrich T, Schriever A, Yamada H (1999). The CLC chloride channel family. *Pflügers Archiv, 437*: 783-795.

527. Jiang M, Xu A, Tokmakejian S, Narayanan N (2000). Thyroid hormone-induced overexpression of functional ryanodine receptors in the rabbit heart. *Am J Physiol, 278*: H1429-1438.

528. Jiang T, Kuznetsov V, Pak E, Zhang H, Robinson RB, Steinberg SF (1996). Thrombin receptor actions in neonatal rat ventricular myocytes. *Circ Res, 78*: 553-563.

529. Johns A, Freay AD, Fraser W, Korach KS, Rubanyi GM (1996). Disruption of estrogen receptor gene prevents 17 beta estradiol-induced angiogenesis in transgenic mice. *Endocrinology, 137*: 4511-4513.

530. Johnson CM, Green KG, Kanter EM, Bou Abboud E, Saffitz JE, Yamada KA (1999). Voltage-gated Na^+ channel activity and connexin expression in Cx43-deficient cardiac myocytes. *J Cardiovasc Electrophysiol, 10*: 1390-1401.

531. Johnson EA, Sommer JR (1967). A strand of cardiac muscle. Its ultrastructure and the electrophysiological implications of its geometry. *J Cell Biol, 33*: 103-129.

532. Johnson TA, Coronel R, Graebner CA, Buchanan JW, Janse MJ, Gettes LS (1987). Relationship between extracellular potassium accumulation and local TQ-segment potential during acute myocardial ischemia in the porcine. *J Mol Cell Cardiol, 19*: 949-952.

533. Jongsma HJ, Wilders R (2000). Gap junctions in cardiovascular disease. *Circ Res, 86*: 1193-1197.

534. Joseph SP, Boehning D, Lin CI (2000). Inositol 1,4,5-trisphosphate receptors: Molecular aspects. In: *Calcium signaling* (ed. JW Putney), pp 203-226. CRC Press, Boca Raton.

535. Josephson IR, Varadi G (1996). The beta subunit increases Ca^{2+} currents and gating charge movements of human cardiac L-type Ca^{2+} channels. *Biophys J, 70*: 1285-1293.

536. Joyner R (1982). Effects of the discrete pattern of electrical coupling on propagation through an electrical syncytium. *Circ Res, 50*: 192-200.

537. Ju Y-K, Saint DA, Gage PW (1996). Hypoxia increases persistent sodium current in rat ventricular myocytes. *J Physiol (Lond), 497*: 337-347.

538. Kaab S, Dixon J, Duc J, Ashen D, Nabauer M, Beuckelmann DJ, Steinbeck G, McKinnon D, Tomaselli GF (1998). Molecular basis of transient outward potassium current downregulation in human heart failure: a decrease in Kv4.3 mRNA correlates with a reduction in current density. *Circulation, 98*: 1383-1393.

539. Kakei M, Noma A, Shibasaki T (1985). Properties of adenosine-triphosphate-regulated potassium channels in guinea-pig ventricular cells. *J Physiol (Lond), 363*: 441-462.

540. Kambouris NG, Hastings LA, Stepanovic S, Marban E, Tomaselli GF, Balser JR (1998). Mechanistic link between lidocaine block and inactivation probed by outer pore mutations in the rat microl skeletal muscle sodium channel. *J Physiol (Lond), 512*: 693-705.

541. Kameyama M, Kakei M, Sato R, Shibasaki T, Matsuda H, Irisawa H (1984). Intracellular Na^+ activates a K^+ channel in mammalian cardiac cells. *Nature, 309*: 354-356.

542. Kameyama M, Kiyosue T, Soejima M (1983). Single channel analysis of the inward rectifier K current in the rabbit ventricular cells. *Jpn J Physiol, 33*: 1039-1056.

543. Kamiya K, Nishiyama A, Yasui K, Hojo M, Sanguinetti MC, Kodama I (2001). Short- and long-term effects of amiodarone on the two components of cardiac delayed rectifier K^+ current. *Circulation, 103*: 1317-1324.

544. Kamkin A, Kiseleva I, Isenberg G (2000). Stretch-activated currents in ventricular myocytes: amplitude and arrhythmogenic effects increase with hypertrophy. *Cardiovasc Res, 48*: 409-420.

545. Kamp TJ, Hell JW (2000). Regulation of cardiac L-type calcium channels by protein kinase A and protein kinase C. *Circ Res, 87*: 1095-1102.

546. Kamp TJ, Hu H, Marban E (2000). Voltage-dependent facilitation of cardiac L-type Ca channels expressed in HEK-293 cells requires beta -subunit. *Am J Physiol, 278*: H126-255.

547. Kaplan P, Hendrikx M, Mattheussen M, Mubagwa K, Flameng W (1992). Effect of ischemia and reperfusion on sarcoplasmic reticulum calcium uptake. *Circ Res, 71*: 1123-1130.

548. Kaplinsky E, Ogawa S, Balke CW, Dreifus LS (1979). Two periods of early ventricular arrhythmia in the canine acute myocardial infarction model. *Circulation, 60*: 397-403.

549. Kaprielian R, Wickenden AD, Kassiri Z, Parker TG, Liu PP, Backx PH (1999). Relationship between K^+ channel down-regulation and $[Ca^{2+}]_i$ in rat ventricular myocytes following myocardial infarction. *J Physiol (Lond), 517*: 229-245.

550. Karmazyn M (1996). The sodium-hydrogen exchange system in the heart: its role in ischemic and reperfusion injury and therapeutic implications. *Can J Cardiol, 12*: 1074-1082.

551. Kasel AM, Faussner A, Pfeifer A, Muller U, Werdan K, Roscher AA (1996). B2 bradykinin receptors in cultured neonatal rat cardiomyocytes mediate a negative chronotropic and negative inotropic response. *Diabetes, 45 Suppl 1*: S44-50.

552. Kass RS, Davies MP (1996). The roles of ion channels in an inherited heart disease: molecular genetics of the long QT syndrome. *Cardiovasc Res, 32*: 443-454.

553. Kass RS, Lederer WJ, Tsien RW, Weingart R (1978). Role of calcium ions in transient inward currents and aftercontractions induced by strophanthidin in cardiac Purkinje fibres. *J Physiol (Lond), 281*: 187-208.

554. Kass RS, Tsien RW, Weingart R (1978). Ionic basis of transient inward current induced by strophanthidin in cardiac Purkinje fibres. *J Physiol (Lond), 281*: 209-226.

555. Kass RS, Wiegers SE (1982). The ionic basis of concentration-related effects of noradrenaline on the action potential of calf cardiac purkinje fibres. *J Physiol (Lond), 322*: 541-558.

556. Katz AM (1992). T wave "Memory": Possible causal relationship to stress-induced changes in cardiac ion channels? *J Cardiovascular Electrophysiology, 3*: 150-159.

557. Katzung BG, Hondeghem LM, Grant AO (1975). Letter: Cardiac ventricular automaticity induced by current of injury. *Pflügers Archiv, 360*: 193-197.

558. Kaupp UB, Seifert R (2001). Molecular diversity of pacemaker ion channels. *Annu Rev Physiol, 63*: 235-257.

559. Kawano S, Hiraoka M (1991). Transient outward currents and action potential alterations in rabbit ventricular myocytes. *J Mol Cell Cardiol, 23*: 681-693.

560. Kawano S, Hirayama Y, Hiraoka M (1995). Activation mechanism of Ca^{2+}-sensitive transient outward current in rabbit ventricular myocytes. *J Physiol (Lond), 486*: 593-604.

561. Kawano S, Nakamura F, Tanaka T, Hiraoka M (1992). Cardiac sarcoplasmic reticulum chloride channels regulated by protein kinase A. *Circ Res, 71*: 585-589.

562. Kedzierski RM, Yanagisawa M (2001). Endothelin system: the double-edged sword in health and disease. *Annu Rev Pharmacol Toxicol, 41*: 851-876.

563. Kent RL, Rozich JD, McCollam PL, McDermott DE, Thacker UF, Menick DR, McDermott PJ, Cooper Gt (1993). Rapid expression of the Na^+-Ca^{2+} exchanger in response to cardiac pressure overload. *Am J Physiol, 265*: H1024-1029.

564. Kentish JC, Barsotti RJ, Lea TJ, Mulligan IP, Patel JR, Ferenczi MA (1990). Calcium release from cardiac sarcoplasmic reticulum induced by photorelease of calcium or Ins(1,4,5)P3. *Am J Physiol, 258*: H610-615.

565. Kiehn J, Karle C, Thomas D, Yao X, Brachmann J, Kubler W (1998). HERG potassium channel activation is shifted by phorbol esters via protein kinase A-dependent pathways. *J Biol Chem, 273*: 25285-25291.

566. Kihara Y, Grossman W, Morgan JP (1989). Direct measurement of changes in intracellular calcium transients during hypoxia, ischemia, and reperfusion of the intact mammalian heart. *Circ Res, 65*: 1029-1044.

567. Kijima Y, Saito A, Jetton TL, Magnuson MA, Fleischer S (1993). Different intracellular localization of inositol 1,4,5-trisphosphate and ryanodine receptors in cardiomyocytes. *J Biol Chem, 268*: 3499-3506.

568. Kim D (1991). Endothelin activation of an inwardly rectifying K^+ current in atrial cells. *Circ Res, 69*: 250-255.

569. Kim D (1992). A mechanosensitive K^+ channel in heart cells. Activation by arachidonic acid. *J Gen Physiol, 100*: 1021-1040.

570. Kim D (1993). Novel cation-selective mechanosensitive ion channel in the atrial cell membrane. *Circ Res, 72*: 225-231.

571. Kim D, Clapham DE (1989). Potassium channels in cardiac cells activated by arachidonic acid and phospholipids. *Science, 244*: 1174-1176.

572. Kim D, Duff RA (1990). Regulation of K^+ channels in cardiac myocytes by free fatty acids. *Circ Res, 67*: 1040-1046.

573.   Kim D, Fujita A, Horio Y, Kurachi Y (1998). Cloning and functional expression of a novel cardiac two-pore background K$^+$ channel (cTBAK-1). *Circ Res, 82*: 513-518.

574.   Kim Y, Bang H, Kim D (1999). TBAK-1 and TASK-1, two-pore K$^+$ channel subunits: kinetic properties and expression in rat heart. *Am J Physiol, 277*: H1669-1678.

575.   Kimura J (2001). Cardiac Na$^+$-Ca^{2+} exchanger: pathophysiology and pharmacology. In: *Heart Physiology and Pathophysiology* (eds. N Sperelakis, Y Kurachi, A Terzic, MV Cohen), pp 417-425. Academic Press, San Diego.

576.   Kimura S, Bassett AL, Kohya T, Kozlovskis PL, Myerburg RJ (1987). Automaticity, triggered activity, and responses to adrenergic stimulation in cat subendocardial Purkinje fibers after healing of myocardial infarction. *Circulation, 75*: 651-660.

577.   Kinnally KW, Antonenko YN, Zorov DB (1992). Modulation of inner mitochondrial membrane channel activity. *J Bioenerg Biomembr, 24*: 99-110.

578.   Kirchhoff S, Kim J-S, Hagendorff A, Thonnissen E, Kruger O, Lamers WH, Willecke K (2000). Abnormal cardiac conduction and morphogenesis in connexin40 and connexin43 double-deficient mice. *Circ Res, 87*: 399-405.

579.   Kiriazis H, Kranias EG (2000). Genetically engineered models with alterations in cardiac membrane Calcium-handling proteins. *Annu Rev Physiol, 62*: 321-350.

580.   Kiss L, Korn SJ (1998). Modulation of C-type inactivation by K$^+$ at the potassium channel selectivity filter. *Biophys J, 74*: 1840-1849.

581.   Kiyosue T, Spindler AJ, Noble SJ, Noble D (1993). Background inward current in ventricular and atrial cells of the guinea-pig. *Proc R Soc Lond B Biol Sci, 252*: 65-74.

582.   Kléber AG (1983). Resting membrane potential, extracellular potassium activity, and intracellular sodium activity during acute global ischemia in isolated perfused guinea pig hearts. *Circ Res, 52*: 442-450.

583.   Kléber AG (1987). Conduction of the impulse in the ischemic myocardium-- implications for malignant ventricular arrhythmias. *Experientia, 43*: 1056-1061.

584.   Kléber AG (1999). Discontinuous propagation of the cardiac impulse and arrhythmogenesis. *J Cardiovasc Electrophysiol, 10*: 1025-1027.

585.   Kléber AG (2000). ST-segment elevation in the electrocardiogram: a sign of myocardial ischemia. *Cardiovasc Res, 45*: 111-118.

586.   Kléber AG, Janse MJ, van Capelle FJ, Durrer D (1978). Mechanism and time course of S-T and T-Q segment changes during acute regional myocardial ischemia in the pig heart determined by extracellular and intracellular recordings. *Circ Res, 42*: 603-613.

587.   Kloner RA, Shook T, Przyklenk K, Davis VG, Junio L, Matthews RV, Burstein S, Gibson M, Poole WK, Cannon CP, et al. (1995). Previous angina alters in-hospital outcome in TIMI 4. A clinical correlate to preconditioning? *Circulation, 91*: 37-45.

588.   Knollmann BC, Knollmann-Ritschel BE, Weissman NJ, Jones LR, Morad M (2000). Remodelling of ionic currents in hypertrophied and failing hearts of transgenic mice overexpressing calsequestrin. *J Physiol (Lond), 525 Pt 2*: 483-498.

589.   Kodama I, Kamiya K, Toyama J (1997). Cellular electropharmacology of amiodarone. *Cardiovasc Res, 35*: 13-29.

590.   Kodama I, Nikmaram MR, Boyett MR, Suzuki R, Honjo H, Owen JM (1997). Regional differences in the role of the Ca^{2+} and Na$^+$ currents in pacemaker activity in the sinoatrial node. *Am J Physiol, 272*: H2793-2806.

591.   Kodama I, Wilde A, Janse MJ, Durrer D, Yamada K (1984). Combined effects of hypoxia, hyperkalemia and acidosis on membrane action potential and excitability of guinea-pig ventricular muscle. *J Mol Cell Cardiol, 16*: 247-259.

592. Kohl P, Hunter P, Noble D (1999). Stretch-induced changes in heart rate and rhythm: clinical observations, experiments and mathematical models. *Prog Biophys Mol Biol, 71*: 91-138.

593. Kokubun S, Nishimura M, Noma A, Irisawa H (1982). Membrane currents in the rabbit atrioventricular node cell. *Pflügers Archiv, 393*: 15-22.

594. Konarzewska H, Peeters GA, Sanguinetti MC (1995). Repolarizing K^+ currents in nonfailing human hearts. Similarities between right septal subendocardial and left subepicardial ventricular myocytes. *Circulation, 92*: 1179-1187.

595. Korichneva I, Puceat M, Millanvoye-Van Brussel E, Geraud G, Vassort G (1995). Aldosterone modulates both the Na/H antiport and Cl/HCO3 exchanger in cultured neonatal rat cardiac cells. *J Mol Cell Cardiol, 27*: 2521-2528.

596. Kostin S, Schaper J (2001). Tissue-specific patterns of gap junctions in adult rat atrial and ventricular cardiomyocytes in vivo and in vitro. *Circ Res, 88*: 933-939.

597. Koumi S, Arentzen CE, Backer CL, Wasserstrom JA (1994). Alterations in muscarinic K^+ channel response to acetylcholine and to G protein-mediated activation in atrial myocytes isolated from failing human hearts. *Circulation, 90*: 2213-2224.

598. Koumi S, Backer CL, Arentzen CE, Sato R (1995). beta-Adrenergic modulation of the inwardly rectifying potassium channel in isolated human ventricular myocytes. Alteration in channel response to beta-adrenergic stimulation in failing human hearts. *J Clin Invest, 96*: 2870-2881.

599. Koumi S, Wasserstrom JA (1994). Acetylcholine-sensitive muscarinic K^+ channels in mammalian ventricular myocytes. *Am J Physiol, 266*: H1812-1821.

600. Kraev A, Chumakov I, Carafoli E (1996). The organization of the human gene NCX1 encoding the sodium-calcium exchanger. *Genomics, 37*: 105-112.

601. Krahn AD, Nguyen-Ho P, Klein GJ, Yee R, Skanes AC, Suskin N (2001). QT dispersion: An electrocardiographic derivative of QT prolongation. *Am Heart J, 141*: 111-116.

602. Krapivinsky G, Gordon EA, Wickman K, Velimirovic B, Krapivinsky L, Clapham DE (1995). The G-protein-gated atrial K^+ channel IKACh is a heteromultimer of two inwardly rectifying K^+-channel proteins. *Nature, 374*: 135-141.

603. Kreuzberg U, Theissen P, Schicha H, Schroder F, Mehlhorn U, de Vivie ER, Boknik P, Neumann J, Grohe C, Herzig S (2000). Single-channel activity and expression of atrial L-type Ca^{2+} channels in patients with latent hyperthyroidism. *Am J Physiol Heart Circ Physiol, 278*: H723-730.

604. Kubo Y, Baldwin TJ, Jan YN, Jan LY (1993). Primary structure and functional expression of a mouse inward rectifier potassium channel. *Nature, 362*: 127-133.

605. Kucera JP, Kléber AG, Rohr S (1998). Slow conduction in cardiac tissue, II: Effects of branching tissue geometry. *Circ Res, 83*: 795-805.

606. Kukreja RC, Hess ML (1992). The oxygen free radical system: from equations through membrane-protein interactions to cardiovascular injury and protection. *Cardiovasc Res, 26*: 641-655.

607. Kunze DL, Lacerda AE, Wilson DL, Brown AM (1985). Cardiac Na currents and the inactivating, reopening, and waiting properties of single cardiac Na channels. *J Gen Physiol, 86*: 691-719.

608. Kupershmidt S, Yang T, Roden DM (1998). Modulation of cardiac Na^+ current phenotype by beta1-subunit expression. *Circ Res, 83*: 441-447.

609. Kurachi Y (1985). Voltage-dependent activation of the inward-rectifier potassium channel in the ventricular cell membrane of guinea-pig heart. *J Physiol (Lond), 366*: 365-385.

610. Kurz T, Tolg R, Richardt G (1997). Bradykinin B2-receptor-mediated stimulation of exocytotic noradrenaline release from cardiac sympathetic neurons. *J Mol Cell Cardiol, 29*: 2561-2569.

611. Kwak BR, Hermans MM, De Jonge HR, Lohmann SM, Jongsma HJ, Chanson M (1995). Differential regulation of distinct types of gap junction channels by similar phosphorylating conditions. *Mol Biol Cell, 6*: 1707-1719.

612. Kwong KF, Schuessler RB, Green KG, Laing JG, Beyer EC, Boineau JP, Saffitz JE (1998). Differential expression of gap junction proteins in the canine sinus node. *Circ Res, 82*: 604-612.

613. Lacampagne A, Duittoz A, Bolanos P, Peineau N, Argibay JA (1995). Effect of sulfhydryl oxidation on ionic and gating currents associated with L-type calcium channels in isolated guinea-pig ventricular myocytes. *Cardiovasc Res, 30*: 799-806.

614. Lacinova L, Hofmann F (2001). Voltage-dependent calcium channels. In: *Heart Physiology and Pathophysiology* (eds. N Sperelakis, Y Kurachi, A Terzic, MV Cohen), pp 247-257. Academic Press, San Diego.

615. Lai LP, Su MJ, Lin JL, Lin FY, Tsai CH, Chen YS, Tseng YZ, Lien WP, Huang SK (1999). Changes in the mRNA levels of delayed rectifier potassium channels in human atrial fibrillation. *Cardiology, 92*: 248-255.

616. Lamb GD, Laver DR, Stephenson DG (2000). Questions about adaptation in ryanodine receptors. *J Gen Physiol, 116*: 883-844.

617. Lamont C, Luther PW, Balke CW, Wier WG (1998). Intercellular Ca^{2+} waves in rat heart muscle. *J Physiol (Lond), 512*: 669-676.

618. Lang F, Busch GL, Ritter M, Volkl H, Waldegger S, Gulbins E, Haussinger D (1998). Functional significance of cell volume regulatory mechanisms. *Physiol Rev, 78*: 247-245.

619. Laskey WK (1999). Beneficial impact of preconditioning during PTCA on creatine kinase release. *Circulation, 99*: 2085-2089.

620. Laurita KR, Rosenbaum DS (2000). Interdependence of modulated dispersion and tissue structure in the mechanism of unidirectional block. *Circ Res, 87*: 922-928.

621. Lawrence C, Rodrigo GC (1999). A Na^{+}-activated K^{+} current (IK,Na) is present in guinea-pig but not rat ventricular myocytes. *Pflügers Archiv, 437*: 831-838.

622. Le Grand B, Deroubaix E, Couetil JP, Coraboeuf E (1992). Effects of atrionatriuretic factor on Ca^{2+} current and Ca_i-independent transient outward K^{+} current in human atrial cells. *Pflügers Archiv, 421*: 486-491.

623. Le Grand BL, Hatem S, Deroubaix E, Couetil JP, Coraboeuf E (1994). Depressed transient outward and calcium currents in dilated human atria. *Cardiovasc Res, 28*: 548-556.

624. le Marec H, Dangman KH, Danilo P, Rosen MR (1985). An evaluation of automaticity and triggered activity in the canine heart one to four days after myocardial infarction. *Circulation, 71*: 1224-1236.

625. Leblanc N, Hume JR (1990). Sodium current-induced release of calcium from cardiac sarcoplasmic reticulum. *Science, 248*: 372-376.

626. Lederer WJ, Nichols CG (1989). Nucleotide modulation of the activity of rat heart ATP-sensitive K^{+} channels in isolated membrane patches. *J Physiol (Lond), 419*: 193-211.

627. Lederer WJ, Niggli E, Hadley RW (1990). Sodium-calcium exchange in excitable cells: fuzzy space. *Science, 248*: 283.

628. Lee KS, Lee EW (1998). Ionic mechanism of ibutilide in human atrium: evidence for a drug-induced Na$^+$ current through a nifedipine inhibited inward channel. *J Pharmacol Exp Ther, 286*: 9-22.

629. Lee KW, Kligfield P, Dower GE, Okin PM (2001). QT Dispersion, T-wave projection, and heterogeneity of repolarization in patients with coronary artery disease. *Am J Cardiol, 87*: 148-151.

630. Leesar MA, Stoddard MF, Dawn B, Jasti VG, Masden R, Bolli R (2001). Delayed preconditioning-mimetic action of nitroglycerin in patients undergoing coronary angioplasty. *Circulation, 103*: 2935-2941.

631. Lei M, Brown HF, Terrar DA (2000). Modulation of delayed rectifier potassium current, iK, by isoprenaline in rabbit isolated pacemaker cells. *Exp Physiol, 85*: 27-35.

632. Lei M, Honjo H, Kodama I, Boyett MR (2000). Characterisation of the transient outward K$^+$ current in rabbit sinoatrial node cells. *Cardiovasc Res, 46*: 433-441.

633. Leifert WR, McMurchie EJ, Saint DA (1999). Inhibition of cardiac sodium currents in adult rat myocytes by n-3 polyunsaturated fatty acids. *J Physiol (Lond), 520 Pt 3*: 671-679.

634. Lemaire S, Piot C, Seguin J, Nargeot J, Richard S (1995). Tetrodotoxin-sensitive Ca^{2+} and Ba^{2+} currents in human atrial cells. *Receptors Channels, 3*: 71-81.

635. Leuranguer V, Monteil A, Bourinet E, Dayanithi G, Nargeot J (2000). T-type calcium currents in rat cardiomyocytes during postnatal development: contribution to hormone secretion. *Am J Physiol, 279*: H2540-2548.

636. Levi R, Malm JR, Bowman FO, Rosen MR (1981). The arrhythmogenic actions of histamine on human atrial fibers. *Circ Res, 49*: 545-550.

637. Levi RC, Alloatti G (1988). Histamine modulates calcium current in guinea pig ventricular myocytes. *J Pharmacol Exp Ther, 246*: 377-383.

638. Levitan ES, Hershman KM, Sherman TG, Takimoto K (1996). Dexamethasone and stress upregulate Kv1.5 K$^+$ channel gene expression in rat ventricular myocytes. *Neuropharmacology, 35*: 1001-1006.

639. Levitsky J, Gurell D, Frishman WH (1998). Sodium ion/hydrogen ion exchange inhibition: a new pharmacologic approach to myocardial ischemia and reperfusion injury. *J Clin Pharmacol, 38*: 887-897.

640. Levy D, Seigneuret M, Bluzat A, Rigaud JL (1990). Evidence for proton countertransport by the sarcoplasmic reticulum Ca^{2+}-ATPase during calcium transport in reconstituted proteoliposomes with low ionic permeability. *J Biol Chem, 265*: 19524-19534.

641. Li D, Benardeau A, Nattel S (2000). Contrasting efficacy of dofetilide in differing experimental models of atrial fibrillation. *Circulation, 102*: 104-112.

642. Li D, Fareh S, Leung TK, Nattel S (1999). Promotion of atrial fibrillation by heart failure in dogs: atrial remodeling of a different sort. *Circulation, 100*: 87-95.

643. Li D, Melnyk P, Feng J, Wang Z, Petrecca K, Shrier A, Nattel S (2000). Effects of experimental heart failure on atrial cellular and ionic electrophysiology. *Circulation, 101*: 2631-2638.

644. Li D, Zhang L, Kneller J, Nattel S (2001). Potential ionic mechanism for repolarization differences between canine right and left atrium. *Circ Res, 88*: 1168-1175.

645. Li GR, Feng J, Wang Z, Fermini B, Nattel S (1995). Comparative mechanisms of 4-aminopyridine-resistant Ito in human and rabbit atrial myocytes. *Am J Physiol, 269*: H463-472.

646. Li GR, Feng J, Wang Z, Fermini B, Nattel S (1996). Adrenergic modulation of ultrarapid delayed rectifier K$^+$ current in human atrial myocytes. *Circ Res, 78*: 903-915.

647. Li GR, Feng J, Yue L, Carrier M (1998). Transmural heterogeneity of action potentials and Ito1 in myocytes isolated from the human right ventricle. *Am J Physiol, 275*: H369-377.

648. Li GR, Feng J, Yue L, Carrier M, Nattel S (1996). Evidence for two components of delayed rectifier K$^+$ current in human ventricular myocytes. *Circ Res, 78*: 689-696.

649. Li GR, Nattel S (1997). Properties of human atrial I$_{Ca}$ at physiological temperatures and relevance to action potential. *Am J Physiol, 272*: H227-235.

650. Li GR, Yang B, Feng J, Bosch RF, Carrier M, Nattel S (1999). Transmembrane I$_{Ca}$ contributes to rate-dependent changes of action potentials in human ventricular myocytes. *Am J Physiol, 276*: H98-H106.

651. Li Q, Zhang J, Loro JF, Pfaffendorf M, van Zwieten PA (1998). Bradykinin B2-receptor-mediated positive chronotropic effect of bradykinin in isolated rat atria. *J Cardiovasc Pharmacol, 32*: 452-456.

652. Li RA, Leppo M, Miki T, Seino S, Marban E (2000). Molecular basis of electrocardiographic ST-segment elevation. *Circ Res, 87*: 837-839.

653. Light PE (1999). Cardiac KATP channels and ischemic preconditioning: current perspectives. *Can J Cardiol, 15*: 1123-1130.

654. Linz KW, Meyer R (2000). Profile and kinetics of L-type calcium current during the cardiac ventricular action potential compared in guinea-pigs, rats and rabbits. *Pflügers Archiv, 439*: 588-599.

655. Linz W, Scholkens BA, Kaiser J, Just M, Qi BY, Albus U, Petry P (1989). Cardiac arrhythmias are ameliorated by local inhibition of angiotensin formation and bradykinin degradation with the converting-enzyme inhibitor ramipril. *Cardiovasc Drugs Ther, 3*: 873-882.

656. Lipp P, Laine M, Tovey SC, Burrell KM, Berridge MJ, Li W, Bootman MD (2000). Functional InsP3 receptors that may modulate excitation-contraction coupling in the heart. *Curr Biol, 10*: 939-942.

657. Lipp P, Mechmann S, Pott L (1987). Effects of calcium release from sarcoplasmic reticulum on membrane currents in guinea pig atrial cardioballs. *Pflügers Archiv, 410*: 121-131.

658. Lipp P, Niggli E (1998). Fundamental calcium release events revealed by two-photon excitation photolysis of caged calcium in Guinea-pig cardiac myocytes. *J Physiol (Lond), 508*: 801-809.

659. Lipsius SL, Huser J, Blatter LA (2001). Intracellular Ca^{2+} release sparks atrial pacemaker activity. *News Physiol Sci, 16*: 101-106.

660. Litovsky SH, Antzelevitch C (1988). Transient outward current prominent in canine ventricular epicardium but not endocardium. *Circ Res, 62*: 116-126.

661. Litwin SE, Bridge JH (1997). Enhanced Na$^+$-Ca^{2+} exchange in the infarcted heart. Implications for excitation-contraction coupling. *Circ Res, 81*: 1083-1093.

662. Litwin SE, Zhang D, Bridge JHB (2000). Dyssynchronous Ca^{2+} sparks in myocytes from infarcted hearts. *Circ Res, 87*: 1040-1047.

663. Liu B, Clanachan AS, Schulz R, Lopaschuk GD (1996). Cardiac efficiency is improved after ischemia by altering both the source and fate of protons. *Circ Res, 79*: 940-948.

664. Liu DW, Antzelevitch C (1995). Characteristics of the delayed rectifier current (IKr and IKs) in canine ventricular epicardial, midmyocardial, and endocardial myocytes. A

weaker IKs contributes to the longer action potential of the M cell. *Circ Res, 76*: 351-365.

665. Liu DW, Gintant GA, Antzelevitch C (1993). Ionic bases for electrophysiological distinctions among epicardial, midmyocardial, and endocardial myocytes from the free wall of the canine left ventricle. *Circ Res, 72*: 671-687.

666. Liu GX, Hanley PJ, Ray J, Daut J (2001). Long-chain acyl-coenzyme A esters and fatty acids directly link metabolism to KATP channels in the heart. *Circ Res*: 918-924.

667. Liu MY, Colombini M (1992). Regulation of mitochondrial respiration by controlling the permeability of the outer membrane through the mitochondrial channel, VDAC. *Biochim Biophys Acta, 1098*: 255-260.

668. Liu P, Fei L, Wu W, Li J, Wang J, Zhang X (1996). Effects of hypothyroidism on the vulnerability to ventricular fibrillation in dogs: a comparative study with amiodarone. *Cardiovasc Drugs Ther, 10*: 369-378.

669. Liu Y, Jurman ME, Yellen G (1996). Dynamic rearrangement of the outer mouth of a K^+ channel during gating. *Neuron, 16*: 859-867.

670. Liu Y, Sato T, O'Rourke B, Marban E (1998). Mitochondrial ATP-dependent potassium channels: novel effectors of cardioprotection? *Circulation, 97*: 2463-2469.

671. Liu Y, Zeng W, Delmar M, Jalife J (1993). Ionic mechanisms of electronic inhibition and concealed conduction in rabbit atrioventricular nodal myocytes. *Circulation, 88*: 1634-1646.

672. Liu YM, Yu H, Li CZ, Cohen IS, Vassalle M (1998). Cesium effects on i_f and i_K in rabbit sinoatrial node myocytes: implications for SA node automaticity. *J Cardiovasc Pharmacol, 32*: 783-790.

673. Lo CW (2000). Role of gap junctions in cardiac conduction and development: insights from the connexin knockout mice. *Circ Res, 87*: 346-348.

674. Lohberger B, Groschner K, Tritthart H, Schreibmayer W (2000). IK.ACh activation by arachidonic acid occurs via a G-protein- independent pathway mediated by the GIRK1 subunit. *Pflügers Archiv, 441*: 251-256.

675. Lopaschuk GD, Wambolt RB, Barr RL (1993). An imbalance between glycolysis and glucose oxidation is a possible explanation for the detrimental effects of high levels of fatty acids during aerobic reperfusion of ischemic hearts. *J Pharmacol Exp Ther, 264*: 135-144.

676. Lopatin AN, Makhina EN, Nichols CG (1994). Potassium channel block by cytoplasmic polyamines as the mechanism of intrinsic rectification. *Nature, 372*: 366-369.

677. Lopes CMB, Gallagher PG, Buck ME, Butler MH, Goldstein SAN (2000). Proton block and voltage gating are potassium-dependent in the cardiac leak channel Kcnk3. *J Biol Chem, 275*: 16969-16978.

678. Loro JF, Zhang J, Pfaffendorf M, van Zwieten PA (1998). Positive chronotropic activity of bradykinin in the pithed normotensive rat. *Fundam Clin Pharmacol, 12*: 77-81.

679. Louch WE, Ferrier GR, Howlett SE (2000). Losartan improves recovery of contraction and inhibits transient inward current in a cellular model of cardiac ischemia and reperfusion. *J Pharmacol Exp Ther, 295*: 697-704.

680. Lu Z, MacKinnon R (1994). Electrostatic tuning of Mg^{2+} affinity in an inward-rectifier K^+ channel. *Nature, 371*: 243-246.

681. Ludwig A, Zong X, Hofmann F, Biel M (1999). Structure and function of cardiac pacemaker channels. *Cell Physiol Biochem, 9*: 179-186.

682. Ludwig A, Zong X, Jeglitsch M, Hofmann F, Biel M (1998). A family of hyperpolarization-activated mammalian cation channels. *Nature, 393*: 587-591.

683. Ludwig A, Zong X, Stieber J, Hullin R, Hofmann F, Biel M (1999). Two pacemaker channels from human heart with profoundly different activation kinetics. *EMBO J, 18*: 2323-2329.

684. Lue WM, Boyden PA (1992). Abnormal electrical properties of myocytes from chronically infarcted canine heart. Alterations in Vmax and the transient outward current. *Circulation, 85*: 1175-1188.

685. Luk HN, Carmeliet E (1990). Na^+-activated K^+ current in cardiac cells: rectification, open probability, block and role in digitalis toxicity. *Pflügers Archiv, 416*: 766-768.

686. Lukas A, Antzelevitch C (1996). Phase 2 reentry as a mechanism of initiation of circus movement reentry in canine epicardium exposed to simulated ischemia. *Cardiovasc Res, 32*: 593-603.

687. Luke RA, Saffitz JE (1991). Remodeling of ventricular conduction pathways in healed canine infarct border zones. *J Clin Invest, 87*: 1594-1602.

688. Luo CH, Rudy Y (1991). A model of the ventricular cardiac action potential. Depolarization, repolarization, and their interaction. *Circ Res, 68*: 1501-1526.

689. Magishi K, Kimura J, Kubo Y, Abiko Y (1996). Exogenous lysophosphatidylcholine increases non-selective cation current in guinea-pig ventricular myocytes. *Pflügers Archiv, 432*: 345-350.

690. Magyar J, Iost N, Kortvely A, Banyasz T, Virag L, Szigligeti P, Varro A, Opincariu M, Szecsi J, Papp JG, Nanasi PP (2000). Effects of endothelin-1 on calcium and potassium currents in undiseased human ventricular myocytes. *Pflügers Archiv, 441*: 144-149.

691. Magyar J, Rusznak Z, Szentesi P, Szucs G, Kovacs L (1992). Action potentials and potassium currents in rat ventricular muscle during experimental diabetes. *J Mol Cell Cardiol, 24*: 841-853.

692. Maisel AS, Motulsky HJ, Insel PA (1985). Externalization of beta-adrenergic receptors promoted by myocardial ischemia. *Science, 230*: 183-186.

693. Makielski JC, Limberis JT, Chang SY, Fan Z, Kyle JW (1996). Coexpression of beta 1 with cardiac sodium channel alpha subunits in oocytes decreases lidocaine block. *Mol Pharmacol, 49*: 30-39.

694. Makielski JC, Sheets MF, Hanck DA, January CT, Fozzard HA (1987). Sodium current in voltage clamped internally perfused canine cardiac Purkinje cells. *Biophys J, 52*: 1-11.

695. Makita N, Bennett PB, Jr., George AL, Jr. (1994). Voltage-gated Na^+ channel beta 1 subunit mRNA expressed in adult human skeletal muscle, heart, and brain is encoded by a single gene. *J Biol Chem, 269*: 7571-7578.

696. Malik M (2000). QT dispersion: time for an obituary? *Eur Heart J, 21*: 955-957.

697. Malinowska B, Godlewski G, Schlicker E (1998). Histamine H3 receptors--general characterization and their function in the cardiovascular system. *J Physiol Pharmacol, 49*: 191-211.

698. Maltsev VA, Wobus AM, Rohwedel J, Bader M, Hescheler J (1994). Cardiomyocytes differentiated in vitro from embryonic stem cells developmentally express cardiac-specific genes and ionic currents. *Circ Res, 75*: 233-244.

699. Mangoni ME, Fontanaud P, Noble PJ, Noble D, Benkemoun H, Nargeot J, Richard S (2000). Facilitation of the L-type calcium current in rabbit sino-atrial cells: effect on cardiac automaticity. *Cardiovasc Res, 48*: 375-392.

700. Mannella CA (1992). The 'ins' and 'outs' of mitochondrial membrane channels. *Trends Biochem Sci, 17*: 315-320.

701. Mansourati J, Le Grand B (1993). Transient outward current in young and adult diseased human atria. *Am J Physiol, 265*: H1466-1470.
702. Marban E, Kitakaze M, Koretsune Y, Yue DT, Chacko VP, Pike MM (1990). Quantification of [Ca^{2+}]$_i$ in perfused hearts. Critical evaluation of the 5F-BAPTA and nuclear magnetic resonance method as applied to the study of ischemia and reperfusion. *Circ Res, 66*: 1255-1267.
703. Marban E, Koretsune Y, Kusuoka H (1994). Disruption of intracellular Ca^{2+} homeostasis in hearts reperfused after prolonged episodes of ischemia. *Ann N Y Acad Sci, 723*: 38-50.
704. Marban E, Yamagishi T, Tomaselli GF (1998). Structure and function of voltage-gated sodium channels. *J Physiol (Lond), 508*: 647-657.
705. Marks AR (1997). Intracellular calcium-release channels: regulators of cell life and death. *Am J Physiol, 272*: H597-605.
706. Marks AR (2000). Cardiac intracellular calcium release channels: role in heart failure. *Circ Res, 87*: 8-11.
707. Marks AR (2001). Ryanodine receptors/calcium release channels in heart failure and sudden cardiac death. *J Mol Cell Cardiol, 33*: 615-624.
708. Maruoka F, Nakashima Y, Takano M, Ono K, Noma A (1994). Cation-dependent gating of the hyperpolarization-activated cation current in the rabbit sino-atrial node cells. *J Physiol (Lond), 477*: 423-435.
709. Maruyama R, Hatta E, Levi R (1999). Norepinephrine release and ventricular fibrillation in myocardial ischemia/reperfusion: roles of angiotensin and bradykinin. *J Cardiovasc Pharmacol, 34*: 913-915.
710. Marx OS, Marks AR (2000). Ryanodine receptors. In: *Calcium signaling* (ed. JW Putney), pp 227-247. CRC Press, Boca Raton.
711. Marx SO, Reiken S, Hisamatsu Y, Jayaraman T, Burkhoff D, Rosemblit N, Marks AR (2000). PKA phosphorylation dissociates FKBP12.6 from the calcium release channel (ryanodine receptor): defective regulation in failing hearts. *Cell, 101*: 365-376.
712. Masaki T (2000). The endothelin family: an overview. *J Cardiovasc Pharmacol, 35*: S3-5.
713. Matherne GP, Linden J, Byford AM, Gauthier NS, Headrick JP (1997). Transgenic A1 adenosine receptor overexpression increases myocardial resistance to ischemia. *Proc Natl Acad Sci USA, 94*: 6541-6546.
714. Mathur A, Hong Y, Kemp BK, Barrientos AA, Erusalimsky JD (2000). Evaluation of fluorescent dyes for the detection of mitochondrial membrane potential changes in cultured cardiomyocytes. *Cardiovasc Res, 46*: 126-138.
715. Matsuda H (1988). Open-state substructure of inwardly rectifying potassium channels revealed by magnesium block in guinea-pig heart cells. *J Physiol (Lond), 397*: 237-258.
716. Matsuda H, Matsuura H, Noma A (1989). Triple-barrel structure of inwardly rectifying K$^+$ channels revealed by Cs$^+$ and Rb$^+$ block in guinea-pig heart cells. *J Physiol (Lond), 413*: 139-157.
717. Matsuda H, Saigusa A, Irisawa H (1987). Ohmic conductance through the inwardly rectifying K channel and blocking by internal Mg^{2+}. *Nature, 325*: 156-159.
718. Matsumoto K, Pappano AJ (1991). Carbachol activates a novel sodium current in isolated guinea pig ventricular myocytes via M2 muscarinic receptors. *Mol Pharmacol, 39*: 359-363.

719. Matsushita T, Oyamada M, Fujimoto K, Yasuda Y, Masuda S, Wada Y, Oka T, Takamatsu T (1999). Remodeling of cell-cell and cell-extracellular matrix interactions at the border zone of rat myocardial infarcts. *Circ Res*, *85*: 1046-1055.

720. Matsushita T, Oyamada M, Fujimoto K, Yasuda Y, Masuda S, Wada Y, Oka T, Takamatsu T (1999). Remodeling of cell-cell and cell-extracellular matrix interactions at the border zone of rat myocardial infarcts. *Circ Res*, *85*: 1046-1055.

721. Matsuura H, Ehara T, Imoto Y (1987). An analysis of the delayed outward current in single ventricular cells of the guinea-pig. *Pflügers Archiv*, *410*: 596-603.

722. Matsuura H, Shattock MJ (1991). Effects of oxidant stress on steady-state background currents in isolated ventricular myocytes. *Am J Physiol*, *261*: H1358-1365.

723. Mays DJ, Foose JM, Philipson LH, Tamkun MM (1995). Localization of the Kv1.5 K$^+$ channel protein in explanted cardiac tissue. *J Clin Invest*, *96*: 282-292.

724. Mazhari R, Greenstein JL, Winslow RL, Marban E, Nuss HB (2001). Molecular interactions between two Long-QT syndrome gene products, HERG and KCNE2, rationalized by In vitro and In silico analysis. *Circ Res*, *89*: 33-38.

725. Mazzanti M, DiFrancesco D (1989). Intracellular Ca modulates K-inward rectification in cardiac myocytes. *Pflügers Archiv*, *413*: 322-324.

726. McDonald TF, Pelzer S, Trautwein W, Pelzer DJ (1994). Regulation and modulation of calcium channels in cardiac, skeletal, and smooth muscle cells. *Physiol Rev*, *74*: 365-507.

727. McHowat J, Creer MH (1997). Lysophosphatidylcholine accumulation in cardiomyocytes requires thrombin activation of Ca^{2+}-independent PLA2. *Am J Physiol*, *272*: H1972-1980.

728. McHowat J, Yamada KA, Wu J, Yan GX, Corr PB (1993). Recent insights pertaining to sarcolemmal phospholipid alterations underlying arrhythmogenesis in the ischemic heart. *J Cardiovasc Electrophysiol*, *4*: 288-310.

729. McManus OB, Blatz AL, Magleby KL (1987). Sampling, log binning, fitting, and plotting durations of open and shut intervals from single channels and the effects of noise. *Pflügers Archiv*, *410*: 530-553.

730. McNeill JH, Verma SC, Tenner TE, Jr. (1980). Cardiac histamine receptors. *Adv Myocardiol*, *1*: 209-216.

731. Meissner G (2001). Calcium release from the cardiac sarcoplasmic reticulum. In: *Heart Physiology and Pathophysiology* (eds. N Sperelakis, Y Kurachi, A Terzic, MV Cohen), pp 461-470. Academic Press, San Diego.

732. Meissner G, McKinley D (1982). Permeability of canine cardiac sarcoplasmic reticulum vesicles to K$^+$, Na$^+$, H$^+$, and Cl$^-$. *J Biol Chem*, *257*: 7704-7711.

733. Mejia Alvarez R, Kettlun C, Rios E, Stern M, Fill M (1999). Unitary Ca^{2+} current through cardiac ryanodine receptor channels under quasi-physiological ionic conditions. *J Gen Physiol*, *113*: 177-186.

734. Mercadier JJ, Lompre AM, Duc P, Boheler KR, Fraysse JB, Wisnewsky C, Allen PD, Komajda M, Schwartz K (1990). Altered sarcoplasmic reticulum Ca^{2+}-ATPase gene expression in the human ventricle during end-stage heart failure. *J Clin Invest*, *85*: 305-309.

735. Mialet J, Berque-Bestel I, Eftekhari P, Gastineau M, Giner M, Dahmoune Y, Donzeau-Gouge P, Hoebeke J, Langlois M, Sicsic S, Fischmeister R, Lezoualc'h F (2000). Isolation of the serotoninergic 5-HT4(e) receptor from human heart and comparative analysis of its pharmacological profile in C6-glial and CHO cell lines. *Br J Pharmacol*, *129*: 771-781.

736. Middleton LM, Harvey RD (1998). PKC regulation of cardiac CFTR Cl⁻ channel function in guinea pig ventricular myocytes. *Am J Physiol, 275*: C293-302.

737. Mihailidou AS, Buhagiar KA, Rasmussen HH (1998). Na⁺ influx and Na⁺-K⁺ pump activation during short-term exposure of cardiac myocytes to aldosterone. *Am J Physiol, 274*: C175-181.

738. Mihailidou AS, Bundgaard H, Mardini M, Hansen PS, Kjeldsen K, Rasmussen HH (2000). Hyperaldosteronemia in rabbits inhibits the cardiac sarcolemmal Na⁺- K⁺ pump. *Circ Res, 86*: 37-42.

739. Mikoshiba K (1997). The InsP3 receptor and intracellular Ca²⁺ signaling. *Curr Opin Neurobiol, 7*: 339-345.

740. Mines GR (1913). On dynamic equilibrium in the heart. *J Physiol (Lond), 46*: 349-383.

741. Mishra SK, Hermsmeyer K (1994). Selective inhibition of T-type Ca²⁺ channels by Ro 40-5967. *Circ Res, 75*: 144-148.

742. Missiaen L, Robberecht W, van den Bosch L, Callewaert G, Parys JB, Wuytack F, Raeymaekers L, Nilius B, Eggermont J, De Smedt H (2000). Abnormal intracellular Ca²⁺ homeostasis and disease. *Cell Calcium, 28*: 1-21.

743. Mitcheson JS, Chen J, Lin M, Culberson C, Sanguinetti MC (2000). A structural basis for drug-induced long QT syndrome. *Proc Natl Acad Sci USA, 97*: 12329-12333.

744. Mitcheson JS, Hancox JC (1999). Characteristics of a transient outward current (sensitive to 4-aminopyridine) in Ca²⁺-tolerant myocytes isolated from the rabbit atrioventricular node. *Pflügers Archiv, 438*: 68-78.

745. Mitcheson JS, Hancox JC (1999). An investigation of the role played by the E-4031-sensitive (rapid delayed rectifier) potassium current in isolated rabbit atrioventricular nodal and ventricular myocytes. *Pflügers Archiv, 438*: 843-850.

746. Mitcheson JS, Sanguinetti MC (1999). Biophysical properties and molecular basis of cardiac rapid and slow delayed rectifier potassium channels. *Cell Physiol Biochem, 9*: 201-216.

747. Mitsuiye T, Noma A (1992). Exponential activation of the cardiac Na⁺ current in single guinea-pig ventricular cells. *J Physiol (Lond), 453*: 261-277.

748. Mitsuiye T, Shinagawa Y, Noma A (2000). Sustained inward current during pacemaker depolarization in mammalian sinoatrial node cells. *Circ Res, 87*: 88-91.

749. Miyata H, Lakatta EG, Stern MD, Silverman HS (1992). Relation of mitochondrial and cytosolic free calcium to cardiac myocyte recovery after exposure to anoxia. *Circ Res, 71*: 605-613.

750. Miyata H, Silverman HS, Sollott SJ, Lakatta EG, Stern MD, Hansford RG (1991). Measurement of mitochondrial free Ca²⁺ concentration in living single rat cardiac myocytes. *Am J Physiol, 261*: H1123-1134.

751. Mogul DJ, Singer DH, Ten Eick RE (1990). Dependence of Na-K pump current on internal Na⁺ in mammalian cardiac myocytes. *Am J Physiol, 259*: H488-496.

752. Moller JV, Juul B, le Maire M (1996). Structural organization, ion transport, and energy transduction of P- type ATPases. *Biochim Biophys Acta, 1286*: 1-51.

753. Moosmang S, Stieber J, Zong X, Biel M, Hofmann F, Ludwig A (2001). Cellular expression and functional characterization of four hyperpolarization-activated pacemaker channels in cardiac and neuronal tissues. *Eur J Biochem, 268*: 1646-1652.

754. Morad M, Ebashi S, Trautwein W, Kurachi Y (1996). Molecular physiology and pharmacology of cardiac ion channels and transporters. Kluwer Academic Publishers, Dordrecht.

755. Moreno AP, Fishman GI, Spray DC (1992). Phosphorylation shifts unitary conductance and modifies voltage dependent kinetics of human connexin43 gap junction channels. *Biophys J, 62*: 51-53.

756. Moreno AP, Rook MB, Fishman GI, Spray DC (1994). Gap junction channels: distinct voltage-sensitive and -insensitive conductance states. *Biophys J, 67*: 113-119.

757. Morgan JM, Cunningham D, Rowland E (1992). Electrical restitution in the endocardium of the intact human right ventricle. *Br Heart J, 67*: 42-46.

758. Morita H, Kimura J, Endoh M (1995). Angiotensin II activation of a chloride current in rabbit cardiac myocytes. *J Physiol (Lond), 483*: 119-130.

759. Morley GE, Jalife J (2000). Cardiac gap junction remodeling by stretch: is it a good thing? *Circ Res, 87*: 272-274.

760. Morley GE, Vaidya D, Samie FH, Lo C, Delmar M, Jalife J (1999). Characterization of conduction in the ventricles of normal and heterozygous Cx43 knockout mice using optical mapping. *J Cardiovasc Electrophysiol, 10*: 1361-1375.

761. Moroni A, Barbuti A, Altomare C, Viscomi C, Morgan J, Baruscotti M, DiFrancesco D (2000). Kinetic and ionic properties of the human HCN2 pacemaker channel. *Pflügers Archiv, 439*: 618-626.

762. Morris AJ, Malbon CC (1999). Physiological regulation of G protein-linked signaling. *Physiol Rev, 79*: 1373-1854.

763. Moschella MC, Marks AR (1993). Inositol 1,4,5-trisphosphate receptor expression in cardiac myocytes. *J Cell Biol, 120*: 1137-1146.

764. Mubagwa K (1995). Sarcoplasmic reticulum function during myocardial ischaemia and reperfusion. *Cardiovasc Res, 30*: 166-175.

765. Mubagwa K, Carmeliet E (1983). Effects of acetylcholine on electrophysiological properties of rabbit cardiac Purkinje fibers. *Circ Res, 53*: 740-751.

766. Mubagwa K, Flameng W, Carmeliet E (1994). Resting and action potentials of nonischemic and chronically ischemic human ventricular muscle. *J Cardiovasc Electrophysiol, 5*: 659-671.

767. Munch G, Bolck B, Sugaru A, Brixius K, Bloch W, Schwinger RHG (2001). Increased expression of isoform 1 of the sarcoplasmic reticulum Ca^{2+}-release channel in failing human heart. *Circulation, 103*: 2739-2744.

768. Munk AA, Adjemian RA, Zhao J, Ogbaghebriel A, Shrier A (1996). Electrophysiological properties of morphologically distinct cells isolated from the rabbit atrioventricular node. *J Physiol (Lond), 493*: 801-818.

769. Murphy JG, Marsh JD, Smith TW (1987). The role of calcium in ischemic myocardial injury. *Circulation, 75*: V15-24.

770. Murry CE, Jennings RB, Reimer KA (1986). Preconditioning with ischemia: a delay of lethal cell injury in ischemic myocardium. *Circulation, 74*: 1124-1136.

771. Murry CE, Richard VJ, Reimer KA, Jennings RB (1990). Ischemic preconditioning slows energy metabolism and delays ultrastructural damage during a sustained ischemic episode. *Circ Res, 66*: 913-931.

772. Nabauer M, Beuckelmann DJ, Uberfuhr P, Steinbeck G (1996). Regional differences in current density and rate-dependent properties of the transient outward current in subepicardial and subendocardial myocytes of human left ventricle. *Circulation, 93*: 168-177.

773. Nagasaki M, Ye L, Duan D, Horowitz B, Hume JR (2000). Intracellular cyclic AMP inhibits native and recombinant volume-regulated chloride channels from mammalian heart. *J Physiol (Lond), 523 Pt 3*: 705-717.

774. Nagashima M, Tohse N, Kimura K, Yamada Y, Fujii N, Yabu H (2001). Alternation of inwardly rectifying background K$^+$ channel during development of rat fetal cardiomyocytes. *J Mol Cell Cardiol, 33*: 533-543.

775. Nagatomo T, January CT, Makielski JC (2000). Preferential block of late sodium current in the LQT3 DeltaKPQ mutant by the class IC antiarrhythmic flecainide. *Mol Pharmacol, 57*: 101-107.

776. Nagaya N, Nishikimi T, Goto Y, Miyao Y, Kobayashi Y, Morii I, Daikoku S, Matsumoto T, Miyazaki S, Matsuoka H, Takishita S, Kangawa K, Matsuo H, Nonogi H (1998). Plasma brain natriuretic peptide is a biochemical marker for the prediction of progressive ventricular remodeling after acute myocardial infarction. *Am Heart J, 135*: 21-28.

777. Nagel G, Hwang TC, Nastiuk KL, Nairn AC, Gadsby DC (1992). The protein kinase A-regulated cardiac Cl$^-$ channel resembles the cystic fibrosis transmembrane conductance regulator. *Nature, 360*: 81-84.

778. Nakai J, Imagawa T, Hakamat Y, Shigekawa M, Takeshima H, Numa S (1990). Primary structure and functional expression from cDNA of the cardiac ryanodine receptor/calcium release channel. *FEBS Lett, 271*: 169-177.

779. Nakajima T, Iwasawa K, Oonuma H, Morita T, Goto A, Wang Y, Hazama H (1999). Antiarrhythmic effect and its underlying ionic mechanism of 17beta-estradiol in cardiac myocytes. *Br J Pharmacol, 127*: 429-440.

780. Nakamura TY, Lee K, Artman M, Rudy B, Coetzee WA (1999). The role of Kir2.1 in the genesis of native cardiac inward-rectifier K$^+$ currents during pre- and postnatal development. *Ann N Y Acad Sci, 868*: 434-437.

781. Nakao M, Gadsby DC (1986). Voltage dependence of Na translocation by the Na/K pump. *Nature, 323*: 628-630.

782. Nakao M, Gadsby DC (1989). [Na] and [K] dependence of the Na/K pump current-voltage relationship in guinea pig ventricular myocytes. *J Gen Physiol, 94*: 539-565.

783. Nakashima H, Kumagai K, Urata H, Gondo N, Ideishi M, Arakawa K (2000). Angiotensin II antagonist prevents electrical remodeling in atrial fibrillation. *Circulation, 101*: 2612-2617.

784. Nakaya H, Takeda Y, Tohse N, Kanno M (1992). Mechanism of the membrane depolarization induced by oxidative stress in guinea-pig ventricular cells. *J Mol Cell Cardiol, 24*: 523-534.

785. Nakayama T, Fozzard HA (1988). Adrenergic modulation of the transient outward current in isolated canine Purkinje cells. *Circ Res, 62*: 162-172.

786. Napolitano C, Priori SG, Schwartz PJ (2000). Significance of QT dispersion in the long QT syndrome. *Prog Cardiovasc Dis, 42*: 345-350.

787. Napolitano C, Schwartz PJ, Brown AM, Ronchetti E, Bianchi L, Pinnavaia A, Acquaro G, Priori SG (2000). Evidence for a cardiac ion channel mutation underlying drug-induced QT prolongation and life-threatening arrhythmias. *J Cardiovasc Electrophysiol, 11*: 691-696.

788. Nargeot J (2000). A Tale of Two (Calcium) Channels. *Circ Res, 86*: 613-615.

789. Nattel S, Bourne G, Talajic M (1997). Insights into mechanisms of antiarrhythmic drug action from experimental models of atrial fibrillation. *J Cardiovasc Electrophysiol, 8*: 469-480.

790. Nattel S, Li D (2000). I Ionic remodeling in the heart: pathophysiological significance and new therapeutic opportunities for atrial fibrillation. *Circ Res, 87*: 440-447.

791. Nattel S, Li D, Yue L (2000). Basic mechanisms of atrial fibrillation--very new insights into very old ideas. *Annu Rev Physiol, 62*: 51-77.

792. Nattel S, Yue L, Wang Z (1999). Cardiac ultrarapid delayed rectifiers: a novel potassium current family o f functional similarity and molecular diversity. *Cell Physiol Biochem, 9*: 217-226.

793. Neely A, Olcese R, Baldelli P, Wei X, Birnbaumer L, Stefani E (1995). Dual activation of the cardiac Ca^{2+} channel alpha 1C-subunit and its modulation by the beta-subunit. *Am J Physiol, 268*: C732-740.

794. Neher E, Sakmann B (1985). Single-Channel Recording. Plenum Press, New York.

795. Neher E, Stevens CF (1977). Conductance fluctuations and ionic pores in membranes. *Annu Rev Biophys Bioeng, 6*: 345-381.

796. Nerbonne JM (2000). Molecular basis of functional voltage-gated K^+ channel diversity in the mammalian myocardium. *J Physiol (Lond), 525 Pt 2*: 285-298.

797. Newton GE, Adelman AG, Lima VC, Seidelin PH, Schampaert E, Parker JD (1997). Cardiac sympathetic activity in response to acute myocardial ischemia. *Am J Physiol, 272*: H2079-2084.

798. Nichols CG (1996). Properties of cardiac ATP-sensitive potassium channels. Kluwer Academic Publishers, Dordrecht.

799. Nichols CG, Ripoll C, Lederer WJ (1991). ATP-sensitive potassium channel modulation of the guinea pig ventricular action potential and contraction. *Circ Res, 68*: 280-287.

800. Niggli E (1999). Localized intracellular calcium signaling in muscle: calcium sparks and calcium quarks. *Annu Rev Physiol, 61*: 311-335.

801. Nilius B, Hess P, Lansman JB, Tsien RW (1985). A novel type of cardiac calcium channel in ventricular cells. *Nature, 316*: 443-446.

802. Nitta J, Furukawa T, Marumo F, Sawanobori T, Hiraoka M (1994). Subcellular mechanism for Ca^{2+}-dependent enhancement of delayed rectifier K^+ current in isolated membrane patches of guinea pig ventricular myocytes. *Circ Res, 74*: 96-104.

803. Noble D, LeGuennec JY, Winslow R (1996). Functional roles of sodium-calcium exchange in normal and abnormal cardiac rhythm. *Ann N Y Acad Sci, 779*: 480-488.

804. Noda T, Takaki H, Kurita T, Taguchi A, Suyama K, Aihara N, Kamakura S, Nakamura K, Ohe T, Towbin JA, Priori SG (2001). Differential response of dynamic ventricular repolarization to sympathetic stimulation in LQT1,LQT2 and LQT3 forms of congenital Long QT syndrome. *PACE, 24*: 589.

805. Noma A (1983). ATP-regulated K^+ channels in cardiac muscle. *Nature, 305*: 147-148.

806. Noma A (1996). Ionic mechanisms of the cardiac pacemaker potential. *Jpn Heart J, 37*: 673-682.

807. Noma A, Kotake H, Irisawa H (1980). Slow inward current and its role mediating the chronotropic effect of epinephrine in the rabbit sinoatrial node. *Pflügers Archiv, 388*: 1-9.

808. Noma A, Morad M, Irisawa H (1983). Does the "pacemaker current" generate the diastolic depolarization in the rabbit SA node cells? *Pflügers Archiv, 397*: 190-194.

809. Noma A, Nakayama T, Kurachi Y, Irisawa H (1984). Resting K conductances in pacemaker and non-pacemaker heart cells of the rabbit. *Jpn J Physiol, 34*: 245-254.

810. Noma A, Trautwein W (1978). Relaxation of the ACh-induced potassium current in the rabbit sinoatrial node cell. *Pflügers Archiv, 377*: 193-200.

811. Noma A, Tsuboi N (1987). Dependence of junctional conductance on proton, calcium and magnesium ions in cardiac paired cells of guinea-pig. *J Physiol (Lond), 382*: 193-211.

812. Nonner W, Catacuzzeno L, Eisenberg B (2000). Binding and selectivity in L-Type Calcium channels: a mean spherical approximation. *Biophys J, 79*: 1976-1992.

813. Nuss HB, Kaab S, Kass DA, Tomaselli GF, Marban E (1999). Cellular basis of ventricular arrhythmias and abnormal automaticity in heart failure. *Am J Physiol, 277*: H80-91.

814. Nuss HB, Kambouris NG, Marban E, Tomaselli GF, Balser JR (2000). Isoform-specific lidocaine block of sodium channels explained by differences in gating. *Biophys J, 78*: 200-210.

815. Nuyens D, Stengl M, Dugarmaa S, Rossenbacker T, Compernolle V, Rudy Y, Smits JF, Flameng W, Clancy CE, Moons L, Vos MA, Dewerchin M, Benndorf K, Collen D, Carmeliet E, Carmeliet P (2001). Sudden heart rate acceleration or premature beats in mice with a long-QT3 syndrome cause life-threatening arrhythmias: suppression by adrenergic agonists. *Submitted for publication.*

816. Nygren A, Fiset C, Firek L, Clark JW, Lindblad DS, Clark RB, Giles WR (1998). Mathematical model of an adult human atrial cell: the role of K^+ currents in repolarization. *Circ Res, 82*: 63-81.

817. Obayashi K, Horie M, Xie L-H, Tsuchiya K, Kubota A, Ishida H, S. S (1997). Angiotensin II inhibits protein kinase A-dependent chloride conductance in heart via pertussis toxin-sensitive G preoteins. *Circulation, 95*: 197-204.

818. Ogden D (1994). Microelectrode Techniques The Plymouth Workshop Handbook. The Company of Biologists Ltd, Cambridge.

819. Okamura M, Kakei M, Ichinari K, Miyamura A, Oketani N, Koriyama N, Tei C (2001). State-dependent modification of ATP-sensitive K^+ channels by phosphatidylinositol 4,5-bisphosphate. *Am J Physiol Cell Physiol, 280*: C303-308.

820. Okazaki Y, Kodama K, Sato H, Kitakaze M, Hirayama A, Mishima M, Hori M, Inoue M (1993). Attenuation of increased regional myocardial oxygen consumption during exercise as a major cause of warm-up phenomenon. *J Am Coll Cardiol, 21*: 1597-1604.

821. Ono K, Arita M (2001). Sodium channels. In: *Heart Physiology and Pathophysiology* (eds. N Sperelakis, Y Kurachi, A Terzic, MV Cohen), pp 229-246. Academic Press, San Diego.

822. Ono K, Ito H (1995). Role of rapidly activating delayed rectifier K^+ current in sinoatrial node pacemaker activity. *Am J Physiol, 269*: H453-462.

823. Ono K, Shibata S, Iijima T (2000). Properties of the delayed rectifier potassium current in porcine sino- atrial node cells. *J Physiol (Lond), 524 Pt 1*: 51-62.

824. Ono K, Shibata S, Iijima T (2000). Properties of the delayed rectifier potassium current in porcine sino-atrial node cells. *J Physiol (Lond), 524 Pt 1*: 51-62.

825. Ono K, Tsujimoto G, Sakamoto A, Eto K, Masaki T, Ozaki Y, Satake M (1994). Endothelin-A receptor mediates cardiac inhibition by regulating calcium and potassium currents. *Nature, 370*: 301-304.

826. Ono K, Yano M, Ohkusa T, Kohno M, Hisaoka T, Tanigawa T, Kobayashi S, Matsuzaki M (2000). Altered interaction of FKBP12.6 with ryanodine receptor as a cause of abnormal Ca^{2+} release in heart failure. *Cardiovasc Res, 48*: 323-331.

827. Ooie T, Takahashi N, Saikawa T, Iwao T, Hara M, Sakata T (2000). Suppression of cesium-induced ventricular tachyarrhythmias by atrial natriuretic peptide in rabbits. *J Card Fail, 6*: 250-256.

828. Opie LH (1998). Heart Physiology from Cell to Circulation. Lippincott-Raven, Philadelphia.

829. Opthof T, Coronel R, Vermeulen JT, Verberne HJ, van Capelle FJ, Janse MJ (1993). Dispersion of refractoriness in normal and ischaemic canine ventricle: effects of sympathetic stimulation. *Cardiovasc Res, 27*: 1954-1960.

830. Opthof T, Dekker LR, Coronel R, Vermeulen JT, van Capelle FJ, Janse MJ (1993). Interaction of sympathetic and parasympathetic nervous system on ventricular refractoriness assessed by local fibrillation intervals in the canine heart. *Cardiovasc Res*, *27*: 753-759.

831. O'Reilly JP, Wang SY, Kallen RG, Wang GK (1999). Comparison of slow inactivation in human heart and rat skeletal muscle Na^+ channel chimaeras. *J Physiol (Lond)*, *515*: 61-73.

832. Orlic D, Kajstura J, Chimenti S, Jakoniuk I, Anderson SM, Li B, Pickel J, McKay R, Nadal-Ginard B, Bodine DM, Leri A, Anversa P (2001). Bone marrow cells regenerate infarcted myocardium. *Nature*, *410*: 701-705.

833. O'Rourke B (2000). Myocardial K(ATP) channels in preconditioning. *Circ Res*, *87*: 845-855.

834. O'Rourke B, Kass DA, Tomaselli GF, Kaab S, Tunin R, Marban E (1999). Mechanisms of altered excitation-contraction coupling in canine tachycardia-induced heart failure, I: experimental studies. *Circ Res*, *84*: 562-570.

835. Otsu K, Willard HF, Khanna VK, Zorzato F, Green NM, MacLennan DH (1990). Molecular cloning of cDNA encoding the Ca^{2+} release channel (ryanodine receptor) of rabbit cardiac muscle sarcoplasmic reticulum. *J Biol Chem*, *265*: 13472-13483.

836. Pacher P, Magyar J, Szigligeti P, Banyasz T, Pankucsi C, Korom Z, Ungvari Z, Kecskemeti V, Nanasi PP (2000). Electrophysiological effects of fluoxetine in mammalian cardiac tissues. *Naunyn Schmiedebergs Arch Pharmacol*, *361*: 67-73.

837. Pachucki J, Burmeister LA, Larsen PR (1999). Thyroid hormone regulates hyperpolarization-activated cyclic nucleotide-gated channel (HCN2) mRNA in the rat heart. *Circ Res*, *85*: 498-503.

838. Page E, Winterfield J, Goings G, Bastawrous A, Upshaw Earley J (1998). Water channel proteins in rat cardiac myocyte caveolae: osmolarity-dependent reversible internalization. *Am J Physiol*, *274*: H1988-2000.

839. Pain T, Yang XM, Critz SD, Yue Y, Nakano A, Liu GS, Heusch G, Cohen MV, Downey JM (2000). Opening of mitochondrial K(ATP) channels triggers the preconditioned state by generating free radicals. *Circ Res*, *87*: 460-466.

840. Pappano AJ, Carmeliet EE (1979). Epinephrine and the pacemaking mechanism at plateau potentials in sheep cardiac Purkinje fibers. *Pflügers Archiv*, *382*: 17-26.

841. Parkes DG, Coghlan JP, Cooper EA, Routley M, McDougall JG, Scoggins BA (1994). Cardiovascular actions of atrial natriuretic factor in sheep with cardiac failure. *Am J Hypertens*, *7*: 905-912.

842. Parratt JR, Vegh A (1999). Coronary vascular endothelium-myocyte interactions in protection of the heart by ischaemic preconditioning. *J Physiol Pharmacol*, *50*: 509-524.

843. Pastore JM, Girouard SD, Laurita KR, Akar FG, Rosenbaum DS (1999). Mechanism linking T-wave alternans to the genesis of cardiac fibrillation. *Circulation*, *99*: 1385-1394.

844. Pastore JM, Rosenbaum DS (2000). Role of structural barriers in the mechanism of alternans-induced reentry. *Circ Res*, *87*: 1157-1164.

845. Patel AJ, Honore E (2001). Properties and modulation of mammalian 2P domain K^+ channels. *Trends Neurosci*, *24*: 339-346.

846. Patel JR, Coronado R, Moss RL (1995). Cardiac sarcoplasmic reticulum phosphorylation increases Ca^{2+} release induced by flash photolysis of nitr-5. *Circ Res*, *77*: 943-949.

847. Patel S, Joseph SK, Thomas AP (1999). Molecular properties of inositol 1,4,5-trisphosphate receptors. *Cell Calcium, 25*: 247-264.

848. Patlak JB, Ortiz M (1985). Slow currents through single sodium channels of the adult rat heart. *J Gen Physiol, 86*: 89-104.

849. Patten RD, Udelson JE, Konstam MA (1998). Ventricular remodeling and its prevention in the treatment of heart failure. *Curr Opin Cardiol, 13*: 162-167.

850. Payet MD, Rousseau E, Sauve R (1985). Single-channel analysis of a potassium inward rectifier in myocytes of newborn rat heart. *J Membr Biol, 86*: 79-88.

851. Perchenet L, Benardeau A, Ertel EA (2000). Pharmacological properties of Ca(V)3.2, a low voltage-activated Ca^{2+} channel cloned from human heart. *Naunyn Schmiedebergs Arch Pharmacol, 361*: 590-599.

852. Perez Garcia MT, Kamp TJ, Marban E (1995). Functional properties of cardiac L-type calcium channels transiently expressed in HEK293 cells. Roles of alpha 1 and beta subunits. *J Gen Physiol, 105*: 289-305.

853. Perez PJ, Ramos-Franco J, Fill M, Mignery GA (1997). Identification and functional reconstitution of the type 2 inositol 1,4,5-trisphosphate receptor from ventricular cardiac myocytes. *J Biol Chem, 272*: 23961-23969.

854. Perez-Reyes E, Cribbs LL, Daud A, Lacerda AE, Barclay J, Williamson MP, Fox M, Rees M, Lee JH (1998). Molecular characterization of a neuronal low-voltage-activated T-type calcium channel. *Nature, 391*: 896-900.

855. Pertsov AM, Davidenko JM, Salomonsz R, Baxter WT, Jalife J (1993). Spiral waves of excitation underlie reentrant activity in isolated cardiac muscle. *Circ Res, 72*: 631-650.

856. Peters NS (1995). Myocardial gap junction organization in ischemia and infarction. *Microsc Res Tech, 31*: 375-386.

857. Peters NS, Coromilas J, Severs NJ, Wit AL (1997). Disturbed connexin43 gap junction distribution correlates with the location of reentrant circuits in the epicardial border zone of healing canine infarcts that cause ventricular tachycardia. *Circulation, 95*: 988-996.

858. Peters NS, Green CR, Poole Wilson PA, Severs NJ (1993). Reduced content of connexin43 gap junctions in ventricular myocardium from hypertrophied and ischemic human hearts. *Circulation, 88*: 864-875.

859. Peters NS, Wit AL (1998). Myocardial architecture and ventricular arrhythmogenesis. *Circulation, 97*: 1746-1754.

860. Petersen KR, Nerbonne JM (1999). Expression environment determines K^+ current properties: Kv1 and Kv4 alpha-subunit-induced K^+ currents in mammalian cell lines and cardiac myocytes. *Pflügers Archiv, 437*: 381-392.

861. Philipson KD, Bersohn MM, Nishimoto AY (1982). Effects of pH on Na^+-Ca^{2+} exchange in canine cardiac sarcolemmal vesicles. *Circ Res, 50*: 287-293.

862. Philipson KD, Nicoll DA (2000). Sodium-Calcium exchange: A molecular perspective. *Annu Rev Physiol, 62*: 111-133.

863. Piacentino V, Dipla K, Gaughan JP, Houser SR (2000). Voltage-dependent Ca^{2+} release from the SR of feline ventricular myocytes is explained by Ca^{2+}-induced Ca^{2+} release. *J Physiol (Lond), 523 Pt 3*: 533-548.

864. Pietrobon D, Hess P (1990). Novel mechanism of voltage-dependent gating in L-type calcium channels. *Nature, 346*: 651-655.

865. Pike MM, Luo CS, Clark MD, Kirk KA, Kitakaze M, Madden MC, Cragoe EJ, Jr., Pohost GM (1993). NMR measurements of Na^+ and cellular energy in ischemic rat heart: role of Na^+-H^+ exchange. *Am J Physiol, 265*: H2017-2026.

866. Pike MM, Luo CS, Yanagida S, Hageman GR, Anderson PG (1995). 23Na and 31P nuclear magnetic resonance studies of ischemia-induced ventricular fibrillation. Alterations of intracellular Na^+ and cellular energy. *Circ Res, 77*: 394-406.

867. Pino R, Cerbai E, Calamai G, Alajmo F, Borgioli A, Braconi L, Cassai M, Montesi GF, Mugelli A (1998). Effect of 5-HT4 receptor stimulation on the pacemaker current I_f in human isolated atrial myocytes. *Cardiovasc Res, 40*: 516-522.

868. Pinter A, Dorian P (2001). Intravenous antiarrhythmic agents. *Curr Opin Cardiol, 16*: 17-22.

869. Pinto JM, Boyden PA (1999). Electrical remodeling in ischemia and infarction. *Cardiovasc Res, 42*: 284-297.

870. Pinto JM, Sosunov EA, Gainullin RZ, Rosen MR, Boyden PA (1999). Effects of mibefradil, a T-type calcium current antagonist, on electrophysiology of Purkinje fibers that survived in the infarcted canine heart. *J Cardiovasc Electrophysiol, 10*: 1224-1235.

871. Pinto JM, Yuan F, Wasserlauf BJ, Bassett AL, Myerburg RJ (1997). Regional gradation of L-type calcium currents in the feline heart with a healed myocardial infarct. *J Cardiovasc Electrophysiol, 8*: 548-560.

872. Piot C, Lemaire S, Albat B, Seguin J, Nargeot J, Richard S (1996). High frequency-induced upregulation of human cardiac calcium currents. *Circulation, 93*: 120-128.

873. Piper HM, Das A (1987). Detrimental actions of endogenous fatty acids and their derivatives. A study of ischaemic mitochondrial injury. *Basic Res Cardiol, 1*: 187-196.

874. Piper HM, Noll T, Siegmund B (1994). Mitochondrial function in the oxygen depleted and reoxygenated myocardial cell. *Cardiovasc Res, 28*: 1-15.

875. Pitt B, Poole-Wilson PA, Segal R, Martinez FA, Dickstein K, Camm AJ, Konstam MA, Riegger G, Klinger GH, Neaton J, Sharma D, Thiyagarajan B (2000). Effect of losartan compared with captopril on mortality in patients with symptomatic heart failure: randomised trial--the Losartan Heart Failure Survival Study ELITE II. *Lancet, 355*: 1582-1587.

876. Pitt B, Zannad F, Remme WJ, Cody R, Castaigne A, Perez A, Palensky J, Wittes J (1999). The effect of spironolactone on morbidity and mortality in patients with severe heart failure. Randomized Aldactone Evaluation Study Investigators. *N Engl J Med, 341*: 709-717.

877. Plonsey R, Rudy Y (1980). Electrocardiogram sources in a 2-dimensional anisotropic activation model. *Med Biol Eng Comput, 18*: 87-94.

878. Poggioli J, Sulpice JC, Vassort G (1986). Inositol phosphate production following alpha 1-adrenergic, muscarinic or electrical stimulation in isolated rat heart. *FEBS Lett, 206*: 292-298.

879. Pogwizd SM, Corr PB (1987). Electrophysiologic mechanisms underlying arrhythmias due to reperfusion of ischemic myocardium. *Circulation, 76*: 404-426.

880. Pogwizd SM, Corr PB (1987). Reentrant and nonreentrant mechanisms contribute to arrhythmogenesis during early myocardial ischemia: results using three-dimensional mapping. *Circ Res, 61*: 352-371.

881. Pogwizd SM, Qi M, Yuan W, Samarel AM, Bers DM (1999). Upregulation of Na^+/Ca^{2+} exchanger expression and function in an arrhythmogenic rabbit model of heart failure. *Circ Res, 85*: 1009-1019.

882. Pogwizd SM, Schlotthauer K, Li L, Yuan W, Bers DM (2001). Arrhythmogenesis and contractile dysfunction in heart failure : Roles of Sodium-Calcium exchange, inward rectifier Potassium current, and residual {beta}-adrenergic responsiveness. *Circ Res, 88*: 1159-1167.

883. Porciatti F, Pelzmann B, Cerbai E, Schaffer P, Pino R, Bernhart E, Koidl B, Mugelli A (1997). The pacemaker current I_f in single human atrial myocytes and the effect of beta-adrenoceptor and A1-adenosine receptor stimulation. *Br J Pharmacol, 122*: 963-969.

884. Potet F, Scott JD, Mohammad-Panah R, Escande D, Baro II (2001). AKAP proteins anchor cAMP-dependent protein kinase to KvLQT1/IsK channel complex. *Am J Physiol Heart Circ Physiol, 280*: H2038-H2045.

885. Powers MJ, Peterson BA, Hardwick JC (2001). Regulation of parasympathetic neurons by mast cells and histamine in the guinea pig heart. *Auton Neurosci, 87*: 37-45.

886. Prestle J, Janssen PML, Janssen AP, Zeitz O, Lehnart SE, Bruce L, Smith GL, Hasenfuss G (2001). Overexpression of FK506-binding protein FKBP12.6 in cardiomyocytes reduces ryanodine receptor-mediated Ca^{2+} leak from the sarcoplasmic reticulum and increases contractility. *Circ Res, 88*: 188-194.

887. Priebe L, Beuckelmann DJ (1998). Simulation study of cellular electric properties in heart failure. *Circ Res, 82*: 1206-1223.

888. Priebe L, Friedrich M, Benndorf K (1996). Functional interaction between K_{ATP} channels and the Na^+-K^+ pump in metabolically inhibited heart cells of the guinea-pig. *J Physiol (Lond), 492*: 405-417.

889. Priori SG, Napolitano C, Cantu F, Brown AM, Schwartz PJ (1996). Differential response to Na^+ channel blockade, beta-adrenergic stimulation, and rapid pacing in a cellular model mimicking the SCN5A and HERG defects present in the long-QT syndrome. *Circ Res, 78*: 1009-1015.

890. Priori SG, Napolitano C, Schwartz PJ, Bloise R, Crotti L, Ronchetti E (2000). The elusive link between LQT3 and Brugada syndrome: the role of flecainide challenge. *Circulation, 102*: 945-947.

891. Protas L, Shen JB, Pappano AJ (1998). Carbachol increases contractions and intracellular Ca^{++} transients in guinea pig ventricular myocytes. *J Pharmacol Exp Ther, 284*: 66-74.

892. Pu J, Boyden PA (1997). Alterations of Na^+ currents in myocytes from epicardial border zone of the infarcted heart. A possible ionic mechanism for reduced excitability and postrepolarization refractoriness. *Circ Res, 81*: 110-119.

893. Puglisi JL, Yuan W, Bassani JWM, Bers DM (1999). Ca^{2+} Influx through Ca^{2+} channels in rabbit ventricular myocytes during action potential clamp : influence of temperature. *Circ Res, 85*: 7e-16e.

894. Qin D, Zhang ZH, Caref EB, Boutjdir M, Jain P, el-Sherif N (1996). Cellular and ionic basis of arrhythmias in postinfarction remodeled ventricular myocardium. *Circ Res, 79*: 461-473.

895. Qu J, Barbuti A, Protas L, Santoro B, Cohen IS, Robinson RB (2001). HCN2 overexpression in newborn and adult ventricular myocytes : distinct effects on gating and excitability. *Circ Res, 89*: 8e-14.

896. Qu J, Cohen IS, Robinson RB (2000). Sympathetic innervation alters activation of pacemaker current I_f in rat ventricle. *J Physiol (Lond), 526 Pt 3*: 561-569.

897. Qu Y, Campbell DL, Strauss HC (1993). Modulation of L-type Ca^{2+} current by extracellular ATP in ferret isolated right ventricular myocytes. *J Physiol (Lond), 471*: 295-317.

898. Qu Y, Campbell DL, Whorton AR, Strauss HC (1993). Modulation of basal L-type Ca^{2+} current by adenosine in ferret isolated right ventricular myocytes. *J Physiol (Lond), 471*: 269-293.

899.   Radermacher M, Wagenknecht T, Grassucci R, Frank J, Inui M, Chadwick C, Fleischer
       S (1992). Cryo-EM of the native structure of the calcium release channel/ryanodine
       receptor from sarcoplasmic reticulum. *Biophys J, 61*: 936-940.
900.   Ramires FJ, Mansur A, Coelho O, Maranhao M, Gruppi CJ, Mady C, Ramires JA
       (2000). Effect of spironolactone on ventricular arrhythmias in congestive heart failure
       secondary to idiopathic dilated or to ischemic cardiomyopathy. *Am J Cardiol, 85*:
       1207-1211.
901.   Ramos-Franco J, Fill M, Mignery GA (1998). Isoform-specific function of single
       inositol 1,4,5-trisphosphate receptor channels. *Biophys J, 75*: 834-839.
902.   Rasmusson RL, Morales MJ, Wang S, Liu S, Campbell DL, Brahmajothi MV, Strauss
       HC (1998). Inactivation of voltage-gated cardiac K^+ channels. *Circ Res, 82*: 739-750.
903.   Ravens U, Wettwer E (1998). Electrophysiological aspects of changes in heart rate.
       Basic Res Cardiol, 93: 60-65.
904.   Reed TD, Babu GJ, Ji Y, Zilberman A, Ver Heyen M, Wuytack F, Periasamy M
       (2000). The expression of SR calcium transport ATPase and the Na^+/Ca^{2+} exchanger
       are antithetically regulated during mouse cardiac development and in
       hypo/hyperthyroidism. *J Mol Cell Cardiol, 32*: 453-464.
905.   Regitz-Zagrosek V, Fielitz J, Fleck E (1998). Myocardial angiotensin receptors in
       human hearts. *Basic Res Cardiol, 93*: 37-42.
906.   Reiffel JA (2000). Drug choices in the treatment of atrial fibrillation. *Am J Cardiol, 85*:
       12D-19D.
907.   Reiffel JA, Reiter MJ, Blitzer M (1998). Antiarrhythmic drugs and devices for the
       management of ventricular tachyarrhythmia in ischemic heart disease. *Am J Cardiol,
       82*: 31I-40I.
908.   Reimann F, Ashcroft FM (1999). Inwardly rectifying potassium channels. *Curr Opin
       Cell Biol, 11*: 503-508.
909.   Reinecke H, Vetter R, Drexler H (1997). Effects of alpha-adrenergic stimulation on the
       sarcolemmal Na^+/Ca^{2+}-exchanger in adult rat ventricular cardiocytes. *Cardiovasc Res,
       36*: 216-222.
910.   Remme WJ (1998). The sympathetic nervous system and ischaemic heart disease. *Eur
       Heart J, 19 Suppl F*: F62-71.
911.   Renaudon B, Lenfant J, Decressac S, Bois P (2000). Thyroid hormone increases the
       conductance density of f-channels in rabbit sino-atrial node cells. *Receptors Channels,
       7*: 1-8.
912.   Ribalet B, John SA, Weiss JN (2000). Regulation of cloned ATP-sensitive K channels
       by phosphorylation, MgADP, and phosphatidylinositol bisphosphate (PIP(2)): a study
       of channel rundown and reactivation. *J Gen Physiol, 116*: 391-410.
913.   Ribuot C, Godin D, Couture R, Regoli D, Nadeau R (1993). In vivo B2-receptor-
       mediated negative chronotropic effect of bradykinin in canine sinus node. *Am J
       Physiol, 265*: H876-879.
914.   Ricard P, Danilo P, Jr., Cohen IS, Burkhoff D, Rosen MR (1999). A role for the renin-
       angiotensin system in the evolution of cardiac memory. *J Cardiovasc Electrophysiol,
       10*: 545-551.
915.   Riccio ML, Koller ML, Gilmour RF, Jr. (1999). Electrical restitution and
       spatiotemporal organization during ventricular fibrillation. *Circ Res, 84*: 955-963.
916.   Rice WJ, Young HS, Martin DW, Sachs JR, Stokes DL (2001). Structure of Na^+,K^+-
       ATPase at 11-A resolution: comparison with Ca^{2+}- ATPase in E1 and E2 states.
       Biophys J, 80: 2187-2197.

917. Richard S, Leclercq F, Lemaire S, Piot C, Nargeot J (1998). Ca^{2+} currents in compensated hypertrophy and heart failure. *Cardiovasc Res, 37*: 300-311.

918. Richmond JE, Featherstone DE, Hartmann HA, Ruben PC (1998). Slow inactivation in human cardiac sodium channels. *Biophys J, 74*: 2945-2952.

919. Riordan JR, Rommens JM, Kerem B, Alon N, Rozmahel R, Grzelczak Z, Zielenski J, Lok S, Plavsic N, Chou JL, et al. (1989). Identification of the cystic fibrosis gene: cloning and characterization of complementary DNA. *Science, 245*: 1066-1073.

920. Robicsek F, Masters TN, Svenson RH, Daniel WG, Daugherty HK, Cook JW, Selle JG (1978). The application of thermography in the study of coronary blood flow. *Surgery, 84*: 858-864.

921. Robinson RB, Yu H, Chang F, Cohen IS (1997). Developmental change in the voltage-dependence of the pacemaker current, i_f, in rat ventricle cells. *Pflügers Archiv, 433*: 533-535.

922. Roden DM (2000). Acquired long QT syndromes and the risk of proarrhythmia. *J Cardiovasc Electrophysiol, 11*: 938-940.

923. Roden DM (2001). Pharmacogenetics and drug-induced arrhythmias. *Cardiovasc Res, 50*: 224-231.

924. Roden DM, George AL, Bennett PB (1995). Recent advances in understanding the molecular mechanisms of the long QT syndrome. *J Cardiovasc Electrophysiol, 6*: 1023-1031.

925. Roden DM, George AL, Jr. (1997). Structure and function of cardiac sodium and potassium channels. *Am J Physiol, 273*: H511-525.

926. Roden DM, Hoffman BF (1985). Action potential prolongation and induction of abnormal automaticity by low quinidine concentrations in canine Purkinje fibers. Relationship to potassium and cycle length. *Circ Res, 56*: 857-867.

927. Roden DM, Wilde AA (1999). Drug-induced J point elevation: a marker for genetic risk of sudden death or ECG curiosity? *J Cardiovasc Electrophysiol, 10*: 219-223.

928. Rodrigo GC (1993). The Na^+-dependence of Na^+-activated K^+-channels (IK(Na)) in guinea pig ventricular myocytes, is different in excised inside/out patches and cell attached patches. *Pflügers Archiv, 422*: 530-532.

929. Rohr S, Kucera JP (1997). Involvement of the calcium inward current in cardiac impulse propagation: induction of unidirectional conduction block by nifedipine and reversal by Bay K 8644. *Biophys J, 72*: 754-766.

930. Rohr S, Kucera JP, Fast VG, Kléber AG (1997). Paradoxical improvement of impulse conduction in cardiac tissue by partial cellular uncoupling. *Science, 275*: 841-844.

931. Rohr S, Kucera JP, Kléber AG (1998). Slow conduction in cardiac tissue, I: effects of a reduction of excitability versus a reduction of electrical coupling on microconduction. *Circ Res, 83*: 781-794.

932. Rook MB, Alshinawi CB, Groenewegen WA, van Gelder IC, van Ginneken AC, Jongsma HJ, Mannens MM, Wilde AA (1999). Human SCN5A gene mutations alter cardiac sodium channel kinetics and are associated with the Brugada syndrome. *Cardiovasc Res, 44*: 507-517.

933. Rosen MR, Bilezikian JP, Cohen IS, Robinson RB, Steinberg SF (1995). Alpha-adrenergic modulation of cardiac rhythm. In: *Cardiac electrophysiology From cell to bedside* (eds. DP.Zipes, J Jalife), pp 435-454. W.B.Saunders Company, Philadelphia.

934. Rosen MR, Cohen IS, Danilo P, Steinberg SF (1998). The heart remembers. *Cardiovasc Res, 40*: 469-482.

935. Rosenbaum MB, Blanco HH, Elizari MV, Lazzari JO, Davidenko JM (1982). Electrotonic modulation of the T wave and cardiac memory. *Am J Cardiol, 50*: 213-222.

936. Rosenberg RL, Hess P, Tsien RW (1988). Cardiac calcium channels in planar lipid bilayers. L-type channels and calcium-permeable channels open at negative membrane potentials. *J Gen Physiol, 92*: 27-54.

937. Rostovtseva T, Colombini M (1997). VDAC channels mediate and gate the flow of ATP: implications for the regulation of mitochondrial function. *Biophys J, 72*: 1954-1962.

938. Roth BJ (2000). Influence of a perfusing bath on the foot of the cardiac action potential. *Circ Res, 86*: 19e-22e.

939. Rousseau E (1989). Single chloride-selective channel from cardiac sarcoplasmic reticulum studied in planar lipid bilayers. *J Membr Biol, 110*: 39-47.

940. Rousseau E, Chabot H, Beaudry C, Muller B (1992). Reconstitution and regulation of cation-selective channels from cardiac sarcoplasmic reticulum. *Mol Cell Biochem, 114*: 109-117.

941. Rousseau E, Smith JS, Meissner G (1987). Ryanodine modifies conductance and gating behavior of single Ca^{2+} release channel. *Am J Physiol, 253*: C364-368.

942. Rozanski GJ, Jalife J, Moe GK (1984). Reflected reentry in nonhomogeneous ventricular muscle as a mechanism of cardiac arrhythmias. *Circulation, 69*: 163-173.

943. Rozanski GJ, Xu Z, Zhang K, Patel KP (1998). Altered K^+ current of ventricular myocytes in rats with chronic myocardial infarction. *Am J Physiol, 274*: H259-265.

944. Rubart M, Lopshire JC, Fineberg NS, Zipes DP (2000). Changes in left ventricular repolarization and ion channel currents following a transient rate increase superimposed on bradycardia in anesthetized dogs. *J Cardiovasc Electrophysiol, 11*: 652-664.

945. Rudy Y (1998). Cardiac conduction: an interplay between membrane and gap junction. *J Electrocardiol, 31 Suppl*: 1-5.

946. Rudy Y (2001). Electrocardiogram and Cardiac Excitation. In: *Heart Physiology and Pathophysiology* (eds. N Sperelakis, Y Kurachi, A Terzic, MV Cohen), pp 133-148. Academic Press, San Diego.

947. Rudy Y, Plonsey R (1980). A comparison of volume conductor and source geometry effects on body surface and epicardial potentials. *Circ Res, 46*: 283-291.

948. Rudy Y, Quan WL (1987). A model study of the effects of the discrete cellular structure on electrical propagation in cardiac tissue. *Circ Res, 61*: 815-823.

949. Rudy Y, Shaw RM (1997). Cardiac excitation: an interactive process of ion channels and gap junctions. *Adv Exp Med Biol, 430*: 269-279.

950. Ruppersberg JP (2000). Intracellular regulation of inward rectifier K^+ channels. *Pflügers Archiv, 441*: 1-11.

951. Rushton WAH (1937). Initiation of the propagated disturbance. *Proc R Soc Lond B Biol Sci, 124*: 201-243.

952. Rusz U, Englert H, Schölkens BA, Gögelein H (1996). Simultaneous recording of ATP-sensitive K^+ current and intracellular Ca^{2+} in anoxic rat ventricular myocytes. Effects of glibenclamide. *Pflügers Archiv, 432*: 75-80.

953. Sabri A, Muske G, Zhang H, Pak E, Darrow A, Andrade-Gordon P, Steinberg SF (2000). Signaling properties and functions of two distinct cardiomyocyte protease-activated receptors. *Circ Res, 86*: 1054-1061.

954. Saez JC, Spray DC, Nairn AC, Hertzberg E, Greengard P, Bennett MV (1986). cAMP increases junctional conductance and stimulates phosphorylation of the 27-kDa principal gap junction polypeptide. *Proc Natl Acad Sci USA, 83*: 2473-2477.

955. Saffitz JE (1999). Electrophysiologic remodeling: what happens to gap junctions? *J Cardiovasc Electrophysiol, 10*: 1684-1687.

956. Saffitz JE, Green KG, Kraft WJ, Schechtman KB, Yamada KA (2000). Effects of diminished expression of connexin43 on gap junction number and size in ventricular myocardium. *Am J Physiol, 278*: H1662-1670.

957. Saffitz JE, Laing JG, Yamada KA (2000). Connexin expression and turnover : implications for cardiac excitability. *Circ Res, 86*: 723-728.

958. Saffitz JE, Schuessler RB, Yamada KA (1999). Mechanisms of remodeling of gap junction distributions and the development of anatomic substrates of arrhythmias. *Cardiovasc Res, 42*: 309-317.

959. Saftenku E, Williams AJ, Sitsapesan R (2001). Markovian models of low and high activity levels of cardiac ryanodine receptors. *Biophys J, 80*: 2727-2714.

960. Sagnella GA (1998). Measurement and significance of circulating natriuretic peptides in cardiovascular disease. *Clin Sci (Colch), 95*: 519-529.

961. Sahu P, Lim PO, Rana BS, Struthers AD (2000). QT dispersion in medicine: electrophysiological holy grail or fool's gold? *QJM, 93*: 425-431.

962. Sakamoto N, Uemura H, Hara Y, Saito T, Masuda Y, Nakaya H (1998). Bradykinin B2-receptor-mediated modulation of membrane currents in guinea-pig cardiomyocytes. *Br J Pharmacol, 125*: 283-292.

963. Sakmann B, Spindler AJ, Bryant SM, Linz KW, Noble D (2000). Distribution of a persistent sodium current across the ventricular wall in guinea pigs. *Circ Res, 87*: 910-914.

964. Sakmann B, Trube G (1984). Conductance properties of single inwardly rectifying potassium channels in ventricular cells from guinea-pig heart. *J Physiol (Lond), 347*: 641-657.

965. Sakmann B, Trube G (1984). Voltage-dependent inactivation of inward-rectifying single-channel currents in the guinea-pig heart cell membrane. *J Physiol (Lond), 347*: 659-683.

966. Sanchez Chapula J, Elizalde A, Navarro Polanco R, Barajas H (1994). Differences in outward currents between neonatal and adult rabbit ventricular cells. *Am J Physiol, 266*: H1184-1194.

967. Sanguinetti MC (1990). Na_i-activated and ATP-sensitive K^+ channels in the heart. Alan R. Liss, Inc.

968. Sanguinetti MC, Curran ME, Zou A, Shen J, Spector PS, Atkinson DL, Keating MT (1996). Coassembly of K_vLQT1 and minK (IsK) proteins to form cardiac I_{ks} potassium channel. *Nature, 384*: 80-83.

969. Sanguinetti MC, Jiang C, Curran ME, Keating MT (1995). A mechanistic link between an inherited and an acquired cardiac arrhythmia: HERG encodes the IKr potassium channel. *Cell, 81*: 299-307.

970. Sanguinetti MC, Jurkiewicz NK (1990). Lanthanum blocks a specific component of IK and screens membrane surface change in cardiac cells. *Am J Physiol, 259*: H1881-1889.

971. Sanguinetti MC, Jurkiewicz NK (1990). Two components of cardiac delayed rectifier K^+ current. Differential sensitivity to block by class III antiarrhythmic agents. *J Gen Physiol, 96*: 195-215.

972.   Sanguinetti MC, Jurkiewicz NK (1992). Role of external Ca^{2+} and K^+ in gating of cardiac delayed rectifier K^+ currents. *Pflügers Archiv, 420*: 180-186.

973.   Sano T, Takayma N, Shimamoto T (1959). Directional influence of conduction velocity in cardiac ventricular syncytium studied by microelectrodes. *Circ Res, 7*: 262-267.

974.   Santana LF, Gomez AM, Lederer WJ (1998). Ca^{2+} flux through promiscuous cardiac Na^+ channels: slip-mode conductance. *Science, 279*: 1027-1033.

975.   Santoro B, Liu DT, Yao H, Bartsch D, Kandel ER, Siegelbaum SA, Tibbs GR (1998). Identification of a gene encoding a hyperpolarization-activated pacemaker channel of brain. *Cell, 93*: 717-729.

976.   Sato C, Ueno Y, Asai K, Takahashi K, Sato M, Engel A, Fujiyoshi Y (2001). The voltage-sensitive sodium channel is a bell-shaped molecule with several cavities. *Nature, 409*: 1048-1051.

977.   Sato N, Tanaka H, Habuchi Y, Giles WR (2000). Electrophysiological effects of ibutilide on the delayed rectifier K^+ current in rabbit sinoatrial and atrioventricular node cells. *Eur J Pharmacol, 404*: 281-288.

978.   Sato R, Koumi S (1995). Modulation of the inwardly rectifying K^+ channel in isolated human atrial myocytes by alpha 1-adrenergic stimulation. *J Membr Biol, 148*: 185-191.

979.   Sato T, Arita M, Kiyosue T (1993). Differential mechanism of block of palmitoyl lysophosphatidylcholine and of palmitoylcarnitine on inward rectifier K^+ channels of guinea-pig ventricular myocytes. *Cardiovasc Drugs Ther, 3*: 575-584.

980.   Sato T, O'Rourke B, Marban E (1998). Modulation of mitochondrial ATP-dependent K^+ channels by protein kinase C. *Circ Res, 83*: 110-114.

981.   Schaapherder AF, Schumacher CA, Coronel R, Fiolet JW (1990). Transmural inhomogeneity of extracellular $[K^+]$ and pH and myocardial energy metabolism in the isolated rat heart during acute global ischemia; dependence on gaseous environment. *Basic Res Cardiol, 85*: 33-44.

982.   Schackow TE, Ten Eick RE (1994). Enhancement of ATP-sensitive potassium current in cat ventricular myocytes by beta-adrenoreceptor stimulation. *J Physiol (Lond), 474*: 131-145.

983.   Schillinger W, Janssen PML, Emami S, Henderson SA, Ross RS, Teucher N, Zeitz O, Philipson KD, Prestle J, Hasenfuss G (2000). Impaired contractile performance of cultured rabbit ventricular myocytes after adenoviral gene transfer of Na^+-Ca^{2+} exchanger. *Circ Res, 87*: 581-539.

984.   Schlotthauer K, Bers DM (2000). Sarcoplasmic reticulum Ca^{2+} release causes myocyte depolarization. Underlying mechanism and threshold for triggered action potentials. *Circ Res, 87*: 774-780.

985.   Schnee JM, Hsueh WA (2000). Angiotensin II, adhesion, and cardiac fibrosis. *Cardiovasc Res, 46*: 264-268.

986.   Schomig A, Fischer S, Kurz T, Richardt G, Schomig E (1987). Nonexocytotic release of endogenous noradrenaline in the ischemic and anoxic rat heart: mechanism and metabolic requirements. *Circ Res, 60*: 194-205.

987.   Schomig A, Haass M, Richardt G (1991). Catecholamine release and arrhythmias in acute myocardial ischaemia. *Eur Heart J, 12*: 38-47.

988.   Schomig A, Richardt G, Kurz T (1995). Sympatho-adrenergic activation of the ischemic myocardium and its arrhythmogenic impact. *Herz, 20*: 169-186.

989.   Schott JJ, Alshinawi C, Kyndt F, Probst V, Hoorntje TM, Hulsbeek M, Wilde AA, Escande D, Mannens MM, Le Marec H (1999). Cardiac conduction defects associate with mutations in SCN5A. *Nat Genet, 23*: 20-21.

990. Schouten VJ, Morad M (1989). Regulation of Ca^{2+} current in frog ventricular myocytes by the holding potential, c-AMP and frequency. *Pflügers Archiv, 415*: 1-11.
991. Schreibmayer W (1999). Isoform diversity and modulation of sodium channels by protein kinases. *Cell Physiol Biochem, 9*: 187-200.
992. Schreieck J, Wang Y, Overbeck M, Schomig A, Schmitt C (2000). Altered transient outward current in human atrial myocytes of patients with reduced left ventricular function. *J Cardiovasc Electrophysiol, 11*: 180-192.
993. Schwartz PJ, Priori SG, Dumaine R, Napolitano C, Antzelevitch C, Stramba-Badiale M, Richard TA, Berti MR, Bloise R (2000). A molecular link between the sudden infant death syndrome and the long-QT syndrome. *N Engl J Med, 343*: 262-267.
994. Schwartz PJ, Priori SG, Locati EH, Napolitano C, Cantu F, Towbin JA, Keating MT, Hammoude H, Brown AM, Chen LS, et al. (1995). Long QT syndrome patients with mutations of the SCN5A and HERG genes have differential responses to Na^+ channel blockade and to increases in heart rate. Implications for gene-specific therapy. *Circulation, 92*: 3381-3386.
995. Schwartz PJ, Priori SG, Spazzolini C, Moss AJ, Vincent GM, Napolitano C, Denjoy I, Guicheney P, Breithardt G, Keating MT, Towbin JA, Beggs AH, Brink P, Wilde AA, Toivonen L, Zareba W, Robinson JL, Timothy KW, Corfield V, Wattanasirichaigoon D, Corbett C, Haverkamp W, Schulze-Bahr E, Lehmann MH, Schwartz K, Coumel P, Bloise R (2001). Genotype-phenotype correlation in the long-QT syndrome : gene-specific triggers for life-threatening arrhythmias. *Circulation , 103*: 89-95.
996. Schwartz PJ, Stramba-Badiale M, Segantini A, Austoni P, Bosi G, Giorgetti R, Grancini F, Marni ED, Perticone F, Rosti D, Salice P (1998). Prolongation of the QT interval and the sudden infant death syndrome. *N Engl J Med, 338*: 1709-1714.
997. Schwinger RH, Wang J, Frank K, Muller-Ehmsen J, Brixius K, McDonough AA, Erdmann E (1999). Reduced sodium pump alpha1, alpha3, and beta1-isoform protein levels and Na^+,K^+-ATPase activity but unchanged Na^+-Ca^{2+} exchanger protein levels in human heart failure. *Circulation, 99*: 2105-2112.
998. Sears SF, Todaro JF, Lewis TS, Sotile W, Conti JB (1999). Examining the psychosocial impact of implantable cardioverter defibrillators: a literature review. *Clin Cardiol, 22*: 481-489.
999. Seifert R, Scholten A, Gauss R, Mincheva A, Lichter P, Kaupp UB (1999). Molecular characterization of a slowly gating human hyperpolarization-activated channel predominantly expressed in thalamus, heart, and testis. *Proc Natl Acad Sci USA, 96*: 9391-9396.
1000. Seino S (1999). ATP-sensitive potassium channels: a model of heteromultimeric potassium channel/receptor assemblies. *Annu Rev Physiol, 61*: 337-362.
1001. Sesti F, Abbott GW, Wei J, Murray KT, Saksena S, Schwartz PJ, Priori SG, Roden DM, George AL, Goldstein SA (2000). A common polymorphism associated with antibiotic-induced cardiac arrhythmia. *Proc Natl Acad Sci USA, 97*: 10613-10618.
1002. Seyedi N, Maruyama R, Levi R (1999). Bradykinin activates a cross-signaling pathway between sensory and adrenergic nerve endings in the heart: a novel mechanism of ischemic norepinephrine release? *J Pharmacol Exp Ther, 290*: 656-663.
1003. Seyedi N, Win T, Lander HM, Levi R (1997). Bradykinin B2-receptor activation augments norepinephrine exocytosis from cardiac sympathetic nerve endings. Mediation by autocrine/paracrine mechanisms. *Circ Res, 81*: 774-784.
1004. Shander GS, Fan Z, Makielski JC (1995). Slowly recovering cardiac sodium current in rat ventricular myocytes: effects of conditioning duration and recovery potential. *J Cardiovasc Electrophysiol, 6*: 786-795.

1005. Shao Y, Pressley TA, Ismail-Beigi F (1999). Na,K-ATPase mRNA beta 1 expression in rat myocardium--effect of thyroid status. *Eur J Biochem*, *260*: 1-8.

1006. Sharma VK, Colecraft HM, Wang DX, Levey AI, Grigorenko EV, Yeh HH, Sheu S-S (1996). Molecular and functional identification of M1 muscarinic acetylcholine receptors in rat ventricular myocytes. *Circ Res*, *79*: 86-93.

1007. Shattock MJ, Matsuura H (1993). Measurement of Na^+-K^+ pump current in isolated rabbit ventricular myocytes using the whole-cell voltage-clamp technique. Inhibition of the pump by oxidant stress. *Circ Res*, *72*: 91-101.

1008. Shattock MJ, Matsuura H, Hearse DJ (1991). Functional and electrophysiological effects of oxidant stress on isolated ventricular muscle: a role for oscillatory calcium release from sarcoplasmic reticulum in arrhythmogenesis? *Cardiovasc Res*, *25*: 645-651.

1009. Shaw RM, Rudy Y (1995). The vulnerable window for unidirectional block in cardiac tissue: characterization and dependence on membrane excitability and intercellular coupling. *J Cardiovasc Electrophysiol*, *6*: 115-131.

1010. Shaw RM, Rudy Y (1997). Electrophysiologic effects of acute myocardial ischemia. A mechanistic investigation of action potential conduction and conduction failure. *Circ Res*, *80*: 124-138.

1011. Shaw RM, Rudy Y (1997). Ionic mechanisms of propagation in cardiac tissue. Roles of the sodium and L-type calcium currents during reduced excitability and decreased gap junction coupling. *Circ Res*, *81*: 727-741.

1012. Sheets MF, Scanley BE, Hanck DA, Makielski JC, Fozzard HA (1987). Open sodium channel properties of single canine cardiac Purkinje cells. *Biophys J*, *52*: 13-22.

1013. Shen JB, Pappano AJ (1995). Palmitoyl-L-carnitine acts like ouabain on voltage, current, and contraction in guinea pig ventricular cells. *Am J Physiol*, *268*: H1027-1036.

1014. Sheridan DJ, Penkoske PA, Sobel BE, Corr PB (1980). Alpha adrenergic contributions to dysrhythmia during myocardial ischemia and reperfusion in cats. *J Clin Invest*, *65*: 161-171.

1015. Shi W, Wymore R, Yu H, Wu J, Wymore RT, Pan Z, Robinson RB, Dixon JE, McKinnon D, Cohen IS (1999). Distribution and prevalence of hyperpolarization-activated cation channel (HCN) mRNA expression in cardiac tissues. *Circ Res*, *85*: e1-6.

1016. Shibasaki T (1987). Conductance and kinetics of delayed rectifier potassium channels in nodal cells of the rabbit heart. *J Physiol (Lond)*, *387*: 227-250.

1017. Shibata EF, Drury T, Refsum H, Aldrete V, Giles W (1989). Contributions of a transient outward current to repolarization in human atrium. *Am J Physiol*, *257*: H1773-1781.

1018. Shieh BH, Xia Y, Sparkes RS, Klisak I, Lusis AJ, Nicoll DA, Philipson KD (1992). Mapping of the gene for the cardiac sarcolemmal Na^+-Ca^{2+} exchanger to human chromosome 2p21-p23. *Genomics*, *12*: 616-617.

1019. Shigekawa M, Iwamoto T (2001). Cardiac Na^+-Ca^{2+} exchange : molecular and pharmacological aspects. *Circ Res*, *88*: 864-876.

1020. Shigematsu S, Maruyama T, Kiyosue T, Arita M (1994). Rate-dependent prolongation of action potential duration in single ventricular myocytes obtained from hearts of rats with streptozotocin-induced chronic diabetes sustained for 30-32 weeks. *Heart Vessels*, *9*: 300-306.

1021. Shimizu W, Antzelevitch C (1998). Cellular basis for the ECG features of the LQT1 form of the long-QT syndrome: effects of beta-adrenergic agonists and antagonists and sodium channel blockers on transmural dispersion of repolarization and torsade de pointes. *Circulation, 98*: 2314-2322.

1022. Shimizu W, Antzelevitch C (1999). Cellular and ionic basis for T-wave alternans under long-QT conditions. *Circulation, 99*: 1499-1507.

1023. Shimizu W, Antzelevitch C (1999). Cellular basis for long QT, transmural dispersion of repolarization, and torsade de pointes in the long QT syndrome. *J Electrocardiol, 32 Suppl*: 177-184.

1024. Shimizu W, Antzelevitch C (2000). Differential effects of beta-adrenergic agonists and antagonists in LQT1, LQT2 and LQT3 models of the long QT syndrome. *J Am Coll Cardiol, 35*: 778-786.

1025. Shimoni Y (1999). Protein kinase C regulation of K^+ currents in rat ventricular myocytes and its modification by hormonal status. *J Physiol (Lond), 520 Pt 2*: 439-449.

1026. Shimoni Y, Clark RB, Giles WR (1992). Role of an inwardly rectifying potassium current in rabbit ventricular action potential. *J Physiol (Lond), 448*: 709-727.

1027. Shimoni Y, Ewart HS, Severson D (1998). Type I and II models of diabetes produce different modifications of K^+ currents in rat heart: role of insulin. *J Physiol (Lond), 507*: 485-496.

1028. Shimoni Y, Ewart HS, Severson D (1999). Insulin stimulation of rat ventricular K^+ currents depends on the integrity of the cytoskeleton. *J Physiol (Lond), 514*: 735-745.

1029. Shimoni Y, Severson DL (1995). Thyroid status and potassium currents in rat ventricular myocytes. *Am J Physiol, 268*: H576-583.

1030. Shin KS, Rothberg BS, Yellen G (2001). Blocker state dependence and trapping in hyperpolarization-activated cation channels. Evidence for an intracellular activation gate. *J Gen Physiol, 117*: 91-102.

1031. Shinagawa Y, Satoh H, Noma A (2000). The sustained inward current and inward rectifier K^+ current in pacemaker cells dissociated from rat sinoatrial node. *J Physiol (Lond), 523 Pt 3*: 593-605.

1032. Shipsey SJ, Bryant SM, Hart G (1997). Effects of hypertrophy on regional action potential characteristics in the rat left ventricle: a cellular basis for T-wave inversion? *Circulation, 96*: 2061-2068.

1033. Shontz RD, Xu Z, Patel KP, Rozanski GJ (2001). Inhibition of K^+ currents by homocysteine in rat ventricular myocytes. *J Cardiovasc Electrophysiol, 12*: 175-182.

1034. Shorofsky SR, Balke CW (2001). Calcium currents and arrhythmias: insights from molecular biology. *Am J Med, 110*: 127-140.

1035. Shorofsky SR, January CT (1992). L- and T-type Ca^{2+} channels in canine cardiac Purkinje cells. Single-channel demonstration of L-type Ca^{2+} window current. *Circ Res, 70*: 456-464.

1036. Shuba YM, Hesslinger B, Trautwein W, McDonald TF, Pelzer D (1990). Whole-cell calcium current in guinea-pig ventricular myocytes dialysed with guanine nucleotides. *J Physiol (Lond), 424*: 205-228.

1037. Shvilkin A, Danilo P, Chevalier P, Chang F, Cohen IS, Rosen MR (1994). Vagal release of vasoactive intestinal peptide can promote vagotonic tachycardia in the isolated innervated rat heart. *Cardiovasc Res, 28*: 1769-1773.

1038. Shvilkin A, Danilo P, Wang J, Burkhoff D, Anyukhovsky EP, Sosunov EA, Hara M, Rosen MR (1998). Evolution and resolution of long-term cardiac memory. *Circulation, 97*: 1810-1817.

1039. Sicouri S, Antzelevitch C (1991). A subpopulation of cells with unique electrophysiological properties in the deep subepicardium of the canine ventricle. The M cell. *Circ Res*, *68*: 1729-1741.

1040. Sicouri S, Antzelevitch C (1993). Drug-induced afterdepolarizations and triggered activity occur in a discrete subpopulation of ventricular muscle cells (M cells) in the canine heart: quinidine and digitalis. *J Cardiovasc Electrophysiol*, *4*: 48-58.

1041. Siegmund B, Zude R, Piper HM (1992). Recovery of anoxic-reoxygenated cardiomyocytes from severe Ca^{2+} overload. *Am J Physiol*, *263*: H1262-1269.

1042. Sigworth FJ (1980). The variance of sodium current fluctuations at the node of Ranvier. *J Physiol (Lond)*, *307*: 97-129.

1043. Sigworth FJ, Sine SM (1987). Data transformations for improved display and fitting of single-channel dwell time histograms. *Biophys J*, *52*: 1047-1054.

1044. Simon AM, Goodenough DA (1998). Diverse functions of vertebrate gap junctions. *Trends Cell Biol*, *8*: 477-483.

1045. Sipido KR (2000). Local Ca^{2+} release in heart failure: timing is important. *Circ Res*, *87*: 966-968.

1046. Sipido KR, Callewaert G, Carmeliet E (1993). $[Ca^{2+}]_i$ transients and $[Ca^{2+}]_i$-dependent chloride current in single Purkinje cells from rabbit heart. *J Physiol (Lond)*, *468*: 641-667.

1047. Sipido KR, Callewaert G, Carmeliet E (1995). Inhibition and rapid recovery of Ca^{2+} current during Ca^{2+} release from sarcoplasmic reticulum in guinea pig ventricular myocytes. *Circ Res*, *76*: 102-109.

1048. Sipido KR, Callewaert G, Porciatti F, Vereecke J, Carmeliet E (1995). $[Ca^{2+}]_i$-dependent membrane currents in guinea-pig ventricular cells in the absence of Na/Ca exchange. *Pflügers Archiv*, *430*: 871-878.

1049. Sipido KR, Carmeliet E, Van de Werf F (1998). T-type Ca^{2+} current as a trigger for Ca^{2+} release from the sarcoplasmic reticulum in guinea-pig ventricular myocytes. *J Physiol (Lond)*, *508*: 439-451.

1050. Sipido KR, Maes M, Van de Werf F (1997). Low efficiency of Ca^{2+} entry through the Na^+-Ca^{2+} exchanger as trigger for Ca^{2+} release from the sarcoplasmic reticulum. A comparison between L-type Ca^{2+} current and reverse-mode Na^+-Ca^{2+} exchange. *Circ Res*, *81*: 1034-1044.

1051. Sipido KR, Stankovicova T, Flameng W, Vanhaecke J, Verdonck F (1998). Frequency dependence of Ca^{2+} release from the sarcoplasmic reticulum in human ventricular myocytes from end-stage heart failure. *Cardiovasc Res*, *37*: 478-488.

1052. Sipido KR, Volders PG, de Groot SH, Verdonck F, Van De Werf F, Wellens HJ, Vos MA (2000). Enhanced Ca^{2+} release and Na/Ca exchange activity in hypertrophied canine ventricular myocytes: potential link between contractile adaptation and arrhythmogenesis. *Circulation*, *102*: 2137-2144.

1053. Sitsapesan R, Williams AJ (2000). Do inactivation mechanisms rather than adaptation hold the key to understanding ryanodine receptor channel gating? *J Gen Physiol*, *116*: 867-844.

1054. Skeberdis VA, Jurevicius J, Fischmeister a R (1997). Beta-2 adrenergic activation of L-type Ca^{++} current in cardiac myocytes. *J Pharmacol Exp Ther*, *283*: 452-461.

1055. Slavik K (1994). Fluorescent Probes in Cellular and Molecular Biology. CRC Press.

1056. Smith JH, Green CR, Peters NS, Rothery S, Severs NJ (1991). Altered patterns of gap junction distribution in ischemic heart disease. An immunohistochemical study of human myocardium using laser scanning confocal microscopy. *Am J Pathol*, *139*: 801-821.

1057. Smith WTt, Fleet WF, Johnson TA, Engle CL, Cascio WE (1995). The Ib phase of ventricular arrhythmias in ischemic in situ porcine heart is related to changes in cell-to-cell electrical coupling. *Circulation, 92*: 3051-3060.

1058. Snyders DJ (1999). Structure and function of cardiac potassium channels. *Cardiovasc Res, 42*: 377-390.

1059. Snyders DJ, Tamkun MM, Bennett PB (1993). A rapidly activating and slowly inactivating potassium channel cloned from human heart. Functional analysis after stable mammalian cell culture expression. *J Gen Physiol, 101*: 513-543.

1060. Sohn HG, Vassalle M (1995). Cesium effects on dual pacemaker mechanisms in guinea pig sinoatrial node. *J Mol Cell Cardiol, 27*: 563-577.

1061. Sommer JR, Johnson EA (1979). Ultrastructure of cardiac muscle. In: *Handbook of Physiology Section 2: The cardiovascular system Vol I The heart* (eds. RM Berne, N Sperelakis, SR Geiger), pp 113-186.

1062. Song DK, Earm YE, Ho W (1999). Blockade of the delayed rectifier K^+ currents, IKr, in rabbit sinoatrial node cells by external divalent cations. *Pflügers Archiv, 438*: 147-153.

1063. Song LS, Wang SQ, Xiao RP, Spurgeon H, Lakatta EG, Cheng H (2001). beta-Adrenergic stimulation synchronizes intracellular Ca^{2+} release during excitation-contraction coupling in cardiac myocytes. *Circ Res, 88*: 794-801.

1064. Song Y, Belardinelli L (1996). Electrophysiological and functional effects of adenosine on ventricular myocytes of various mammalian species. *Am J Physiol, 271*: C1233-C1243.

1065. Song Y, Thedford S, Lerman BB, Belardinelli L (1992). Adenosine-sensitive afterdepolarizations and triggered activity in guinea pig ventricular myocytes. *Circ Res, 70*: 743-753.

1066. Sorgato MC, Keller BU, Stuhmer W (1987). Patch-clamping of the inner mitochondrial membrane reveals a voltage-dependent ion channel. *Nature, 330*: 498-500.

1067. Sorota S (1992). Swelling-induced chloride-sensitive current in canine atrial cells revealed by whole-cell patch-clamp method. *Circ Res, 70*: 679-687.

1068. Sorota S (1999). Insights into the structure, distribution and function of the cardiac chloride channels. *Cardiovasc Res, 42*: 361-376.

1069. Sorrentino V, Barone V, Rossi D (2000). Intracellular Ca^{2+} release channels in evolution. *Curr Opin Genet Dev, 10*: 662-667.

1070. Spach MS (1983). The discontinuous nature of electrical propagation in cardiac muscle. Consideration of a quantitative model incorporating the membrane ionic properties and structural complexities. The ALZA distinguished lecture. *Ann Biomed Eng, 11*: 209-261.

1071. Spach MS (2001). Mechanisms of the dynamics of reentry in a fibrillating myocardium: Developing a genes-to-rotors paradigm. *Circ Res, 88*: 753-755.

1072. Spach MS, Barr RC (1972). The use of isopotential surface maps in understanding clinical ECGs. *Am J Dis Child, 124*: 359-363.

1073. Spach MS, Barr RC (2000). Effects of cardiac microstructure on propagating electrical waveforms. *Circ Res, 86*: 23e-28e.

1074. Spach MS, Barr RC, Johnson EA, Kootsey JM (1973). Cardiac extracellular potentials. Analysis of complex wave forms about the Purkinje networks in dogs. *Circ Res, 33*: 465-473.

1075. Spach MS, Dolber PC (1986). Relating extracellular potentials and their derivatives to anisotropic propagation at a microscopic level in human cardiac muscle. Evidence for electrical uncoupling of side-to-side fiber connections with increasing age. *Circ Res*, *58*: 356-371.

1076. Spach MS, Dolber PC, Heidlage JF (1989). Interaction of inhomogeneities of repolarization with anisotropic propagation in dog atria. A mechanism for both preventing and initiating reentry. *Circ Res*, *65*: 1612-1631.

1077. Spach MS, Dolber PC, Heidlage JF (1990). Properties of discontinuous anisotropic propagation at a microscopic level. *Ann N Y Acad Sci*, *591*: 62-74.

1078. Spach MS, Dolber PC, Sommer JR (1985). Discontinuous propagation: an hypothesis based on known cardiac structural complexities. *Int J Cardiol*, *7*: 167-174.

1079. Spach MS, Heidlage JF (1995). The stochastic nature of cardiac propagation at a microscopic level. Electrical description of myocardial architecture and its application to conduction. *Circ Res*, *76*: 366-380.

1080. Spach MS, Heidlage JF, Darken ER, Hofer E, Raines KH, Starmer CF (1992). Cellular Vmax reflects both membrane properties and the load presented by adjoining cells. *Am J Physiol*, *263*: H1855-1863.

1081. Spach MS, Heidlage JF, Dolber PC, Barr RC (1998). Extracellular discontinuities in cardiac muscle: evidence for capillary effects on the action potential foot. *Circ Res*, *83*: 1144-1164.

1082. Spach MS, Heidlage JF, Dolber PC, Barr RC (2000). Electrophysiological effects of remodeling cardiac gap junctions and cell size: experimental and model studies of normal cardiac growth. *Circ Res*, *86*: 302-301.

1083. Spach MS, Kootsey JM (1983). The nature of electrical propagation in cardiac muscle. *Am J Physiol*, *244*: H3-22.

1084. Spach MS, Miller WTd, Dolber PC, Kootsey JM, Sommer JR, Mosher CE, Jr. (1982). The functional role of structural complexities in the propagation of depolarization in the atrium of the dog. Cardiac conduction disturbances due to discontinuities of effective axial resistivity. *Circ Res*, *50*: 175-191.

1085. Spach MS, Miller WTd, Geselowitz DB, Barr RC, Kootsey JM, Johnson EA (1981). The discontinuous nature of propagation in normal canine cardiac muscle. Evidence for recurrent discontinuities of intracellular resistance that affect the membrane currents. *Circ Res*, *48*: 39-54.

1086. Spector PS, Curran ME, Keating MT, Sanguinetti MC (1996). Class III antiarrhythmic drugs block HERG, a human cardiac delayed rectifier K^+ channel. Open-channel block by methanesulfonanilides. *Circ Res*, *78*: 499-503.

1087. Sperelakis N, Kurachi Y, Terzic A, Cohen MV (2001). Heart Physiology and Pathophysiology. Academic Press, San Diego.

1088. Splawski I, Tristani Firouzi M, Lehmann MH, Sanguinetti MC, Keating MT (1997). Mutations in the hminK gene cause long QT syndrome and suppress IKs function. *Nat Genet*, *17*: 338-340.

1089. Spray DC, Fishmann GI (1996). Physiological and molecular properties of cardiac gap junctions. Kluwer Academic Publishers, Dordrecht.

1090. Spray DC, Suadicani SO, Vink MJ, Srinivas M (2001). Gap-junction channels and healing-over of injury. In: *Heart Physiology and Pathophysiology* (eds. N Sperelakis, Y Kurachi, A Terzic, MV Cohen), pp 149-172. Academic Press, San Diego.

1091. Spruce AE, Standen NB, Stanfield PR (1987). Studies of the unitary properties of adenosine-5'-triphosphate-regulated potassium channels of frog skeletal muscle. *J Physiol (Lond)*, *382*: 213-236.

1092. Stankovicova T, Szilard M, De Scheerder I, Sipido KR (2000). M cells and transmural heterogeneity of action potential configuration in myocytes from the left ventricular wall of the pig heart. *Cardiovasc Res, 45*: 952-960.

1093. Starmer CF, Grant AO, Strauss HC (1984). Mechanisms of use-dependent block of sodium channels in excitable membranes by local anesthetics. *Biophys J, 46*: 15-27.

1094. Starmer CF, Lastra AA, Nesterenko VV, Grant AO (1991). Proarrhythmic response to sodium channel blockade. Theoretical model and numerical experiments. *Circulation, 84*: 1364-1377.

1095. Steinberg SF (1999). The molecular basis for distinct beta-adrenergic receptor subtype actions in cardiomyocytes. *Circ Res, 85*: 1101-1111.

1096. Steinberg SF, Alter A (1993). Enhanced receptor-dependent inositol phosphate accumulation in hypoxic myocytes. *Am J Physiol, 265*: H691-699.

1097. Steinberg SF, Robinson RB, Lieberman HB, Stern DM, Rosen MR (1991). Thrombin modulates phosphoinositide metabolism, cytosolic calcium, and impulse initiation in the heart. *Circ Res, 68*: 1216-1229.

1098. Steinfath M, Chen YY, Lavicky J, Magnussen O, Nosc M, Rosswag S, Schmitz W, Scholz H (1992). Cardiac alpha 1-adrenoceptor densities in different mammalian species. *Br J Pharmacol, 107*: 185-188.

1099. Stengl M, Bartak F (2000). Calcitonin gene-related peptide suppresses the transient outward current in rat ventricular myocytes. *Pflügers Archiv, 441*: 138-143.

1100. Stengl M, Carmeliet E, Mubagwa K, Flameng W (1998). Modulation of transient outward current by extracellular protons and Cd^{2+} in rat and human ventricular myocytes. *J Physiol (Lond), 511*: 827-836.

1101. Stern MD (1992). Theory of excitation-contraction coupling in cardiac muscle. *Biophys J, 63*: 497-517.

1102. Stern MD, Song LS, Cheng H, Sham JS, Yang HT, Boheler KR, Rios E (1999). Local control models of cardiac excitation-contraction coupling. A possible role for allosteric interactions between ryanodine receptors. *J Gen Physiol, 113*: 469-489.

1103. Stimers JR (2001). Cardiac Na^+/K^+ pump. In: *Heart Physiology and Pathophysiology* (eds. N Sperelakis, Y Kurachi, A Terzic, MV Cohen), pp 407-416. Academic Press, San Diego.

1104. Stimers JR, Liu S, Kinard TA (1993). Effect of Na_i on activity and voltage dependence of the Na/K pump in adult rat cardiac myocytes. *J Membr Biol, 135*: 39-47.

1105. Stimers JR, Liu S, Lieberman M (1991). Apparent affinity of the Na/K pump for ouabain in cultured chick cardiac myocytes. Effects of Nai and Ko. *J Gen Physiol, 98*: 815-833.

1106. Stramba-Badiale M, Priori SG, Napolitano C, Locati EH, Vinolas X, Haverkamp W, Schulze-Bahr E, Goulene K, Schwartz PJ (2000). Gene-specific differences in the circadian variation of ventricular repolarization in the long QT syndrome: a key to sudden death during sleep? *Ital Heart J, 1*: 323-328.

1107. Strauss HC, Morales MJ, Wang S, Brahmajothi MV, Campbell DL (2001). Voltage-dependent K^+ channels. In: *Heart Physiology and Pathophysiology* (eds. N Sperelakis, Y Kurachi, A Terzic, MV Cohen), pp 259-280. Academic Press, San Diego.

1108. Streeter DR (1979). Gross morphology and fiber geometry of the heart. In: *Handbook of Physiology Section 2: The cardiovascular system Vol I The heart* (eds. RM Berne, N Sperelakis, SR Geiger), pp 61-112.

1109. Striessnig J (1999). Pharmacology, structure and function of cardiac L-type Ca^{2+} channels. *Cell Physiol Biochem, 9*: 242-269.

1110. Su Z, Sugishita K, Ritter M, Li F, Spitzer KW, Barry WH (2001). The sodium pump modulates the influence of I_{Na} on $[Ca^{2+}]_i$ transients in mouse ventricular myocytes. *Biophys J, 80*: 1230-1237.

1111. Sudhof TC, Newton CL, Archer BT, Ushkaryov YA, Mignery GA (1991). Structure of a novel InsP3 receptor. *Embo J, 10*: 3199-3206.

1112. Sun H, Chartier D, Leblanc N, Nattel S (2001). Intracellular calcium changes and tachycardia-induced contractile dysfunction in canine atrial myocytes. *Cardiovasc Res, 49*: 751-761.

1113. Sun H, Leblanc N, Nattel S (1997). Mechanisms of inactivation of L-type calcium channels in human atrial myocytes. *Am J Physiol, 272*: H1625-1635.

1114. Sun ZQ, Ojamaa K, Coetzee WA, Artman M, Klein I (2000). Effects of thyroid hormone on action potential and repolarizing currents in rat ventricular myocytes. *Am J Physiol Endocrinol Metab, 278*: E302-307.

1115. Surawicz B (1998). U wave: facts, hypotheses, misconceptions, and misnomers. *J Cardiovasc Electrophysiol, 9*: 1117-1128.

1116. Swynghedauw B (1999). Molecular mechanisms of myocardial remodeling. *Physiol Rev, 79*: 215-262.

1117. Szabo I, Bernardi P, Zoratti M (1992). Modulation of the mitochondrial megachannel by divalent cations and protons. *J Biol Chem, 267*: 2940-2946.

1118. Szabo I, Zoratti M (1992). The mitochondrial megachannel is the permeability transition pore. *J Bioenerg Biomembr, 24*: 111-117.

1119. Szokodi I, Horkay F, Merkely B, Solti F, Geller L, Kiss P, Selmeci L, Kekesi V, Vuolteenaho O, Ruskoaho H, Juhasz-Nagy A, Toth M (1998). Intrapericardial infusion of endothelin-1 induces ventricular arrhythmias in dogs. *Cardiovasc Res, 38*: 356-364.

1120. Szymanska G, Stromer H, Kim DH, Lorell BH, Morgan JP (2000). Dynamic changes in sarcoplasmic reticulum function in cardiac hypertrophy and failure. *Pflügers Archiv, 439*: 339-348.

1121. Taggart P, Sutton PMI, Opthof T, Coronel R, Trimlett R, Pugsley W, Kallis P (2001). Transmural repolarisation in the left ventricle in humans during normoxia and ischaemia. *Cardiovasc Res, 50*: 454-462.

1122. Takagi G, Kiuchi K, Endo T, Yamamoto T, Sato N, Nejima J, Takano T (2000). Alpha-human atrial natriuretic peptide, carperitide, reduces infarct size but not arrhythmias after coronary occlusion/reperfusion in dogs. *J Cardiovasc Pharmacol, 36*: 22-30.

1123. Takata Y, Hirayama Y, Kiyomi S, Ogawa T, Iga K, Ishii T, Nagai Y, Ibukiyama C (1996). The beneficial effects of atrial natriuretic peptide on arrhythmias and myocardial high-energy phosphates after reperfusion. *Cardiovasc Res, 32*: 286-293.

1124. Takens Kwak BR, Jongsma HJ (1992). Cardiac gap junctions: three distinct single channel conductances and their modulation by phosphorylating treatments. *Pflügers Archiv, 422*: 198-200.

1125. Takimoto K, Levitan ES (1994). Glucocorticoid induction of Kv1.5 K^+ channel gene expression in ventricle of rat heart. *Circ Res, 75*: 1006-1013.

1126. Tamaddon HS, Vaidya D, Simon AM, Paul DL, Jalife J, Morley GE (2000). High-Resolution Optical Mapping of the Right Bundle Branch in Connexin40 Knockout Mice Reveals Slow Conduction in the Specialized Conduction System. *Circ Res, 87*: 929-936.

1127. Tan HL, Bink-Boelkens MT, Bezzina CR, Viswanathan PC, Beaufort-Krol GC, van Tintelen PJ, van den Berg MP, Wilde AA, Balser JR (2001). A sodium-channel mutation causes isolated cardiac conduction disease. *Nature, 409*: 1043-1047.

1128. Tan RC, Osaka T, Joyner RW (1991). Experimental model of effects on normal tissue of injury current from ischemic region. *Circ Res, 69*: 965-974.

1129. Tanabe S, Hata T, Hiraoka M (1999). Effects of estrogen on action potential and membrane currents in guinea pig ventricular myocytes. *Am J Physiol, 277*: H826-833.

1130. Tanaka H, Habuchi Y, Nishio M, Yamamoto T, Suto F, Yoshimura M (1998). Endothelin-1 inhibits pacemaker currents in rabbit SA node cells. *J Cardiovasc Pharmacol, 31*: S440-442.

1131. Tanemoto M, Fujita A, Kurachi Y (2001). Inwardly-rectifying K$^+$ channels. In: *Heart Physiology and Pathophysiology* (eds. N Sperelakis, Y Kurachi, A Terzic, MV Cohen), pp 281-308. Academic Press, San Diego.

1132. Tani M, Neely JR (1989). Role of intracellular Na$^+$ in Ca^{2+} overload and depressed recovery of ventricular function of reperfused ischemic rat hearts. Possible involvement of H$^+$-Na$^+$ and Na$^+$-Ca^{2+} exchange. *Circ Res, 65*: 1045-1056.

1133. Tareen FM, Ono K, Noma A, Ehara T (1991). Beta-adrenergic and muscarinic regulation of the chloride current in guinea-pig ventricular cells. *J Physiol (Lond), 440*: 225-241.

1134. Tarr M, Arriaga E, Goertz KK, Valenzeno DP (1994). Properties of cardiac I(leak) induced by photosensitizer-generated reactive oxygen. *Free Radic Biol Med, 16*: 477-484.

1135. ten Velde I, de Jonge B, Verheijck EE, van Kempen MJ, Analbers L, Gros D, Jongsma HJ (1995). Spatial distribution of connexin43, the major cardiac gap junction protein, visualizes the cellular network for impulse propagation from sinoatrial node to atrium. *Circ Res, 76*: 802-811.

1136. Terracciano CM, Philipson KD, MacLeod KT (2001). Overexpression of the Na$^+$/Ca^{2+} exchanger and inhibition of the sarcoplasmic reticulum Ca^{2+}-ATPase in ventricular myocytes from transgenic mice. *Cardiovasc Res, 49*: 38-47.

1137. Terzic A, Jahangir A, Kurachi Y (1995). Cardiac ATP-sensitive K$^+$ channels: regulation by intracellular nucleotides and K$^+$ channel-opening drugs. *Am J Physiol, 269*: C525-545.

1138. Tesfamariam B, Allen GT, Powell JR (1995). Bradykinin B2 receptor-mediated chronotropic effect of bradykinin in isolated guinea pig atria. *Eur J Pharmacol, 281*: 17-20.

1139. Teshima Y, Takahashi N, Saikawa T, Hara M, Yasunaga S, Hidaka S, Sakata T (2000). Diminished expression of sarcoplasmic reticulum Ca^{2+}-ATPase and ryanodine sensitive Ca^{2+} channel mRNA in streptozotocin-induced diabetic rat heart. *J Mol Cell Cardiol, 32*: 655-664.

1140. Thiemann A, Grunder S, Pusch M, Jentsch TJ (1992). A chloride channel widely expressed in epithelial and non-epithelial cells. *Nature, 356*: 57-60.

1141. Thomas CJ, Head GA, Woods RL (1998). ANP and bradycardic reflexes in hypertensive rats: influence of cardiac hypertrophy. *Hypertension, 32*: 548-555.

1142. Thomas GP, Sims SM, Karmazyn M (1997). Differential effects of endothelin-1 on basal and isoprenaline-enhanced Ca^{2+} current in guinea-pig ventricular myocytes. *J Physiol (Lond), 503*: 55-65.

1143. Thomas L, Kocsis E, Colombini M, Erbe E, Trus BL, Steven AC (1991). Surface topography and molecular stoichiometry of the mitochondrial channel, VDAC, in crystalline arrays. *J Struct Biol, 106*: 161-171.

1144. Thome U, Berger F, Borchard U, Hafner D (1992). Electrophysiological characterization of histamine receptor subtypes in sheep cardiac Purkinje fibers. *Agents Actions, 37*: 30-38.

1145. Thuringer D, Lauribe P, Escande D (1992). A hyperpolarization-activated inward current in human myocardial cells. *J Mol Cell Cardiol, 24*: 451-455.

1146. Tiaho F, Nerbonne JM (1996). VIP and secretin augment cardiac L-type calcium channel currents in isolated adult rat ventricular myocytes. *Pflügers Archiv, 432*: 821-830.

1147. Tinker A, Williams AJ (1992). Divalent cation conduction in the ryanodine receptor channel of sheep cardiac muscle sarcoplasmic reticulum. *J Gen Physiol, 100*: 479-493.

1148. Tiso N, Stephan DA, Nava A, Bagattin A, Devaney JM, Stanchi F, Larderet G, Brahmbhatt B, Brown K, Bauce B, Muriago M, Basso C, Thiene G, Danieli GA, Rampazzo A (2001). Identification of mutations in the cardiac ryanodine receptor gene in families affected with arrhythmogenic right ventricular cardiomyopathy type 2 (ARVD2). *Hum Mol Genet, 10*: 189-194.

1149. Tohse N, Kameyama M, Irisawa H (1987). Intracellular Ca^{2+} and protein kinase C modulate K^+ current in guinea pig heart cells. *Am J Physiol, 253*: H1321-1324.

1150. Tomaselli GF, Marban E (1999). Electrophysiological remodeling in hypertrophy and heart failure. *Cardiovasc Res, 42*: 270-283.

1151. Toyama J, Honjo H, Osaka T, Anno T, Hirai M, Ohta T, Kodama I, Yamada K (1987). Endocardial excitation and conduction during reperfusion arrhythmias. *Jpn Circ J, 51*: 163-171.

1152. Toyofuku T, Yabuki M, Otsu K, Kuzuya T, Tada M, Hori M (1999). Functional role of c-Src in gap junctions of the cardiomyopathic heart. *Circ Res, 85*: 672-681.

1153. Trafford AW, Diaz ME, Eisner DA (1998). Ca-activated chloride current and Na-Ca exchange have different timecourses during sarcoplasmic reticulum Ca release in ferret ventricular myocytes. *Pflügers Archiv, 435*: 743-745.

1154. Tseng GN (1988). Calcium current restitution in mammalian ventricular myocytes is modulated by intracellular calcium. *Circ Res, 63*: 468-482.

1155. Tseng GN (1992). Cell swelling increases membrane conductance of canine cardiac cells: evidence for a volume-sensitive Cl channel. *Am J Physiol, 262*: C1056-1068.

1156. Tseng GN, Boyden PA (1991). Different effects of intracellular Ca and protein kinase C on cardiac T and L Ca currents. *Am J Physiol, 261*: H364-379.

1157. Tseng GN, Hoffman BF (1989). Two components of transient outward current in canine ventricular myocytes. *Circ Res, 64*: 633-647.

1158. Tseng GN, Robinson RB, Hoffman BF (1987). Passive properties and membrane currents of canine ventricular myocytes. *J Gen Physiol, 90*: 671-701.

1159. Tsien RW, Bean BP, Hess P, Lansman JB, Nilius B, Nowycky MC (1986). Mechanisms of calcium channel modulation by beta-adrenergic agents and dihydropyridine calcium agonists. *J Mol Cell Cardiol, 18*: 691-710.

1160. Tsien RW, Giles W, Greengard P (1972). Cyclic AMP mediates the effects of adrenaline on cardiac purkinje fibres. *Nature New Biol, 240*: 181-183.

1161. Tsien RW, Hess P, McCleskey EW, Rosenberg RL (1987). Calcium channels: mechanisms of selectivity, permeation, and block. *Annu Rev Biophys Biophys Chem, 16*: 265-290.

1162. Tsuchiya K, Horie M, Watanuki M, Albrecht CA, Obayashi K, Fujiwara H, Sasayama S (1997). Functional compartmentalization of ATP is involved in angiotensin II-mediated closure of cardiac ATP-sensitive K^+ channels. *Circulation, 96*: 3129-3135.

1163. Tu Q, Velez P, Cortes Gutierrez M, Fill M (1994). Surface charge potentiates conduction through the cardiac ryanodine receptor channel. *J Gen Physiol, 103*: 853-867.

1164. Tunwell RE, Wickenden C, Bertrand BM, Shevchenko VI, Walsh MB, Allen PD, Lai FA (1996). The human cardiac muscle ryanodine receptor-calcium release channel: identification, primary structure and topological analysis. *Biochem J, 318*: 477-487.

1165. Tytgat J, Nilius B, Carmeliet E (1990). Modulation of the T-type cardiac Ca channel by changes in proton concentration. *J Gen Physiol, 96*: 973-990.

1166. Tytgat J, Nilius B, Vereecke J, Carmeliet E (1988). The T-type Ca channel in guinea-pig ventricular myocytes is insensitive to isoproterenol. *Pflügers Archiv, 411*: 704-706.

1167. Ulens C, Tytgat J (2001). Functional heteromerization of HCN1 and HCN2 pacemaker channels. *J Biol Chem, 276*: 6069-6072.

1168. Undrovinas AI, Fleidervish IA, Makielski JC (1992). Inward sodium current at resting potentials in single cardiac myocytes induced by the ischemic metabolite lysophosphatidylcholine. *Circ Res, 71*: 1231-1241.

1169. Ungerer M, Kessebohm K, Kronsbein K, Lohse MJ, Richardt G (1996). Activation of ß-adrenergic receptor kinase during myocardial ischemia. *Circ Res, 79*: 455-460.

1170. Unsold B, Kerst G, Brousos H, Hubner M, Schreiber R, Nitschke R, Greger R, Bleich M (2000). KCNE1 reverses the response of the human K$^+$ channel KCNQ1 to cytosolic pH changes and alters its pharmacology and sensitivity to temperature. *Pflügers Archiv, 441*: 368-378.

1171. Ursell PC, Gardner PI, Albala A, Fenoglio JJ, Wit AL (1985). Structural and electrophysiological changes in the epicardial border zone of canine myocardial infarcts during infarct healing. *Circ Res, 56*: 436-451.

1172. Uzzaman M, Honjo H, Takagishi Y, Emdad L, Magee AI, Severs NJ, Kodama I (2000). Remodeling of gap junctional coupling in hypertrophied right ventricles of rats with monocrotaline-induced pulmonary hypertension. *Circ Res, 86*: 871-878.

1173. Vaccari T, Moroni A, Rocchi M, Gorza L, Bianchi ME, Beltrame M, DiFrancesco D (1999). The human gene coding for HCN2, a pacemaker channel of the heart. *Biochim Biophys Acta, 1446*: 419-425.

1174. Valderrabano M, Lee MH, Ohara T, Lai AC, Fishbein MC, Lin SF, Karagueuzian HS, Chen PS (2001). Dynamics of intramural and transmural reentry during ventricular fibrillation in isolated swine ventricles. *Circ Res, 88*: 839-848.

1175. Valiunas V, Weingart R, Brink PR (2000). Formation of heterotypic gap junction channels by connexins 40 and 43. *Circ Res, 86*: 42e-49e.

1176. van der Velden HM, Ausma J, Rook MB, Hellemons AJ, van Veen TA, Allessie MA, Jongsma HJ (2000). Gap junctional remodeling in relation to stabilization of atrial fibrillation in the goat. *Cardiovasc Res, 46*: 476-486.

1177. van der Vusse GJ, van Bilsen M, Reneman RS (1994). Ischemia and reperfusion induced alterations in membrane phospholipids: an overview. *Ann N Y Acad Sci, 723*: 1-14.

1178. Van Emous JG, Schreur JH, Ruigrok TJ, Van Echteld CJ (1998). Both Na$^+$-K$^+$ ATPase and Na$^+$-H$^+$ exchanger are immediately active upon post-ischemic reperfusion in isolated rat hearts. *J Mol Cell Cardiol, 30*: 337-348.

1179. Van Gelder IC, Brugemann J, Crijns HJ (1998). Current treatment recommendations in antiarrhythmic therapy. *Drugs, 55*: 331-346.

1180. van Ginneken AC, Giles W (1991). Voltage clamp measurements of the hyperpolarization-activated inward current I$_f$ in single cells from rabbit sino-atrial node. *J Physiol (Lond), 434*: 57-83.

1181. van Ginneken AC, Veldkamp MW (1999). Implications of inhomogeneous distribution of IKS and IKr channels in ventricle with respect to effects of class III agents and beta-agonists. *Cardiovasc Res, 43*: 20-22.

1182. van Os CH, Kamsteeg EJ, Marr N, Deen PM (2000). Physiological relevance of aquaporins: luxury or necessity? *Pflügers Archiv, 440*: 513-520.

1183. van Rijen HV, van Veen TA, Hermans MM, Jongsma HJ (2000). Human connexin40 gap junction channels are modulated by cAMP. *Cardiovasc Res, 45*: 941-951.

1184. Van Wagoner DR, Nerbonne JM (2001). Molecular mechanisms of atrial fibrillation. In: *Heart Physiology and Pathophysiology* (eds. N Sperelakis, Y Kurachi, A Terzic, MV Cohen), pp 1107-1124. Academic Press, San Diego.

1185. Van Wagoner DR, Pond AL, Lamorgese M, Rossie SS, McCarthy PM, Nerbonne JM (1999). Atrial L-type Ca^{2+} currents and human atrial fibrillation. *Circ Res, 85*: 428-436.

1186. Van Wagoner DR, Pond AL, McCarthy PM, Trimmer JS, Nerbonne JM (1997). Outward K^+ current densities and Kv1.5 expression are reduced in chronic human atrial fibrillation. *Circ Res, 80*: 772-781.

1187. Vandecasteele G, Verde I, Rucker-Martin C, Donzeau-Gouge P, Fischmeister R (2001). Cyclic GMP regulation of the L-type Ca^{2+} channel current in human atrial myocytes. *J Physiol (Lond), 533*: 329-340.

1188. Vandenberg CA (1987). Inward rectification of a potassium channel in cardiac ventricular cells depends on internal magnesium ions. *Proc Natl Acad Sci USA, 84*: 2560-2564.

1189. Vandenberg JI, Bett GC, Powell T (1997). Contribution of a swelling-activated chloride current to changes in the cardiac action potential. *Am J Physiol, 273*: C541-547.

1190. Vandenberg JI, Rees SA, Wright AR, Powell T (1996). Cell swelling and ion transport pathways in cardiac myocytes. *Cardiovasc Res, 32*: 85-97.

1191. Vanoli E, De Ferrari GM, Stramba-Badiale M, Hull SS, Foreman RD, Schwartz PJ (1991). Vagal stimulation and prevention of sudden death in conscious dogs with a healed myocardial infarction. *Circ Res, 68*: 1471-1481.

1192. Varro A, Balati B, Iost N, Takacs J, Virag L, Lathrop DA, Csaba L, Talosi L, Papp JG (2000). The role of the delayed rectifier component IKs in dog ventricular muscle and Purkinje fibre repolarization. *J Physiol (Lond), 523 Pt 1*: 67-81.

1193. Vassalle M (1970). Electrogenic suppression of automaticity in sheep and dog Purkinje fibres. *Circ Res, 27*: 361-377.

1194. Vassalle M (1995). The pacemaker current (I_f) does not play an important role in regulating SA node pacemaker activity. *Cardiovasc Res, 30*: 309-310.

1195. Vassort G (2001). Adenosine 5'-triphosphate: a P2-purinergic agonist in the myocardium. *Physiol Rev, 81*: 767-806.

1196. Vassort G, Alvarez J (1994). Cardiac T-type calcium current: pharmacology and roles in cardiac tissues. *J Cardiovasc Electrophysiol, 5*: 376-393.

1197. Vassort G, Pucéat M, Alvarez J (1996). Regulation of cardiac activity by ATP, a purine agonist. In: *Molecular physiology and pharmacology of cardiac ion channels and transporters* (eds. M Morad, S Ebashi, W Trautwein, Y Kurachi), pp 231-238. Kluwer Academic Publishers, Dordrecht / Boston / London.

1198. Vassort G, Scamps F, Pucéat M, Clément O (1992). Multiple site effects of extracellular ATP in cardiac tissues. *NIPS, 7*: 212-215.

1199. Vedantham V, Cannon SC (1999). The position of the fast-inactivation gate during lidocaine block of voltage-gated Na^+ channels. *J Gen Physiol, 113*: 7-16.

1200. Veenstra RD, DeHaan RL (1986). Measurement of single channel currents from cardiac gap junctions. *Science, 233*: 972-974.

1201. Veenstra RD, DeHaan RL (1988). Cardiac gap junction channel activity in embryonic chick ventricle cells. *Am J Physiol, 254*: H170-180.

1202. Veldkamp MW (1998). Is the slowly activating component of the delayed rectifier current, IKs' absent from undiseased human ventricular myocardium? *Cardiovasc Res, 40*: 433-435.

1203. Veldkamp MW, van Ginneken AC, Opthof T, Bouman LN (1995). Delayed rectifier channels in human ventricular myocytes. *Circulation, 92*: 3497-3504.

1204. Veldkamp MW, Viswanathan PC, Bezzina C, Baartscheer A, Wilde AA, Balser JR (2000). Two distinct congenital arrhythmias evoked by a multidysfunctional Na^+ channel. *Circ Res, 86*: 91e-97e.

1205. Vera Z, Pride HP, Zipes DP (1995). Reperfusion arrhythmias: role of early afterdepolarizations studied by monophasic action potential recordings in the intact canine heart during autonomically denervated and stimulated states. *J Cardiovasc Electrophysiol, 6*: 532-543.

1206. Verdonck F (1995). How high does intracellular sodium rise during acute myocardial ischaemia? *Cardiovasc Res, 29*: 278.

1207. Vereecke J, Carmeliet E (2000). The effect of external pH on the delayed rectifying K^+ current in cardiac ventricular myocytes. *Pflügers Archiv, 439*: 739-751.

1208. Verheijck EE, van Ginneken AC, Bourier J, Bouman LN (1995). Effects of delayed rectifier current blockade by E-4031 on impulse generation in single sinoatrial nodal myocytes of the rabbit. *Circ Res, 76*: 607-615.

1209. Verheijck EE, van Ginneken AC, Wilders R, Bouman LN (1999). Contribution of L-type Ca^{2+} current to electrical activity in sinoatrial nodal myocytes of rabbits. *Am J Physiol, 276*: H1064-1077.

1210. Verheule S, van Kempen MJA, Postma S, Rook MB, Jongsma HJ (2001). Gap junctions in the rabbit sinoatrial node. *Am J Physiol, 280*: H2103-2115.

1211. Verkerk AO, Veldkamp MW, Bouman LN, van Ginneken AC (2000). Calcium-activated Cl^- current contributes to delayed afterdepolarizations in single Purkinje and ventricular myocytes. *Circulation, 101*: 2639-2644.

1212. Verkerk AO, Veldkamp MW, Ginneken ACGv, Bouman LN (1996). Biphasic response of action potential duration to metabolic inhibition in rabbit and human ventricular myocytes: Role of transient outward current and ATP-regulated potassium current. *J Mol Cell Cardiol, 28*: 2443-2456.

1213. Viatchenko-Karpinski S, Györke S (2001). Modulation of the Ca^{2+}-induced Ca^{2+} release cascade by {beta}-adrenergic stimulation in rat ventricular myocytes. *J Physiol (Lond), 533*: 837-848.

1214. Vigne P, Lazdunski M, Frelin C (1989). The inotropic effect of endothelin-1 on rat atria involves hydrolysis of phosphatidylinositol. *FEBS Lett, 249*: 143-146.

1215. Vilin YY, Fujimoto E, Ruben PC (2001). A single residue differentiates between human cardiac and skeletal muscle Na^+ channel slow inactivation. *Biophys J, 80*: 2221-2230.

1216. Viscomi C, Altomare C, Bucchi A, Camatini E, Baruscotti M, Moroni A, DiFrancesco D (2001). C-terminus-mediated control of voltage- and cAMP-gating of HCN channels. *J Biol Chem, In press*.

1217. Viskin S, Fish R, Zeltser D, Belhassen B, Heller K, Brosh D, Laniado S, Barron HV (2000). Arrhythmias in the congenital long QT syndrome: how often is torsade de pointes pause dependent? *Heart, 83*: 661-666.

1218. Viswanathan PC, Rudy Y (1999). Pause induced early afterdepolarizations in the long QT syndrome: a simulation study. *Cardiovasc Res, 42*: 530-542.

1219. Viswanathan PC, Rudy Y (2000). Cellular arrhythmogenic effects of congenital and acquired long-QT syndrome in the heterogeneous myocardium. *Circulation, 101*: 1192-1198.

1220. Vites AM, Pappano A (1990). Inositol 1,4,5-trisphosphate releases intracellular Ca^{2+} in permeabilized chick atria. *Am J Physiol, 258*: H1745-1752.

1221. Volders PG, Kulcsar A, Vos MA, Sipido KR, Wellens HJ, Lazzara R, Szabo B (1997). Similarities between early and delayed afterdepolarizations induced by isoproterenol in canine ventricular myocytes. *Cardiovasc Res, 34*: 348-359.

1222. Volders PG, Sipido KR, Carmeliet E, Spatjens RL, Wellens HJ, Vos MA (1999). Repolarizing K^+ currents I_{to1} and I_{Ks} are larger in right than left canine ventricular midmyocardium. *Circulation, 99*: 206-210.

1223. Volders PG, Sipido KR, Vos MA, Kulcsar A, Verduyn SC, Wellens HJ (1998). Cellular basis of biventricular hypertrophy and arrhythmogenesis in dogs with chronic complete atrioventricular block and acquired torsade de pointes. *Circulation, 98*: 1136-1147.

1224. Volders PG, Sipido KR, Vos MA, Spatjens RL, Leunissen JD, Carmeliet E, Wellens HJ (1999). Downregulation of delayed rectifier K^+ currents in dogs with chronic complete atrioventricular block and acquired torsades de pointes. *Circulation, 100*: 2455-2461.

1225. Wagenknecht T, Radermacher M (1997). Ryanodine receptors: structure and macromolecular interactions. *Curr Opin Struct Biol, 7*: 258-265.

1226. Wahler GM (2001). Cardiac action potentials. In: *Heart Physiology and Pathophysiology* (eds. N Sperelakis, Y Kurachi, A Terzic, MV Cohen), pp 199-211. Academic Press, San Diego.

1227. Wahler GM, Dollinger SJ, Smith JM, Flemal KL (1994). Time course of postnatal changes in rat heart action potential and in transient outward current is different. *Am J Physiol, 267*: H1157-1166.

1228. Wainger BJ, DeGennaro M, Santoro B, Siegelbaum SA, Tibbs GR (2001). Molecular mechanism of cAMP modulation of HCN pacemaker channels. *Nature, 411*: 805 - 810.

1229. Waldegger S, Jentsch TJ (2000). From tonus to tonicity: physiology of CLC chloride channels. *J Am Soc Nephrol, 11*: 1331-1339.

1230. Wallert MA, Ackerman MJ, Kim D, Clapham DE (1991). Two novel cardiac atrial K^+ channels, IK.AA and IK.PC. *J Gen Physiol, 98*: 921-939.

1231. Walsh KB, Kass RS (1988). Regulation of a heart potassium channel by protein kinase A and C. *Science, 242*: 67-69.

1232. Walsh KB, Kass RS (1991). Distinct voltage-dependent regulation of a heart-delayed IK by protein kinases A and C. *Am J Physiol, 261*: C1081-1090.

1233. Wang D, Armstrong DL (2000). Tetraethylammonium potentiates the activity of muscarinic potassium channels in guinea-pig atrial myocytes. *J Physiol (Lond), 529*: 699-466.

1234. Wang DW, Makita N, Kitabatake A, Balser JR, George AL (2000). Enhanced Na^+ channel intermediate inactivation in Brugada syndrome. *Circ Res, 87*: E37-43.

1235. Wang DW, Yazawa K, Makita N, George AL, Bennett PB (1997). Pharmacological targeting of long QT mutant sodium channels. *J Clin Invest, 99*: 1714-1720.

1236. Wang HZ, Li J, Lemanski LF, Veenstra RD (1992). Gating of mammalian cardiac gap junction channels by transjunctional voltage. *Biophys J, 63*: 139-151.

1237. Wang J, Schwinger RH, Frank K, Muller Ehmsen J, Martin Vasallo P, Pressley TA, Xiang A, Erdmann E, McDonough AA (1996). Regional expression of sodium pump subunits isoforms and Na⁺-Ca⁺⁺ exchanger in the human heart. *J Clin Invest, 98*: 1650-1658.

1238. Wang L, Duff HJ (1996). Identification and characteristics of delayed rectifier K⁺ current in fetal mouse ventricular myocytes. *Am J Physiol, 270*: H2088-2093.

1239. Wang L, Duff HJ (1997). Developmental changes in transient outward current in mouse ventricle. *Circ Res, 81*: 120-127.

1240. Wang L, Feng ZP, Duff HJ (1999). Glucocorticoid regulation of cardiac K⁺ currents and L-type Ca²⁺ current in neonatal mice. *Circ Res, 85*: 168-173.

1241. Wang L, Feng Z-P, Kondo CS, Sheldon RS, Duff HJ (1996). Developmental changes in the delayed rectifier K⁺ channels in mouse heart. *Circ Res, 79*: 79-85.

1242. Wang Q, Curran ME, Splawski I, Burn TC, Millholland JM, VanRaay TJ, Shen J, Timothy KW, Vincent GM, de Jager T, Schwartz PJ, Toubin JA, Moss AJ, Atkinson DL, Landes GM, Connors TD, Keating MT (1996). Positional cloning of a novel potassium channel gene: KVLQT1 mutations cause cardiac arrhythmias. *Nat Genet, 12*: 17-23.

1243. Wang S-Q, Song L-S, Lakatta E, Cheng H (2001). Ca²⁺ signalling between single L-type Ca²⁺ channels and ryanodine receptors in heart cells. *Nature, 410*: 592 - 596.

1244. Wang SY, Clague JR, Langer GA (1995). Increase in calcium leak channel activity by metabolic inhibition or hydrogen peroxide in rat ventricular myocytes and its inhibition by polycation. *J Mol Cell Cardiol, 27*: 211-222.

1245. Wang TL, Tseng YZ, Chang H (2000). Regulation of connexin 43 gene expression by cyclical mechanical stretch in neonatal rat cardiomyocytes. *Biochem Biophys Res Commun, 267*: 551-557.

1246. Wang Y, Rudy Y (2000). Action potential propagation in inhomogeneous cardiac tissue: safety factor considerations and ionic mechanism. *Am J Physiol, 278*: H1019-1029.

1247. Wang YG, Huser J, Blatter LA, Lipsius SL (1997). Withdrawal of acetylcholine elicits Ca²⁺-induced delayed afterdepolarizations in cat atrial myocytes. *Circulation, 96*: 1275-1281.

1248. Wang YG, Lipsius SL (1995). Acetylcholine activates a glibenclamide-sensitive K⁺ current in cat atrial myocytes. *Am J Physiol, 268*: H1322-1334.

1249. Wang Z, Feng J, Shi H, Pond A, Nerbonne JM, Nattel S (1999). Potential molecular basis of different physiological properties of the transient outward K⁺ current in rabbit and human atrial myocytes. *Circ Res, 84*: 551-561.

1250. Wang Z, Fermini B, Nattel S (1993). Sustained depolarization-induced outward current in human atrial myocytes. Evidence for a novel delayed rectifier K⁺ current similar to Kv1.5 cloned channel currents. *Circ Res, 73*: 1061-1076.

1251. Wang Z, Fermini B, Nattel S (1994). Rapid and slow components of delayed rectifier current in human atrial myocytes. *Cardiovasc Res, 28*: 1540-1546.

1252. Wang Z, Kimitsuki T, Noma A (1991). Conductance properties of the Na⁺-activated K⁺ channel in guinea-pig ventricular cells. *J Physiol (Lond), 433*: 241-257.

1253. Wang ZG, Fermini B, Nattel S (1991). Repolarization differences between guinea pig atrial endocardium and epicardium: evidence for a role of Ito. *Am J Physiol, 260*: H1501-1506.

1254. Warmke JW, Ganetzky B (1994). A family of potassium channel genes related to eag in Drosophila and mammals. *Proc Natl Acad Sci USA, 91*: 3438-3442.

1255. Washizuka T, Horie M, Watanuki M, Sasayama S (1997). Endothelin-1 inhibits the slow component of cardiac delayed rectifier K⁺ currents via a pertussis toxin-sensitive mechanism. *Circ Res, 81*: 211-218.

1256. Watanabe A, Endoh M (1998). Relationship between the increase in Ca^{2+} transient and contractile force induced by angiotensin II in aequorin-loaded rabbit ventricular myocardium. *Cardiovasc Res*, *37*: 524-531.

1257. Watanabe E-I, Honjo H, Boyett MR, Kodama I, Toyama J (1996). Inactivation of the calcium current is involved in overdrive suppression of rabbit sinoatrial node cells. *Am J Physiol*, *271*: H2097-H2107.

1258. Watanabe Y (1975). Purkinje repolarization as a possible cause of the U wave in the electrocardiogram. *Circulation*, *51*: 1030-1037.

1259. Watano T, Harada Y, Harada K, Nishimura N (1999). Effect of Na^+/Ca^{2+} exchange inhibitor, KB-R7943 on ouabain-induced arrhythmias in guinea-pigs. *Br J Pharmacol*, *127*: 1846-1850.

1260. Watano T, Kimura J, Morita T, Nakanishi H (1996). A novel antagonist, No. 7943, of the Na^+/Ca^{2+} exchange current in guinea-pig cardiac ventricular cells. *Br J Pharmacol*, *119*: 555-563.

1261. Watson CL, Gold MR (1995). Effect of intracellular and extracellular acidosis on sodium current in ventricular myocytes. *Am J Physiol*, *268*: H1749-1756.

1262. Weber C, Ginsburg K, Philipson K, Shannon T, Bers D (2001). Allosteric regulation of Na/Ca exchange current by cytosolic Ca in intact cardiac myocytes. *J Gen Physiol*, *117*: 119-132.

1263. Wei SK, Colecraft HM, DeMaria CD, Peterson BZ, Zhang R, Kohout TA, Rogers TB, Yue DT (2000). Ca^{2+} channel modulation by recombinant auxiliary beta subunits expressed in young adult heart cells. *Circ Res*, *86*: 175-184.

1264. Weidmann S (1952). The electrical constants of Purkinje fibers. *J Physiol (Lond)*, *118*: 348-360.

1265. Weiss JN, Chen PS, Qu Z, Karagueuzian HS, Garfinkel A (2000). Ventricular fibrillation: how do we stop the waves from breaking? *Circ Res*, *87*: 1103-1107.

1266. Weiss JN, Lamp ST (1989). Cardiac ATP-sensitive K^+ channels. Evidence for preferential regulation by glycolysis. *J Gen Physiol*, *94*: 911-935.

1267. Weiss JN, Weiss JN, Chen PS, Qu Z, Karagueuzian HS, Garfinkel A (2000). Ventricular fibrillation: how do we stop the waves from breaking? *Circ Res*, *87*: 1103-1107.

1268. Wellens HJ (1994). Atrial fibrillation--the last big hurdle in treating supraventricular tachycardia. *N Engl J Med*, *331*: 944-945.

1269. Wendt Gallitelli MF, Voigt T, Isenberg G (1993). Microheterogeneity of subsarcolemmal sodium gradients. Electron probe microanalysis in guinea-pig ventricular myocytes. *J Physiol (Lond)*, *472*: 33-44.

1270. Wettwer E, Amos GJ, Posival H, Ravens U (1994). Transient outward current in human ventricular myocytes of subepicardial and subendocardial origin. *Circ Res*, *75*: 473-482.

1271. Weylandt KH, Valverde MA, Nobles M, Raguz S, Amey JS, Diaz M, Nastrucci C, Higgins CF, Sardini A (2001). Human ClC-3 is not the swelling-activated chloride channel involved in cell volume regulation. *J Biol Chem*, *276*: 17461-17467.

1272. White RL, Doeller JE, Verselis VK, Wittenberg BA (1990). Gap junctional conductance between pairs of ventricular myocytes is modulated synergistically by H^+ and Ca^{++}. *J Gen Physiol*, *95*: 1061-1075.

1273. White TW, Paul DL (1999). Genetic diseases and gene knockouts reveal diverse connexin functions. *Annu Rev Physiol*, *61*: 283-310.

1274. Wible BA, De Biasi M, Majumder K, Taglialatela M, Brown AM (1995). Cloning and functional expression of an inwardly rectifying K$^+$ channel from human atrium. *Circ Res, 76*: 343-350.

1275. Wibo M, Kilar F, Zheng L, Godfraind T (1995). Influence of thyroid status on postnatal maturation of calcium channels, beta-adrenoceptors and cation transport ATPases in rat ventricular tissue. *J Mol Cell Cardiol, 27*: 1731-1743.

1276. Wickenden AD, Kaprielian R, Parker TG, Jones OT, Backx PH (1997). Effects of development and thyroid hormone on K$^+$ currents and K$^+$ channel gene expression in rat ventricle. *J Physiol (Lond), 504*: 271-286.

1277. Wickman K, Clapham DE (1995). Ion channel regulation by G proteins. *Physiol Rev, 75*: 865-885.

1278. Wier WG, Balke CW (1999). Ca^{2+} release mechanisms, Ca^{2+} sparks, and local control of excitation-contraction coupling in normal heart muscle. *Circ Res, 85*: 770-776.

1279. Wijffels MC, Kirchhof CJ, Dorland R, Allessie MA (1995). Atrial fibrillation begets atrial fibrillation. A study in awake chronically instrumented goats. *Circulation, 92*: 1954-1968.

1280. Wijffels MC, Kirchhof CJ, Dorland R, Power J, Allessie MA (1997). Electrical remodeling due to atrial fibrillation in chronically instrumented conscious goats: roles of neurohumoral changes, ischemia, atrial stretch, and high rate of electrical activation. *Circulation, 96*: 3710-3720.

1281. Wilde AA (1994). K$^+$ ATP-channel opening and arrhythmogenesis. *J Cardiovasc Pharmacol, 24*: S35-40.

1282. Wilde AA, Aksnes G (1995). Myocardial potassium loss and cell depolarisation in ischaemia and hypoxia. *Cardiovasc Res, 29*: 1-15.

1283. Wilders R, Jongsma HJ, van Ginneken AC (1991). Pacemaker activity of the rabbit sinoatrial node. A comparison of mathematical models. *Biophys J, 60*: 1202-1216.

1284. Willette RN, Minehart H, Ellison J, Simons T, Short B, Pullen M, Ohlstein EH, Nambi P (1998). Effects of endothelin receptor antagonism and angiotensin-converting enzyme inhibition on cardiac and renal remodeling in the rat. *J Cardiovasc Pharmacol, 31*: S277-283.

1285. Winslow RL, Rice J, Jafri S, Marban E, O'Rourke B (1999). Mechanisms of altered excitation-contraction coupling in canine tachycardia-induced heart failure, II: model studies. *Circ Res, 84*: 571-586.

1286. Wit AL, Cranefield PF (1977). Triggered and automatic activity in the canine coronary sinus. *Circ Res, 41*: 434-445.

1287. Wit AL, Janse MJ (1992). Experimental models of ventricular tachycardia and fibrillation caused by ischemia and infarction. *Circulation, 85*: I32-42.

1288. Wit AL, Janse MJ (1993). The Ventricular Arrhythmias of Ischemia and Infarction. Futura Publishing Company, Inc, Mount Kisco, New York.

1289. Wit AL, Rosen MR (1992). Afterdepolarizations and triggered activity: Distinction from automaticity as an arrhythmogenic mechanism. Raven Press New-York.

1290. Witchel HJ, Hancox JC (2000). Familial and acquired long QT syndrome and the cardiac rapid delayed rectifier potassium current. *Clin Exp Pharmacol Physiol, 27*: 753-766.

1291. Wollert KC, Studer R, Doerfer K, Schieffer E, Holubarsch C, Just H, Drexler H (1997). Differential effects of kinins on cardiomyocyte hypertrophy and interstitial collagen matrix in the surviving myocardium after myocardial infarction in the rat. *Circulation, 95*: 1910-1917.

1292. Wolska BM, Averyhart-Fullard V, Omachi A, Stojanovic MO, Kallen RG, Solaro RJ
(1997). Changes in thyroid state affect pH_i and Na_i^+ homeostasis in rat ventricular
myocytes. *J Mol Cell Cardiol, 29*: 2653-2663.

1293. Woo SH, Lee CO (1999). Effects of endothelin-1 on Ca^{2+} signaling in guinea-pig
ventricular myocytes: role of protein kinase C. *J Mol Cell Cardiol, 31*: 631-643.

1294. Woo SH, Lee CO (1999). Role of PKC in the effects of alpha1-adrenergic stimulation
on Ca^{2+} transients, contraction and Ca^{2+} current in guinea-pig ventricular myocytes.
Pflügers Archiv, 437: 335-344.

1295. Woodhull AM (1973). Ionic blockage of sodium channels in nerve. *J Gen Physiol, 61*:
687-708.

1296. Wu CF, Bishopric NH, Pratt RE (1997). Atrial natriuretic peptide induces apoptosis in
neonatal rat cardiac myocytes. *J Biol Chem, 272*: 14860-14866.

1297. Wu J, McHowat J, Saffitz JE, Yamada KA, Corr PB (1993). Inhibition of gap
junctional conductance by long-chain acylcarnitines and their preferential
accumulation in junctional sarcolemma during hypoxia. *Circ Res, 72*: 879-889.

1298. Wu JY, Lipsius SL (1990). Effects of extracellular Mg^{2+} on T- and L-type Ca^{2+}
currents in single atrial myocytes. *Am J Physiol, 259*: H1842-1850.

1299. Wu Y, Anderson ME (2000). Ca^{2+}-activated non-selective cation current in rabbit
ventricular myocytes. *J Physiol (Lond), 522 Pt 1*: 51-57.

1300. Wu Y, MacMillan LB, McNeill RB, Colbran RJ, Anderson ME (1999). CaM kinase
augments cardiac L-type Ca^{2+} current: a cellular mechanism for long Q-T arrhythmias.
Am J Physiol, 276: H2168-2178.

1301. Wu Y, Roden DM, Anderson ME (1999). Calmodulin kinase inhibition prevents
development of the arrhythmogenic transient inward current. *Circ Res, 84*: 906-912.

1302. Xiao RP, Cheng H, Zhou YY, Kuschel M, Lakatta EG (1999). Recent advances in
cardiac beta(2)-adrenergic signal transduction. *Circ Res, 85*: 1092-1100.

1303. Xu L, Mann G, Meissner G (1996). Regulation of cardiac Ca^{2+} release channel
(ryanodine receptor) by Ca^{2+}, H^+, Mg^{2+}, and adenine nucleotides under normal and
simulated ischemic conditions. *Circ Res, 79*: 1100-1109.

1304. Xu X, Best PM (1992). Postnatal changes in T-type calcium current density in rat atrial
myocytes. *J Physiol (Lond), 454*: 657-672.

1305. Yamada KA, McHowat J, Yan GX, Donahue K, Peirick J, Kléber AG, Corr PB (1994).
Cellular uncoupling induced by accumulation of long-chain acylcarnitine during
ischemia. *Circ Res, 74*: 83-95.

1306. Yamaguchi H, Sakamoto N, Watanabe Y, Saito T, Masuda Y, Nakaya H (1997). Dual
effects of endothelins on the muscarinic K^+ current in guinea pig atrial cells. *Am J
Physiol, 273*: H1745-1753.

1307. Yamaoka K, Yakehiro M, Yuki T, Fujii H, Seyama I (2000). Effect of sulfhydryl
reagents on the regulatory system of the L-type Ca channel in frog ventricular
myocytes. *Pflügers Archiv, 440*: 207-215.

1308. Yamashita T, Nakajima T, Hazama H, Hamada E, Murakawa Y, Sawada K, Omata M
(1995). Regional differences in transient outward current density and inhomogeneities
of repolarization in rabbit right atrium. *Circulation, 92*: 3061-3069.

1309. Yamashita T, Nakaya H, Tohse N, Kusaka M, Uemura H, Sakuma I, Yasuda H, Kanno
M, Kitabatake A (1994). Depressed responsiveness to angiotensin II in ventricular
myocytes of hypertrophic cardiomyopathic Syrian hamster. *J Mol Cell Cardiol, 26*:
1429-1438.

1310. Yan GX, Antzelevitch C (1996). Cellular basis for the electrocardiographic J wave.
Circulation, 93: 372-379.

1311. Yan GX, Antzelevitch C (1998). Cellular basis for the normal T wave and the electrocardiographic manifestations of the long-QT syndrome. *Circulation, 98*: 1928-1936.

1312. Yan G-X, Chen J, Yamada KA, Kléber AG, Corr PB (1996). Contribution of shrinkage of extracellular space to extracellular K$^+$ accumulation in myocardial ischaemia of the rabbit. *J Physiol (Lond), 490*: 215-228.

1313. Yan GX, Park TH, Corr PB (1995). Activation of thrombin receptor increases intracellular Na$^+$ during myocardial ischemia. *Am J Physiol, 268*: H1740-1748.

1314. Yan GX, Shimizu W, Antzelevitch C (1998). Characteristics and distribution of M cells in arterially perfused canine left ventricular wedge preparations. *Circulation, 98*: 1921-1927.

1315. Yanagihara K, Irisawa H (1980). Potassium current during the pacemaker depolarization in rabbit sinoatrial node cell. *Pflügers Archiv, 388*: 255-260. .

1316. Yang JM, Chu CH, Yang SN, Jao MJ (1993). Effects of histamine on intracellular Na$^+$ activity and twitch tension in guinea pig papillary muscles. *Jpn J Physiol, 43*: 207-220.

1317. Yang T, Roden DM (1996). Extracellular potassium modulation of drug block of IKr. Implications for torsade de pointes and reverse use-dependence. *Circulation, 93*: 407-411.

1318. Yang T, Snyders DJ, Roden DM (1997). Rapid inactivation determines the rectification and [K$^+$]$_o$ dependence of the rapid component of the delayed rectifier K$^+$ current in cardiac cells. *Circ Res, 80*: 782-789.

1319. Yano M, Ono K, Ohkusa T, Suetsugu M, Kohno M, Hisaoka T, Kobayashi S, Hisamatsu Y, Yamamoto T, Noguchi N, Takasawa S, Okamoto H, Matsuzaki M (2000). Altered stoichiometry of FKBP12.6 versus ryanodine receptor as a cause of abnormal Ca^{2+} leak through ryanodine receptor in heart failure. *Circulation, 102*: 2131-2136.

1320. Yasui K, Liu W, Opthof T, Kada K, Lee JK, Kamiya K, Kodama I (2001). I$_f$ current and spontaneous activity in mouse embryonic ventricular myocytes. *Circ Res, 88*: 536-542.

1321. Yasutake M, Haworth RS, King A, Avkiran M (1996). Thrombin activates the sarcolemmal Na$^+$-H$^+$ exchanger. Evidence for a receptor-mediated mechanism involving protein kinase C. *Circ Res, 79*: 705-715.

1322. Yatani A, Bahinski A, Mikala G, Yamamoto S, Schwartz A (1994). Single amino acid substitutions within the ion permeation pathway alter single-channel conductance of the human L-type cardiac Ca^{2+} channel. *Circ Res, 75*: 315-323.

1323. Yeager M (1998). Structure of cardiac gap junction intercellular channels. *J Struct Biol, 121*: 231-245.

1324. Yellon DM, Baxter GF (1995). A second window of protection; or delayed preconditioning phenomenon: future horizons for myocardial protection? *J Mol Cell Cardiol, 27*: 1023-1034.

1325. Yokoshiki H, Tohse N (2001). Developmental changes of ion channels. In: *Heart Physiology and Pathophysiology* (eds. N Sperelakis, Y Kurachi, A Terzic, MV Cohen), pp 719-735. Academic Press, San Diego.

1326. Yorikane R, Koike H, Miyake S (1991). Electrophysiological effects of endothelin-1 on canine myocardial cells. *J Cardiovasc Pharmacol, 17*: S159-162.

1327. Yoshida H, Zhang JJ, Chao L, Chao J (2000). Kallikrein gene delivery attenuates myocardial infarction and apoptosis after myocardial ischemia and reperfusion. *Hypertension, 35*: 25-31.

1328. Yu H, Chang F, Cohen IS (1993). Pacemaker current exists in ventricular myocytes. *Circ Res, 72*: 232-236.

1329. Yu H, Chang F, Cohen IS (1995). Pacemaker current i_f in adult canine cardiac ventricular myocytes. *J Physiol (Lond), 485*: 469-483.

1330. Yu H, Gao J, Wang H, Wymore R, Steinberg S, McKinnon D, Rosen MR, Cohen IS (2000). Effects of the renin-angiotensin system on the current I_{to} in epicardial and endocardial ventricular myocytes from the canine heart. *Circ Res, 86*: 1062-1068.

1331. Yu H, McKinnon D, Dixon JE, Gao J, Wymore R, Cohen IS, Danilo P, Jr., Shvilkin A, Anyukhovsky EP, Sosunov EA, Hara M, Rosen MR (1999). Transient outward current, I_{to1}, is altered in cardiac memory. *Circulation, 99*: 1898-1905.

1332. Yu H, Wu J, Potapova I, Wymore RT, Holmes B, Zuckerman J, Pan Z, Wang H, Shi W, Robinson RB, El-Maghrabi MR, Benjamin W, Dixon J, McKinnon D, Cohen IS, Wymore R (2001). MinK-Related Peptide 1 : A {beta} subunit for the HCN ion channel subunit family enhances expression and speeds activation. *Circ Res, 88*: 84e-87e.

1333. Yuan F, Pinto JM, Li Q, Wasserlauf BJ, Yang X, Bassett AL, Myerburg RJ (1999). Characteristics of I_K and its response to quinidine in experimental healed myocardial infarction. *J Cardiovasc Electrophysiol, 10*: 844-854.

1334. Yue DT, Marban E (1990). Permeation in the dihydropyridine-sensitive calcium channel. Multi-ion occupancy but no anomalous mole-fraction effect between Ba^{2+} and Ca^{2+}. *J Gen Physiol, 95*: 911-939.

1335. Yue L, Feng J, Gaspo R, Li GR, Wang Z, Nattel S (1997). Ionic remodeling underlying action potential changes in a canine model of atrial fibrillation. *Circ Res, 81*: 512-525.

1336. Yue L, Feng J, Li G-R, Nattel S (1996). Characterization of an ultrarapid delayed rectifier potassium channel involved in canine atrial repolarization. *J Physiol (Lond), 496*: 647-662.

1337. Yue L, Melnyk P, Gaspo R, Wang Z, Nattel S (1999). Molecular mechanisms underlying ionic remodeling in a dog model of atrial fibrillation. *Circ Res, 84*: 776-784.

1338. Yue L, Wang Z, Rindt H, Nattel S (2000). Molecular evidence for a role of Shaw (Kv3) potassium channel subunits in potassium currents of dog atrium. *J Physiol (Lond), 527*: 467-478.

1339. Zaritsky JJ, Redell JB, Tempel BL, Schwarz TL (2001). The consequences of disrupting cardiac inwardly rectifying K^+ current (I_{K1}) as revealed by the targeted deletion of the murine Kir2.1 and Kir2.2 genes. *J Physiol (Lond), 533*: 697-710.

1340. Zaza A (2000). The cardiac action potential. In: *An introduction to Cardiac Cellular Electrophysiology* (eds. A Zaza, MR Rosen), pp 59-82. Harwood Academic Publishers.

1341. Zaza A, Micheletti M, Brioschi A, Rocchetti M (1997). Ionic currents during sustained pacemaker activity in rabbit sino- atrial myocytes. *J Physiol (Lond), 505*: 677-688.

1342. Zaza A, Robinson RB, DiFrancesco D (1996). Basal responses of the L-type Ca^{2+} and hyperpolarization-activated currents to autonomic agonists in the rabbit sino-atrial node. *J Physiol (Lond), 491*: 347-355.

1343. Zaza A, Rocchetti M, DiFrancesco D (1996). Modulation of the hyperpolarization-activated current (I_f) by adenosine in rabbit sinoatrial myocytes. *Circulation, 94*: 734-741.

1344. Zaza A, Rosen MR (2000). An introduction to Cardiac Cellular Electrophysiology. Harwood Academic Publishers.

1345. Zeng J, Rudy Y (1995). Early afterdepolarizations in cardiac myocytes: mechanism and rate dependence. *Biophys J, 68*: 949-964.

1346. Zeng T, Bett GC, Sachs F (2000). Stretch-activated whole cell currents in adult rat cardiac myocytes. *Am J Physiol, 278*: H548-557.

1347. Zhang JF, Siegelbaum SA (1991). Effects of external protons on single cardiac sodium channels from guinea pig ventricular myocytes. *J Gen Physiol, 98*: 1065-1083.

1348. Zhang M, Jiang M, Tseng G-N (2001). MinK-Related Peptide 1 associates with Kv4.2 and modulates its gating function : potential role as {beta} subunit of cardiac transient outward channel? *Circ Res, 88*: 1012-1019.

1349. Zhang Y, Cribbs LL, Satin J (2000). Arachidonic acid modulation of alpha 1H, a cloned human T-type calcium channel. *Am J Physiol, 278*: H184-210.

1350. Zhang YH, Youm JB, Sung HK, Lee SH, Ryu SY, Ho WK, Earm YE (2000). Stretch-activated and background non-selective cation channels in rat atrial myocytes. *J Physiol (Lond), 523 Pt 3*: 607-619.

1351. Zhou Z, Bers DM (2000). Ca^{2+} influx via the L-type Ca^{2+} channel during tail current and above current reversal potential in ferret ventricular myocytes. *J Physiol (Lond), 523 Pt 1*: 57-66.

1352. Zhou Z, January CT (1998). Both T- and L-type Ca^{2+} channels can contribute to excitation-contraction coupling in cardiac Purkinje cells. *Biophys J, 74*: 1830-1839.

1353. Zhou Z, Lipsius SL (1994). T-type calcium current in latent pacemaker cells isolated from cat right atrium. *J Mol Cell Cardiol, 26*: 1211-1219.

1354. Zhu Y, Nosek TM (1991). Inositol trisphosphate enhances Ca^{2+} oscillations but not Ca^{2+}-induced Ca^{2+} release from cardiac sarcoplasmic reticulum. *Pflügers Archiv, 418*: 1-6.

1355. Zhuang J, Yamada KA, Saffitz JE, Kléber AG (2000). Pulsatile stretch remodels cell-to-cell communication in cultured myocytes. *Circ Res, 87*: 316-322.

1356. Zipes DP, Jalife J (1999). Cardiac Electrophysiology. From Cell to Bedside. W.b. Saunders Co, Philadelphia.

1357. Zipes DP, Wellens HJ (2000). What have we learned about cardiac arrhythmias? *Circulation, 102*: IV52-57.

1358. Zuanetti G, De Ferrari GM, Priori SG, Schwartz PJ (1987). Protective effect of vagal stimulation on reperfusion arrhythmias in cats. *Circ Res, 61*: 429-435.

1359. Zuanetti G, Hoyt RH, Corr PB (1990). Beta-adrenergic-mediated influences on microscopic conduction in epicardial regions overlying infarcted myocardium. *Circ Res, 67*: 284-302.

1360. Zuhlke RD, Pitt GS, Deisseroth K, Tsien RW, Reuter H (1999). Calmodulin supports both inactivation and facilitation of L-type calcium channels. *Nature, 399*: 159-162.

1361. Zuhlke RD, Pitt GS, Tsien RW, Reuter H (2000). Ca^{2+}-sensitive inactivation and facilitation of L-type Ca^{2+} channels both depend on specific amino acid residues in a consensus calmodulin- binding motif in the(alpha)1C subunit. *J Biol Chem, 275*: 21121-21129.

1362. Zygmunt AC (1994). Intracellular calcium activates a chloride current in canine ventricular myocytes. *Am J Physiol, 267*: H1984-1995.

1363. Zygmunt AC, Gibbons WR (1991). Calcium-activated chloride current in rabbit ventricular myocytes. *Circ Res, 68*: 424-437.

1364. Zygmunt AC, Goodrow RJ, Antzelevitch C (2000). I(NaCa) contributes to electrical heterogeneity within the canine ventricle. *Am J Physiol Heart Circ Physiol, 278*: H1671-1678.

1365. Zygmunt AC, Goodrow RJ, Weigel CM (1998). INaCa and ICl(Ca) contribute to isoproterenol-induced delayed after depolarizations in midmyocardial cells. *Am J Physiol, 275*: H1979-1992.

Abbreviations

4-AP:	4-aminopyridine
5-HT:	5-hydroxytryptamine (serotonin)
A1:	Adenosine type 1 receptor
AA:	Arachidonic acid
AC:	Adenylate cyclase
ACE:	Angiotensin converting enzyme
ACh:	Acetylcholine
ACTH:	Adrenocorticotropic hormone
Ado:	Adenosine
ADP:	Adenosine-5'-diphosphate
AF	Atrial fibrillation
AMP:	Adenosine-5'-monophosphate
Ang II	Angiotensine II
ANP:	Atrial natriuretic peptide
APD:	Action potential duration
ATII:	Angiotensin type II receptor
ATP:	Adenosine-5'-triphosphate
AVN:	Atrioventricular node
BNP:	Brain natriuretic peptide
cAMP:	Adenosine 3',5'-cyclic monophosphate
CAT:	Carnitine acyltransferase
CFTR:	Cystic fibrosis transmembrane conductance regulator
cGMP:	guanosine 3',5'-cyclic monophosphate
CHF:	Chronic heart failure
CICR:	Calcium-induced calcium release
CL:	Cycle length
CNG:	Cyclic nucleotide gated

DAD:	Delayed afterdepolarisation
DAG:	1,2-diacylglycerol
DHP:	Dihydropyridine
DHPR:	Dihydropyridine receptor
DIDS:	4,4'-diisothiocyanostilbene-2,2'-disulphonic acid
EAD:	Early afterdepolarisation
ENDO:	Endocardial
EPI:	Epicardial
ERF:	Effective refractory period
ES:	Extracellular space
ET-1:	Endothelin 1
ETA:	Endothelin type A receptor
FA:	Fatty acid
GC:	Guanylate cyclase
GDP:	Guanosine-5'-diphosphate
GJIC:	Gap junctional intercellular communication
GTP:	Guanosine-5'-triphosphate
H1:	Histamine type 1 receptor
H2:	Histamine type 2 receptor
HEPES:	N-(hydroxyethyl)piperazine-N'-(2-ethanesulfonic acid)
IP3:	Inositol 1,4,5-trisphosphate
IP3R:	Inositol 1,4,5-trisphosphate receptor
LCAC:	Long chain acylcarnitines
LPC:	Lysophosphatidylcholine
LPG:	Lysophosphoglycerides
LQT:	Long QT
LT:	Leukotrienes
LV:	Left ventricle
M2:	Muscarinic type 2 receptor
MAP:	Monophasic action potential
MAPK:	Mitogen-activated protein (MAP) kinase
NA:	Noradrenaline
NAD:	Nicotinamide adenine dinucleotide
NMR:	Nuclear magnetic resonance
NO:	Nitric oxide
NOS:	NO synthase
NSC:	Non-selective cation channel
P1:	Purinergic type 1 receptor
P2:	Purinergic type 2 receptor
PAR:	Protease-activated receptor
PDE:	Cyclic nucleotide phosphodiesterase
PKA:	Protein kinase A

PKC:	Protein kinase C
PKD:	Protein kinase D
PKG:	Protein kinase G
PLA2:	Phospholipase A2
PLC:	Phospholipase C
PtdIP2:	Phosphatidylinositol 4,5-bisphosphate
PTK:	Protein tyrosine kinase
RyR:	Ryanodine receptor
SAN:	Sino-atrial node
SITS:	4-acetamido-4'-isothiocyanatostilbene 2,2' disulphonic acid
SR:	Sarcoplasmic reticulum
TdP:	Torsades de pointes
TEA:	Tetraethylammonium
PTK:	Protein tyrosine kinase
TM:	Transmembrane
TTX:	Tetrodotoxin
TWIK:	Two-pore inward rectifier K^+ channel
VF:	Ventricular fibrillation
VIP:	Vasoactive intestinal peptide
VT:	Ventricular tachycardia

Index